Cardiac Arrhythmias
A Practical Guide for the Clinician
Second Edition

Cardiac Arrhythmias
A Practical Guide for the Clinician
Second Edition

Robert A. Waugh, M.D.
Associate Professor of Medicine
Director
Cardiac Diagnostic Unit
Duke University Medical Center
Durham, North Carolina

Barry W. Ramo, M.D.
Clinical Professor of Medicine
University of New Mexico School of Medicine
Director, Cardiology Education
Presbyterian Hospital
Albuquerque, New Mexico

Galen S. Wagner, M.D.
Associate Professor of Medicine
Department of Medicine
Duke University Medical Center
Durham, North Carolina

Marcel Gilbert, M.D.
Director
Electrophysiology Laboratory
Institut de Cardiologie de Québec
Ste-Foy, Quebec, Canada

 F. A. DAVIS COMPANY • Philadelphia

F. A. Davis Company
1915 Arch Street
Philadelphia, PA 19103

Printed in the United States of America

Last digit indicates print number: 10 9 8 7 6 5 4 3 2 1

Medical Editor: Robert W. Reinhardt
Medical Developmental Editor: Bernice M. Wissler
Production Editor: Gail Shapiro
Cover Illustration By: Donald B. Freggens, Jr. and Christopher M. Wagner, BFA

As new scientific information becomes available through basic and clinical research, recommended treatments and drug therapies undergo changes. The author(s) and publisher have done everything possible to make this book accurate, up to date, and in accord with accepted standards at the time of publication. The authors, editors, and publisher are not responsible for errors or omissions or for consequences from application of the book, and make no warranty, expressed or implied, in regard to the contents of the book. Any practice described in this book should be applied by the reader in accordance with professional standards of care used in regard to the unique circumstances that may apply in each situation. The reader is advised always to check product information (package inserts) for changes and new information regarding dose and contraindications before administering any drug. Caution is especially urged when using new or infrequently ordered drugs.

Dedicated to:

Andrew G. Wallace, M.D.

FOREWORD

I am deeply grateful to the editors for dedicating this book to me. It is a remarkably practical and useful guide to understanding the electrocardiogram, especially in recognizing disturbances of rhythm and guiding treatment.

It was my opportunity and pleasure to guide many of the contributors to this book while they were trainees in the Cardiology Division at Duke University Medical Center. I had developed an early fascination with the electrocardiogram as a medical student working with E. Harvey Estes who was and is a great teacher. The field of electrocardiography had developed principally on the basis of pattern recognition. Estes' work represented a major step in the quantitative analysis of the electrocardiogram. At about the same time (actually a few years earlier), remarkable work was going on in Chicago under the direction of Louis Katz, Alfred Pick, and Richard Langendorf. Their work focused principally on the creation of testable hypotheses regarding disturbances of cardiac rhythm.

During my cardiology training, I had the unique opportunity to work with Brian Hoffman in New York in whose laboratory the microelectrode and intracavitary recording of electrograms from the conduction system were used to explore the mechanisms of cardiac arrhythmias. Brian introduced me to Gordon Moe, whose laboratory was involved in using both of these methods to test hypotheses of arrhythmias, many of which had been developed by Katz, Pick, and Langendorf. Most of their hypotheses proved correct.

When I became Chief of Cardiology at Duke, we began to extend some of these techniques to an understanding of the electrocardiogram and disturbances of cardiac rhythm in the operating room. It was a productive period for all of us, and as trainees came through our laboratory, I encouraged them to spend time in the heart station interpreting electrocardiograms, to work in basic electrophysiology laboratories, to collaborate with us in the operating room, and importantly, to go to Chicago and to benefit from the extraordinary course taught by Katz, Pick, and Langendorf. Most of the contributors to this book had that combination of experiences. Their subsequent contributions and their chapters in this book reflect this relatively unique exposure.

The eletrocardiogram has been a remarkable bridge between basic science and clinical diagnosis. Much of what we know about the electrocardiogram is based on correlation. The electrocardiogram has also generated numerous hypotheses which have been tested in the laboratory, and understandings from the laboratory have become increasingly important to the interpretation of the electrocardiogram. The ability to enjoy the practice of cardiology and electrocardiography is enhanced by positioning oneself on this bridge, applying one's knowledge of physiology to the interpretation of the ECG and translating observations in the heart station into productive experiments in the laboratory. Each of the contributors to this book enjoys that position and it is reflected in their enthusiasm for the electrocardiogram as a diagnostic tool.

I am proud to be associated with this book. However, my principal pleasure comes from knowing these individuals as friends and colleagues and having played a role in making the use of the electrocardiogram a rewarding and productive experience for them.

Andrew G. Wallace, M.D.
Vice President for Health Affairs
  and
Dean
Dartmouth School of Medicine

PREFACE

In the mid 1960s, Andrew G. Wallace established the Cardiac Care Unit at Duke University Medical Center and began his studies of basic electrophysiology in Will Sealey's laboratory. These clinical and research activities formed the foundations for the subsequent training of many individuals. Andy's first research fellows were Rick Schaal and Doug Zipes, who are currently electrophysiologists at Ohio State University and the University of Indiana, respectively. The four editors/authors and five contributing authors to this text, *Cardiac Arrhythmias: A Practical Guide For The Clinician*, were also participants in one or another of these various experiences. Many additional clinical and research fellows in coronary care, basic arrhythmia research, and the medical and surgical management of arrhythmia problems continue to pursue the study of cardiac arrhythmias in academic medical centers and in practice, through collaborative clinical research efforts coordinated by the DUCCS (Duke University Clinical Cardiology Studies) consortium. The Duke program has been responsible for major advances in the understanding and management of cardiac arrhythmias, beginning with pioneering work in the surgical management of the Wolff-Parkinson-White syndrome. The laboratories of Ray Ideker, Gus Grant, Ed Pritchett, Harold Strauss, and Marcus Wharton continue to train the next generation of basic and clinical investigators of cardiac arrhythmias.

Our goal has been to produce a book that is different from existing arrhythmia texts. The extensive figures have been reproduced where possible, at full size. Contrasting examples are presented in a single figure to provide the most dramatic illustration of particularly important principles. We have tried to simplify the terminology regarding cardiac arrhythmias as much as possible and present practical classification systems. This book is written primarily for nonelectrophysiologists and does not attempt to cover all aspects of cardiac arrhythmias. It emphasizes a "How To" approach regarding the history, physical examination, manipulation of the autonomic nervous system, and use of ECG monitoring techniques.

The first chapter by Galen Wagner and Barry Ramo covers basic principles and a systematic approach. Barry Ramo's years of experience in using the patient's history in the evaluation of arrhythmias is reflected in Chapter 2. Bob Waugh continues to investigate optimal ways of using the physical examination to teach medical students about cardiovascular physiology including arrhythmias (Chapter 3). Menashe Waxman and his colleagues at the University of Toronto have developed methods for fine-tuning the balance between the sympathetic and parasympathetic components of the autonomic nervous system for the diagnosis and management of cardiac arrhythmias (Chapter 4). Bob Waugh and Galen Wagner relied heavily on Wanda Bride, the head nurse of Duke's Coronary Care Unit, for the section of ECG monitoring (Chapter 5). The greater than 20 years of experience in the performance of clinical electrophysiologic studies by Barry Ramo in Albuquerque and Marcel Gilbert in Quebec City were key to the preparation of Chapter 6.

There are only a small number of major cardiac arrhythmia problems and each is presented, using a common format, in Chapters 7 through 14. The editors wrote most of these chapters. Mike Rotman's extensive research and clinical experience with AV conduction problems at Duke, in the Air Force, and in Austin, Texas, contributed importantly to the preparation of Chapter 14.

Chapter 15, on the use of drugs to manage arrhythmias, is the result of the combined experiences of Kathy Murray at Vanderbilt, of Jodie Hurwitz at the University of Pennsylvania, and of Barry Ramo. Larry German's extensive experience in basic and clinical electrophysiology, including the directorships of electrophysiology laboratories at Duke and at St. Thomas's Hospital in Nashville, are reflected in Chapters 16 and 17.

We believe this book will be useful to anyone who is responsible for the clinical management of patients with cardiac arrhythmias and for those who want to develop a practical understanding of the principles governing their diagnosis and management.

We wish to acknowledge the extensive contributions of Sheila Y. Gainey in preparing the original and numerous revisions of the manuscript. Rick Klausner and Mal Thaler were vital to the production of the first edition of this book (*Cardiac Arrhythmias*. Wagner GS, Waugh RA, and Ramo BW (eds): Churchill Livingstone, New York, 1983), which served as an important foundation for this revision. Finally, we wish to thank Bernice Wissler and her colleagues at the F. A. Davis Company for their guidance, patience, and editorial expertise in producing this second edition.

Robert A. Waugh
Galen S. Wagner

CONTRIBUTORS

Lawrence D. German, M.D.
Cardiology Consultants, P.C.
Nashville, Tennessee

Marcel Gilbert, M.D.
Director
Electrophysiology Laboratory
Institut de Cardiologie de Québec
Ste-Foy, Quebec, Canada

Jodie L. Hurwitz, M.D.
Assistant Professor of Medicine
Hospital of the University of Pennsylvania
Philadelphia, Pennsylvania

Katherine T. Murray, M.D.
Assistant Professor of Medicine and Pharmacology
Cardiac Arrhythmia Service
Vanderbilt University Medical Center
Nashville, Tennessee

Barry W. Ramo, M.D.
Clinical Professor of Medicine
University of New Mexico School of Medicine
Director, Cardiology Education
Presbyterian Hospital
Albuquerque, New Mexico

Michael Rotman, M.D.
Central Texas Cardiology Associates
Consultant in Cardiology
Seaton Hospital
St. David's Hospital
Brackenridge Hospital
Austin, Texas

Galen S. Wagner, M.D.
Associate Professor of Medicine
Department of Medicine
Duke University Medical Center
Durham, North Carolina

Robert A. Waugh, M.D.
Associate Professor of Medicine
Director, Cardiac Diagnostic Unit
Duke University Medical Center
Durham, North Carolina

Menashe B. Waxman, M.D.
Professor of Medicine
University of Toronto
Physician, Department of Medicine
The Toronto Hospital General Division
Toronto, Ontario, Canada

CONTENTS

Chapter 4   Autonomic Maneuvers 72
Menashe B. Waxman, MD

Chapter 11 Atrioventricular Junctional Tachycardias 238
Barry W. Ramo, MD

Chapter 12 Ventricular Tachycardias 262
Marcel Gilbert, M.D., Galen S. Wagner, M.D., and Barry W. Ramo, MD

Chapter 14   Bradycardias Due to Failure of Atrioventricular Conduction .320
Robert A. Waugh, MD, and Michael Rotman, MD

Section Four
Drugs and Devices in the Treatment of Cardiac Arrhythmias 345

Chapter 15   Clinical Pharmacology and Use of Antiarrhythmic Drugs 347
Katherine T. Murray, MD, Barry W. Ramo, MD, and Jodie L. Hurwitz, MD

Chapter 16   Cardiac Pacing for Bradycardia 392
Lawrence D. German, MD

Chapter 17.   The Nonpharmacologic Therapy of Tachyarrhythmias 412
Lawrence D. German, MD

THE TOOLS FOR UNDERSTANDING AND DIAGNOSING ARRHYTHMIAS

CHAPTER 1

The Physiology of Normal and Abnormal Rhythms

BARRY W. RAMO, MD, and
GALEN S. WAGNER, MD

NORMAL CELLULAR ELECTROPHYSIOLOGY

The heart has two principal types of cells: (1) those that are responsible for contraction, and (2) those that are responsible for impulse formation or conduction, or both. Cells of the first group, the working myocardial cells of the atria and ventricles, are passive participants in the electrical activation of the heart. Cells of the second group—specialized cells in the sinus node, atria, atrioventricular (AV) node, and His-Purkinje system—are the active participants in the initiation and organized spread of depolarization throughout the heart. Both types of cells are important in the genesis and maintenance of a variety of cardiac rhythm disturbances.

Cardiac cells are electrically polarized in the resting state so that the inside of the cell is negative with respect to the outside.[1] Electrical activation of these cells requires depolarization with loss of intracellular negativity. This process initiates the mechanical action of shortening or contraction of cardiac cells. Following electrical activation, the cell remains in a depolarized state for a period of time during which it cannot be further depolarized. This nonexcitable period is called the *refractory period*. Following this refractory period, the cardiac cell "repolarizes" and is then capable of being depolarized again.

The action potential is the "electrocardiogram" ("ECG") of a single cardiac cell, which can be recorded by placing a microelectrode inside the cell. Figure 1–1 shows an action potential from a single working myocardial cell. The action potential is divided into five phases. Phase 0 occurs during initial cell depolarization and reflects a rapid change in intracellular polarity from -90 mV to $+20$ mV. During phases 1 and 2, the cell remains depolarized. Since it cannot be further stimulated, these phases are termed, collectively, the *absolute refractory period (ARP)*. During phase 3, repolarization (recovery) occurs and the cell returns to its resting state; the cell can be further depolarized, but more energy than normal is required. This phase is called the *relative refractory period (RRP)*. Any new action potential that is generated during the RRP is of lower amplitude and serves as a weaker electrical impulse to depolarize adjacent cells, causing slower-than-normal conduction from one cell to the next. Phase 4 is the resting phase for working myocardial cells, during which the membrane potential remains constant. The cell will not be reactivated until it is again depolarized by the spread of electrical current from an adjacent cell. Pacemaker cells, on the other hand, spontaneously become less negative (or depolarize) during phase 4, resulting in a gradual reduction in the membrane potential until it reaches a threshold potential and rapid phase 0 begins. This spontaneous phase 4 (or diastolic) depolarization is referred to as *automaticity*. A more detailed discussion of the action potential is found in Chapter 15.

The surface ECG represents the sum of the action potentials from all of the electrically active cardiac cells. Figure 1–1 also shows the correspondence between the action potential and the surface ECG.

The rate of depolarization of a group of cells determines the speed of impulse conduction through them. The speed of rapid depolarization is described by the maximum voltage change per unit time, or maximum dV/dT of phase 0, termed $\dot{V}_{max}$. Both His-Purkinje cells and working myocardial cells use fast sodium channels for depolarization and are referred to as *fast-response cells*. Sinus and atrioventricular (AV) nodal cells undergo depolarization, due to a slow inward flow of calcium ions (Ca^{2+}) through calcium channels. These calcium-dependent cells are called *slow-response cells*. This slower rate of depolarization results in a smaller action potential than that of the fast-response cell, causing a slower rate of impulse conduction.

Fast-response cells can take on the characteristics of slow-response cells if depolarized at a lower membrane potential (closer to zero) or if the sodium channels are not functioning. All cells depolarized during their RRPs produce an action potential similar to the slow-response cell (Fig. 1–2). When slowed conduction occurs in one part of the heart while the re-

FIGURE 1–1. The various phases of depolarization and repolarization of a nonpacemaking, working cardiac cell are depicted in relation to the surface electrocardiogram (ECG), which is the electrical sum over time of all the activity of the heart's depolarizing and repolarizing cells. The top horizontal line is at zero or reference voltage, whereas the bottom horizontal line represents resting transmembrane potential. Phase 0 depicts cell depolarization; phases 1 to 3 correspond with various phases of repolarization. During phases 1 and 2, the cell is refractory to further stimulation (absolute refractory period). During phase 3, a greater-than-normal stimulus can elicit depolarization (relative refractory period). During phase 4, the cell is fully recovered. (From Singer DH and Ten Eick RE: Pharmacology of cardiac arrhythmias. Prog Cardiovasc Dis 11:489, 1969, with permission.)

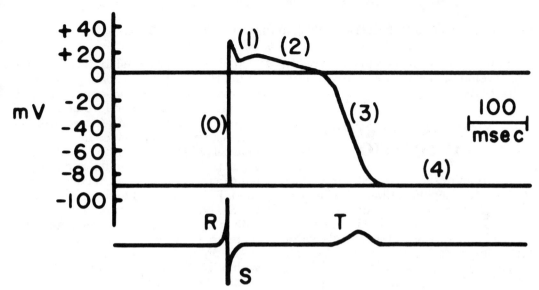

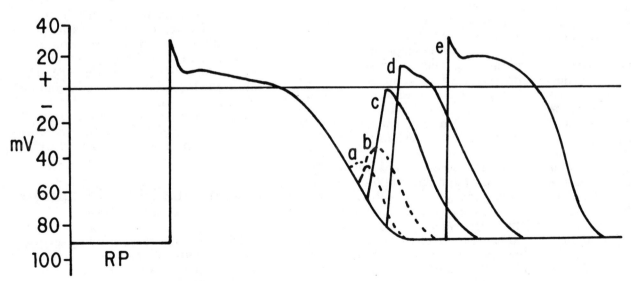

FIGURE 1–2. A Purkinje fiber is stimulated at progressively later periods during its recovery period (a,b,c,d) and after it has fully repolarized (e). The earlier in the refractory period the cell is depolarized, the smaller the amplitude of the generated action potential and the slower its rate of rise of phase 0 (or $\dot{V}_{max}$). The action potentials generated by the earliest stimulations (e.g., a and b) mimic those of slow-response cells. RP = resting potential. (From Singer DH and Ten Eick RE: Pharmacology of cardiac arrhythmias. Prog Cardiovasc Dis 11:489, 1969, with permission.)

mainder of the heart conducts normally, the development of reentrant arrhythmias is facilitated.[2]

NORMAL CARDIAC ACTIVATION

The relationship between the surface ECG and the depolarization of various cardiac structures is shown in Figure 1–3. The normal cardiac rhythm is initiated by the spontaneous activation of cells within the sinus node located high in the right atrium. This event is silent on the surface ECG. The P wave begins when the electrical impulse starts to spread through the right atrial myocardium. By the time approximately one half of the P wave has been inscribed and the impulse has just begun to advance through the left atrium, the AV node is entered. The latter portion of the P wave is produced solely by left atrial activation. In the normal heart, the electrical impulse exits from the atria only through the AV node, and slow conduction through this structure accounts for the majority of the PR interval. After emerging from the AV node, the impulse conducts through the His bundle, right and left bundle branches, their fascicles, and the Purkinje network. This fast infranodal conduction accounts for the remainder of the PR interval. When the ventricular myocardium is engaged, the onset of the QRS begins.

All the areas proximal to the branching of the His bundle are capable of producing rhythms with normal-appearing QRS complexes and are therefore considered *supraventricular*. These supraventricular areas can be further divided into atrial (sinoatrial [SA] node and atria) and AV junctional (AV node, His bundle, and the rare congenital anomaly of an accessory pathway). The areas distal to the branching of the His bundle cannot produce a rhythm with a normal QRS complex and are therefore considered *ventricular*.

The AV node has a posterior location within the AV connective tissue, and the exiting Purkinje fibers form the His bundle. As the His bundle then moves anteriorly, some fibers exit to form the posterior fascicle of the left bundle that travels toward the posterior papillary muscle of the mitral valve. On the left side of the septum, some of the remaining fibers continue anteriorly to form the anterior fascicle of the left bundle, which extends toward the anterior papillary muscle of the mitral valve, while others directly enter the midportion of septal myocardium. These latter fibers initiate ventricular activation and produce left-to-right septal depolarization with an initial positive (R) wave in lead V_1 and an initial negative (Q) wave in lead V_6.

The right bundle separates from the fibers of the anterior aspect of the left bundle at the top of the interventricular septum and proceeds as an intact bundle toward the apex of the right ventricle. Normally, the thinner-walled right ventricle is completely activated during the first half of the QRS complex, and it exerts minimal, if any, effect on the shape of the QRS. This elaborate impulse conduction system provides an efficient mechanism for ventricular activation, but it is vulnerable to AV block at three levels: (1) the AV node, (2) the His bundle, and (3) the bundle branches.

MECHANISMS OF ARRHYTHMIAS

The mechanisms responsible for the genesis of cardiac arrhythmias are (1) abnormalities of impulse formation, or (2) abnormalities of impulse conduction. Our present clinical tools do not allow us always to be certain of the electrophysiologic mechanism of an arrhythmia.[3] This classification system, nevertheless, is clinically useful and provides the framework for the diagnosis and treatment of arrhythmias.

Abnormalities of Impulse Formation

Impulse formation, or automaticity, is found in cells capable of spontaneous diastolic depolarization. These are principally located in the sinus node and the

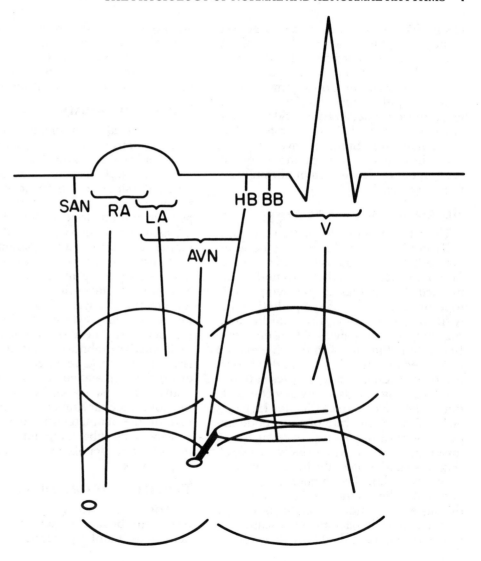

FIGURE 1–3. The relationship between depolarization of various cardiac structures and the surface ECG is shown. The depolarization of the sinoatrial (SA) node (depicted in this diagram as SAN) is "silent." During the time from the beginning of the P wave to the onset of the QRS complex, several areas of the heart are activated, including the right atrium (RA), left atrium (LA), atrioventricular (AV) node (depicted as AVN), His (common) bundle (HB), and the bundle branches (BB). The electrical impulse enters the left atrium and the AV node almost simultaneously, but a much longer time is required to traverse the AV node. In the absence of a bundle branch block, activation of the ventricles (V) is relatively synchronous.

His-Purkinje system but are also scattered throughout the atria and the distal AV node. Diseased cardiac cells that normally do not demonstrate pacemaker function may also take on automatic properties. Impulse formation is abnormal when there is acceleration or depression beyond the normal discharge rate for that particular site. Sinus tachycardia and sinus bradycardia are examples of enhancement or depression of normally automatic cells.

DEPRESSED AUTOMATICITY

The rate of impulse formation is continually modulated by the balance between sympathetic and parasympathetic tone. Automatic activity in the sinus node is depressed by increased parasympathetic tone or withdrawal of sympathetic tone, with resulting sinus bradycardia and, sometimes, sinus pauses of long duration. In addition, the rate of sinus firing may be depressed by intrinsic sinus node disease, premature activation (overdrive suppression), or drug effects, or by any combination of these factors (see Chapter 13, pages 304 to 310). If the rate of sinus node impulse formation slows excessively, a lower pacemaker will usually "escape" (Fig. 1–4) and protect the heart from stopping (asystole). The higher the escape pacemaker lies in the conduction system, the faster and more reliable its escape rate. His bundle pacemakers escape at a rate between 40 and 60 beats per minute

and are influenced to some degree by autonomic tone. Bundle branch or fascicular pacemakers escape at a slower rate (30 to 40 per minute or less) and are not significantly influenced by autonomic tone.

ENHANCED AUTOMATICITY

Tachycardias or premature beats can result both from increased activity of normal pacemakers and from abnormal pacemakers. Increased impulse formation in the sinus node is due to an increase in sympathetic tone or withdrawal of parasympathetic tone, or to both mechanisms, rather than to an intrinsic abnormality. Similarly, latent pacemakers in other areas may develop enhanced automaticity, resulting in an "automatic (or ectopic) atrial tachycardia," "accelerated AV junctional rhythm," or "accelerated idioventricular rhythm." Normal working cells may develop abnormal pacemaker activity (abnormal automaticity) in response to drugs (e.g., catecholamines, electrolyte imbalance) and when they are injured (e.g., ischemia, hypoxia). Abnormal ionic mechanisms cause these cells to take on the characteristics described for slow-response fibers, including spontaneous diastolic depolarization and a slow $\dot{V}_{max}$ of phase 0.[3]

TRIGGERED AUTOMATICITY

"Triggered activity" may also cause premature beats and tachycardias and is defined as impulse generation caused by

either early or late afterdepolarizations. Triggered activity is initiated by oscillations in the cell's membrane potential of sufficient magnitude to cause cell depolarization (Fig. 1–5).[4] "Early" afterdepolarizations occur during repolarization, and "late" afterdepolarizations occur following complete repolarization. Once triggered, the initial afterdepolarization can induce a burst of action potentials that continue in the absence of further driving impulses. The role of afterdepolarizations in the genesis of clinical arrhythmias has not yet been completely defined, but early afterdepolarizations may be responsible for torsades de pointes. Late or delayed afterpotentials may cause multifocal atrial tachycardias, digitalis-induced automatic atrial tachycardias, and verapamil-sensitive ventricular tachycardia.[5] The latter arrhythmias may be facilitated by increased catecholamines and xanthines (see Chapter 9, pages 182–183 and Chapter 12, pages 264, 289, and 295).

Abnormalities of Impulse Conduction

Abnormalities of impulse conduction may take one of two forms: (1) failure of an impulse to be transmitted from one region of the heart to another, resulting in block; and (2) reentry of an impulse back into a previously activated area, resulting

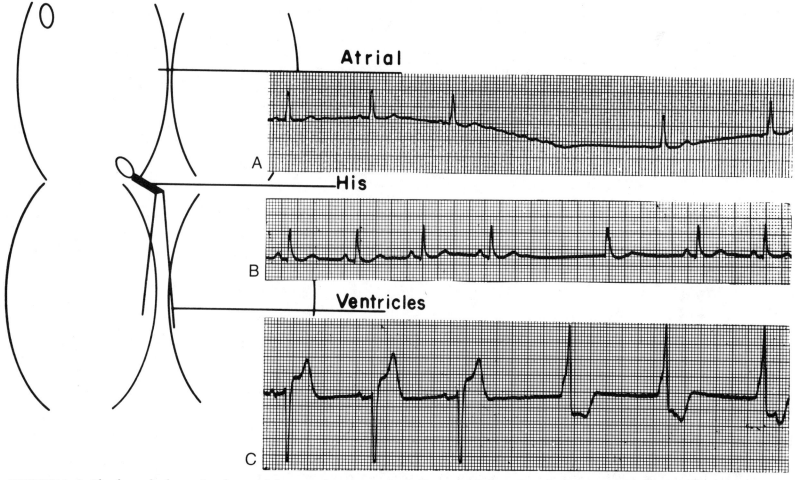

FIGURE 1-4. The three rhythm strips show atrial pauses that are terminated by escape beats at three different levels. (*A*) The escape beat is from the atrium, as evidenced by the ectopic P wave (small and inverted) that precedes the apparently normal QRS complex terminating the pause. (*B*) The escape beat is from the His bundle, as evidenced by the absence of atrial activity preceding the apparently normal QRS complex that terminates the pause. (*C*) The escape beat is from the ventricle, as evidenced by the absence of atrial activity preceding the wide, different QRS complex terminating the pause.

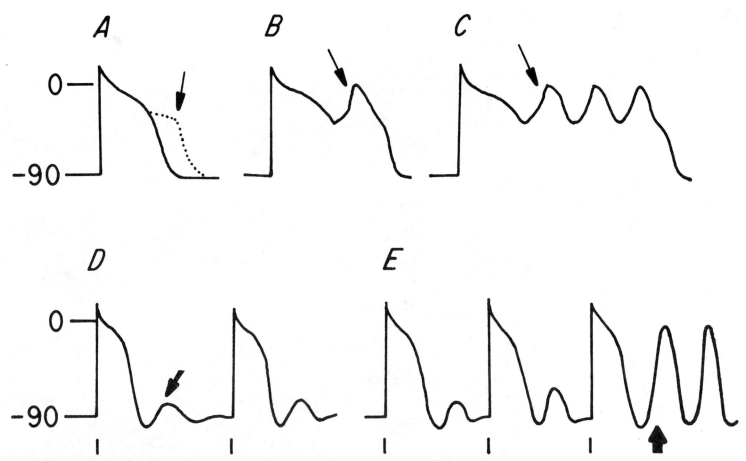

FIGURE 1–5. Afterdepolarizations are classified as early (EAD) or late (LAD). EADs occur during the period of repolarization of cardiac cells. (*A*) A low-amplitude EAD (dotted line and arrow) produces only a local response. (*B*) An EAD triggers a single extra beat (arrow). (*C*) An EAD triggers a run of three triggered action potentials. (The arrow indicates the first beat of this run.) LADs arise after the completion of repolarization and may also "trigger" a single action potential or runs of action potentials. (*D*) The LADs (arrow) do not reach threshold. (*E*) An increased rate increases the amplitude of the LADs, allowing them to reach threshold and trigger a rhythm (broad arrow). (From Wit AL and Rosen MR: Cellular electrophysiology of cardiac arrhythmias. I. Arrhythmias caused by abnormal impulse generation. Modern Concepts of Cardiovascular Disease 50:5, 1981, with permission.)

in a premature beat(s) or a tachyarrhythmia.

FAILURE OF IMPULSE CONDUCTION

Failure of conduction can occur between a pacemaker and the surrounding myocardium *(exit block)*, between the atria and the ventricles *(AV block)*, or within the ventricles *(fascicular or bundle branch block)*. Exit block may explain the sudden offset of some pacemaker tachycardias but is, for the most part, a diagnosis of exclusion. Although it may reflect many of the same causal factors as AV block, it is rarely associated with clinically important arrhythmias. AV block is by far the more important disorder of impulse conduction.[6] Chapters 13 and 14 discuss the clinical problems associated with abnormalities of impulse conduction.

The level of AV block is described by the terms *nodal* (AV node) and *infranodal* (His bundle and bundle branches). Almost all infranodal block is due to block in both right and left bundle branches rather than in the His bundle itself.

The AV nodal cells are slow conducting, with a prolonged RRP, whereas infranodal cells are fast conducting, with a very brief RRP. The clinician can often determine the level of AV block by understanding these differing electrophysiologic properties of the nodal versus the infranodal tissues. The determination of the level of block provides insight into the natural history and optimal therapies.

AV block is characterized by amount and location (Fig. 1–6). The amount of AV block is indicated by the term "degree." *First-degree AV block* indicates slow conduction through one or more of the three levels of the conduction system of sufficient magnitude to produce a prolongation of the PR interval greater than 0.20 seconds. *Second-degree AV block* indicates conduction of only some atrial impulses. *Third-degree AV block* indicates no conduction at all and is referred to as complete AV block.

The clinical diagnosis of the location of AV block is based on two features—the width of the QRS complex and the behavior of the PR interval during conducted beats. Intra–His bundle block is so rare that, for all practical purposes, only the AV node or bundle branches should be considered as the locations for AV block. The localization of the level of third-degree block is based solely on determining the origin of the escape pacemaker. If the escape QRS complex is narrow (less than 0.12 seconds), then the block is in the AV node. If the escape QRS complex is wide (greater than 0.12 seconds) in a patient without preexisting bundle branch block, the site of AV block is distal to the His bundle. In the presence of a preexisting bundle branch block, the site of complete AV block is difficult to determine clinically (see Chapter 14, pages 327 to 336).

The second feature to help localize the level of AV block is the "type," a characterization that is based on the behavior of the PR interval during conducted beats (Fig. 1–7). There is an ARP in both the AV node and the His bundle and its branches. During this time, the cells cannot be excited. The RRP is long in the AV node and virtually nonexistent in the His–bundle-branch system. This functional difference in the two action potentials accounts for the different clinical behavior; the AV node shows variability in conduction times depending on how early in the RRP the impulse occurs, and the His–bundle-branch system shows either normal conduction of premature impulses or complete block with no preceding, gradual change in the PR interval. The physiologic differences in behavior of AV block in the AV node versus AV block in His-Purkinje system are outlined in Table 1–1.

Type I AV block (A Wenckebach sequence is the pure or classic form) is due to the slow-channel conduction properties of the AV node. It rarely occurs in its pure or classic form, however (regular PP, increasing PR, decreasing RR, and a pause less than twice the shortest RR), and it is more helpful to look for variations in the PR interval, which typically result from reciprocal RP-PR relationships. The interval from the last conducted QRS complex to the next conducted P wave is the *RP interval*. The long RRP in the AV node affords the opportunity for marked variation in its conduction time. The earlier the atrial impulse

1st°: PR > 0.20 seconds; all P waves conducted

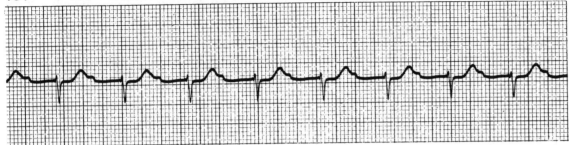

2nd°: Some P waves not conducted

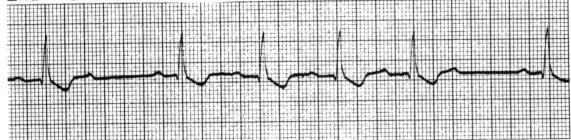

3rd°: All P waves not conducted

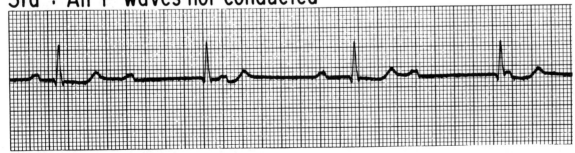

FIGURE 1–6. The three degrees of AV block are defined and illustrated. *(Top)* All P waves are conducted, but with a greater-than-normal PR interval (in this case, 0.32 seconds), typical of first-degree AV block. *(Middle)* Second-degree AV block is shown with conduction of some, but not all, P waves. The constant PP intervals with varying PR and RR intervals imply at least some AV association and, therefore, conduction of at least some P waves. *(Bottom)* Third-degree AV block is evidenced by complete AV dissociation, with P waves that should have conducted but did not (i.e., occurring after the preceding T wave and more than 0.2 seconds before the next QRS complex).

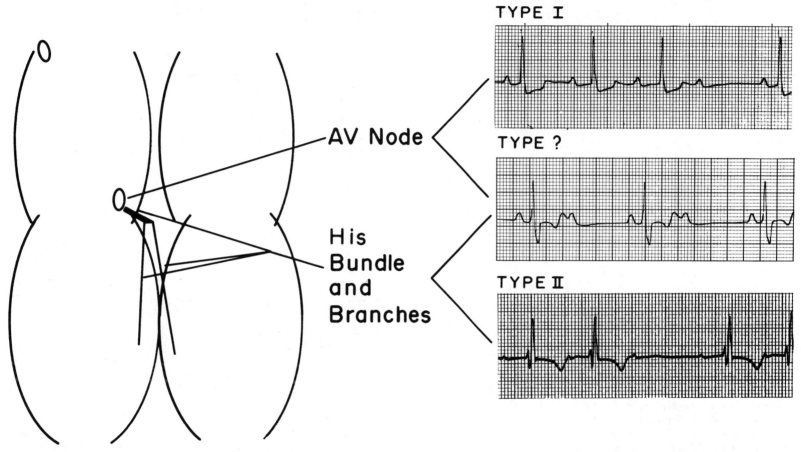

FIGURE 1–7. Type of AV block. *(Top)* Type I second-degree AV block is defined by a prolonging of the PR interval before the blocked P wave and pause, with a shortening of the PR interval following the pause (i.e., there is an inverse relationship between any given RP interval and the subsequent PR interval [see also next strip]). *(Middle)* The RP interval is fixed when there is 2:1 block; therefore, the PR interval is constant, and the block cannot be "typed." In order to diagnose the site of block in this instance, observation must be repeated following an intervention (e.g., vagal maneuvers) or during a longer monitoring period. *(Bottom)* When the PR interval is constant before the pause and remains constant after the pause, type II second-degree AV block is present (i.e., despite a varying RP interval, the PR interval remains constant). Type II block is usually due to block in the His or bundle branch system; the latter cause is much more common.

Table 1–1. DIFFERENTIAL DIAGNOSIS OF AV BLOCK: BEHAVIOR OF AV NODE VS. HIS-PURKINJE SYSTEM

	ANATOMIC SITE	
PHYSIOLOGIC VARIABLE	**AV NODE**	**HIS-PURKINJE**
Type of block	Type I	Type II
Conduction velocity	Slow	Fast
Relative refractory period	Long	Clinically nonexistent
Premature atrial beats	Increased PR	No change in PR
Automatic atrial tachycardias and atrial pacing	Type I block induced	No block induced
Sympathetic stimulation	Speeds conduction	No effect
Parasympathetic stimulation	Slows conduction	No effect
Digitalis, verapamil, β-blockers, adenosine	Slow conduction	No effect

AV = atrioventricular.

engages the AV node in its RRP, the shorter the RP interval, the slower the conduction, and the longer the PR interval. Hence the rule, "There is an inverse relationship between the RP and PR intervals in type I or AV nodal block." A very early impulse (i.e., a very short RP interval) may block completely in the AV node, whereas a very late impulse (long RP) may conduct normally (shorter PR interval). The long RRP of the AV node varies considerably with changes in autonomic tone, with enhanced sympathetic tone speeding conduction, and with enhanced parasympathetic tone slowing conduction.

Type II AV block is more difficult to identify clinically. It is possible to diagnose only when the PR intervals remain constant despite variations in the preceding RP intervals. When constant PR intervals occur only in the presence of constant RP intervals, typing of the AV block is impossible. When there is a 2:1, 3:1, 4:1, and so forth, AV relationship, there is a great temptation to diagnose "type II" block simply because the PR is constant. Because there is no variation in the RP that precedes the constant PR interval, however, a constant conduction time would be expected even in the AV node and such blocks cannot be "typed."

The cells in the His-Purkinje system have a very rapid rate of depolarization, rapid conduction, and a very short RRP. Indeed, for clinical purposes they have no RRP, so that a P wave will either be conducted as usual or not at all. Unlike block in the AV node (particularly given the slow recording speed of surface ECG rhythm strips), the PR does not vary but remains constant until a P wave is suddenly blocked. This relatively short RRP does not vary with changes in autonomic tone. Thus the conduction time through the His bundle and its branches remains constant despite progressively more premature activation. When, with extremely premature stimulation, the ARP is encountered, no conduction results. The His bundle and its branches thereby exhibit essentially "all-or-none" conduction capability.

In normal sinus rhythm, changes in autonomic balance may affect AV nodal conduction and, therefore, the PR interval. During sleep, when parasympathetic tone is high, type I second-degree AV block may be seen in normal subjects and is even more likely in conditioned athletes. When sympathetic activity predominates, as with exercise, the sinus rate is increased, as is the speed of AV nodal conduction (i.e., the PR interval shortens), causing the ventricular rate to increase by a 1:1 relationship with the atrial rate. Conversely, when the atrial rate is increased by a factor other than increased sympathetic activity (e.g., atrial pacing), AV nodal conduction remains under baseline sympathetic-parasympathetic balance. As the atrial rate accelerates, PR interval prolongation (first-degree AV block) occurs; with further acceleration, some atrial impulses may block in the AV node and fail to conduct to the ventricles, resulting in second-degree AV block with type I characteristics. With further atrial rate increases, 2:1, 3:1, or even higher ratios of AV block may occur. This increasing AV block and decreasing ventricular rate occur because the faster atrial rates result in more impulses partially penetrating and depolarizing the AV node, making it more refractory to the next atrial impulse. This AV conduction is "concealed" because there is no direct evidence of its occurrence on the surface ECG. The only evidence of its occurrence is indirect through its effects on subsequent AV conduction. Concealed conduction into the AV node is the reason that patients with atrial fibrillation have some degree of AV block even without drugs that slow AV conduction.

REENTRY

The second major abnormality of impulse conduction is *reentry,* a phenomenon that occurs when a given impulse enters tissue, depolarizes it, and then reenters the tissue to depolarize it a second time. This process can lead to a single reactivation (premature beat) or repetitive reactivation (a tachycardia) and may occur in the atria, AV junction, or ventricles, or in any of these structures in some combination. For reentry to occur, there must be at least two pathways, with unidirectional absence of conduction in one and slowed conduction in the other (Fig. 1–8). Definition of these pathways may be anatomic or physiologic, or both.

In ventricular preexcitation, two anatomically distinct pathways connect the atria to the ventricles: the normal AV node–His-Purkinje pathway and the accessory pathway, which is formed from an abnormal muscle bridge. If conduction proceeds in an anterograde manner through both pathways, there will be a short PR interval with a slow initial portion (delta wave) of the QRS complex. The PR interval is short because conduction through the accessory pathway is faster than through the normal pathway. The QRS, on the other hand, is a fusion beat because the initial part of the QRS (the delta wave) reflects the relatively slow muscle-to-muscle spread of ventricular activation resulting from the accessory pathway "short circuit," whereas the latter part of the QRS complex results from activation of the ventricles through the more rapidly conducting "normal" His-Purkinje pathway (Fig. 1–9). The model of reentry with preexcitation (called *atrioventricular reciprocating tachycardia* [*AVRT*]) is a paradigm for reentry and is easy to visualize because the reentrant circuit includes several discrete macroscopic areas of the heart (macroreentry).[7]

Two pathways may also exist in similar and anatomically contiguous tissue because of different electrophysiologic behavior. For example, one area of the ventricular myocardium may demonstrate slowed conduction because of ischemia, while an adjacent area may conduct normally, facilitating reentry. This may occur at a local level (microreentry) or throughout both ventricles (macroreentry). A similar phenomenon can occur within the AV node (microreentry) when two functionally separate pathways are exposed by a premature beat (see Fig. 11–3). The differing electrophysiologic characteristics of the A and B pathways are identical to the situation in the example of preexcitation. The A pathway has a slow conduction velocity but a short recovery time (analogous to the normal AV node–His-Purkinje

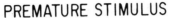

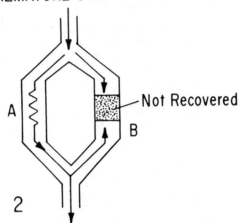

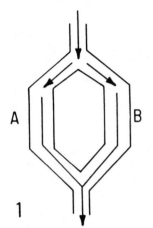

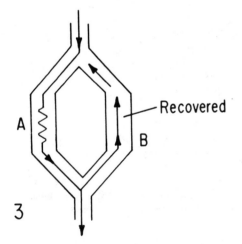

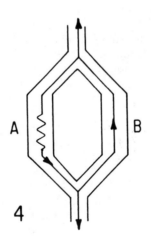

FIGURE 1-8. Two potential pathways, A and B, are shown schematically. (*1*) During normal activation, both pathways are activated homogeneously. (*2*) A premature stimulus arrives when pathway B is refractory (stippled area), where the impulse blocks. If pathway A is only partially refractory, the impulse conducts more slowly than normal (crooked line) and then enters the B pathway from a retrograde direction. (*3*) If the B pathway recovers by the time the impulse reaches the previously blocked area, then the impulse continues to activate pathway B in a retrograde direction. (*4*) If the impulse encounters excitable tissue as it exits from the proximal end of pathway B, it can reactivate (or "reenter") pathway A and establish a reentry loop.

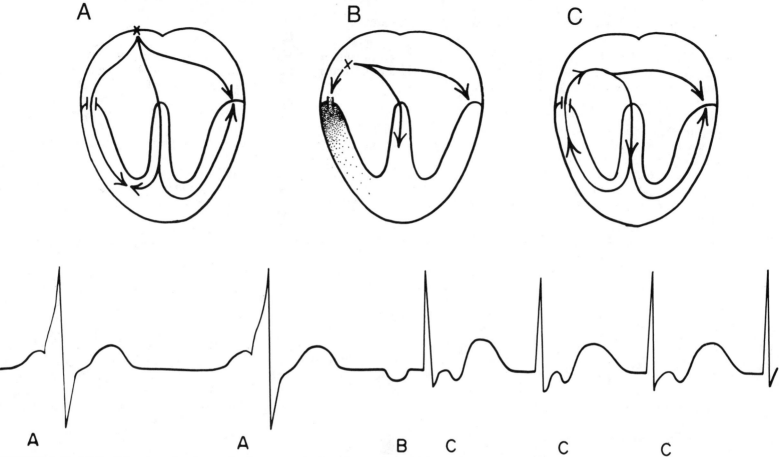

FIGURE 1–9. (*A*) In this example of ventricular preexcitation due to the Wolff-Parkinson-White syndrome, an accessory pathway (Kent bundle) connects the right atrium and ventricle; during normal sinus rhythm, ventricular fusion beats occur (ECG complexes A). (*B*) A premature beat (x) blocks in the accessory pathway, but conducts normally, or is only slightly slowed, in the normal pathway. The block in the accessory pathway occurs because its refractory period is longer than that of the AV node. (Note the loss of the delta wave in ECG complex B.) (*C*) A reentry loop develops when the impulse travels to the ventricle, engages the recovered accessory pathway, and conducts to the atrium in a retrograde direction. (Note the retrograde P waves following the QRS in ECG complexes (C). A reentry loop is established when antegrade conduction to the ventricles through the normal AV node–His-Purkinje pathway and retrograde conduction to the atrium through the accessory pathway become self-perpetuating (ECG complexes C).

limb), and the B pathway has a long recovery time but a fast conduction velocity (analogous to the accessory pathway). A premature atrial beat that arrives at the AV node when the B pathway is refractory causes the impulse to conduct down the A pathway and subsequently reenter the recovered B pathway in a retrograde direction. A reentry circuit that travels down the A pathway (antegrade) to activate the His bundle and back up the B pathway (retrograde) to activate the atrium causes a tachycardia that is called *atrioventricular nodal reentry (AVNR)* (see also Chapter 11, pages 240 to 245).

In the case of both anatomic and physiologic pathways, reentry is allowed because of the differences in recovery times or conduction velocities, or in both. Once initiated, the tachycardias continue as long as the conduction velocity is sufficiently slow and the recovery time sufficiently short to permit the recycling electrical impulse to encounter repolarized or receptive tissue continuously.

These electrophysiologic characteristics dictate three important behavioral aspects of reentry:

1. Reentry is usually initiated by a single premature beat that dissociates two functionally separate pathways.
2. Once a reentry loop has developed, there need not be a persistent abnormality for the resultant tachycardia to continue.

3. A reentrant tachycardia will terminate abruptly if conduction in any portion of the loop fails.

ARRHYTHMIA DIAGNOSIS

Arrhythmia diagnosis involves a systematic approach that begins with the application of standard definitions for the various arrhythmias and accurate measurement of important intervals of beats, followed by the use of clinical and electrocardiographic data to determine what the atria are doing, what the ventricles are doing, and whether they are acting dependently or independently of each other. The following sections review the important definitions and principles that can provide the clinician with answers to these questions and facilitate accurate arrhythmia diagnosis.

Abnormal Heart Rates

A *bradycardia* is generally defined by a ventricular rate of less than 60 beats per minute, and a *tachycardia*, by a ventricular rate exceeding 100 beats per minute. These limits, however, are arbitrary. A pathologic tachycardia might be appropriately designated even when the rate is less than 100 beats per minute if a rhythm is initiated by a ventricular pacemaker (whose normal escape function occurs at a rate of 30 to 40 beats per minute) that becomes abnormally accelerated to a rate between 60 and 100 beats per minute. Rate limits for both bradycardias and tachycardias, therefore, should be considered as only relative guidelines.

The terms *bradycardia* and *tachycardia* may sound ominous and falsely lead to the assumption that there is an abnormality of the heart. Appropriate physiologic slowing to a rate less than 60 beats per minute, however, may occur in athletes or result from parasympathetic predominance during sleep, even though appropriate physiologic acceleration due to sympathetic predominance is the norm with exercise or various other forms of stress.

BRADYCARDIA

When the pacing rate falls to less than 60 beats per minute, a bradycardia is present. The bradycardia is usually named according to the appearance of the P wave, the QRS complex, and the relationship between the P wave and the QRS complex (Fig. 1–10). If normal P waves precede the slower QRS complex with normal AV conduction, sinus bradycardia is present. If no preceding P waves are present, but the QRS complex is narrow (less than 0.12 seconds), the term *junctional rhythm* is used. If there is no preceding P wave and the QRS complex is broad (0.12 seconds or more), then the term *idioventricular*

A "Sinus Bradycardia"

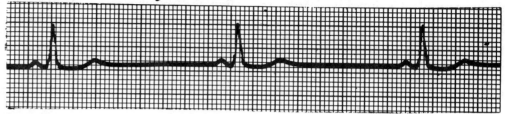

B "Junctional Rhythm"

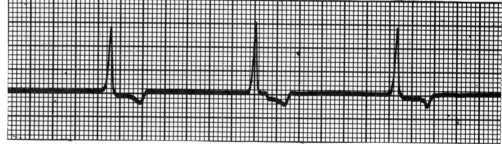

C "Idio-Ventricular Rhythm"

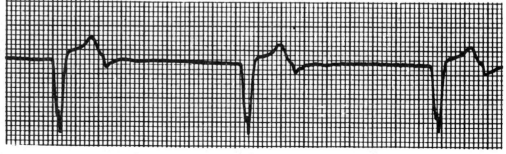

FIGURE 1–10. These three different arrhythmias are all due to atrial slowing. (*A*) The sinus rate has slowed to 38 beats per minute, but because no lower pacemaker site has a faster escape rate, the rhythm remains sinus bradycardia. (*B*) Although somewhat variable, the atrial rate is about 42 beats per minute. A slightly faster AV junctional pacemaker at a rate of 48 beats per minute supervenes. This similarity between atrial and ventricular rates produces isorhythmic AV dissociation. (*C*) There is an idioventricular escape rhythm at about 32 beats per minute. Continuing retrograde ventriculoatrial (VA) conduction, indicated by the inverted P waves in the terminal portion of the T waves, contributes to the continuing suppression of the sinus node.

rhythm is used. In all of the examples with no preceding P waves, however, the underlying problem is sinus bradycardia, regardless of whether the observed rhythm is sinus in origin or whether one of the lower areas has emerged as an escape focus. This is an important consideration, because the use of one of these other terms might lead one to assume that the problem is in these lower areas rather than in the failure of sinus impulse formation.

Bradycardias with isolated ventricular rate slowing result when second- or third-degree block at some level in the AV conduction system prevents the atrial impulse from reaching the ventricles. In this situation, it is important to localize the level of block to gain insight into the cause and the prognosis (see Chapter 14.).

TACHYCARDIA

A single premature beat can be viewed as potentially representing the first beat of a sustained tachycardia. The electrophysiologic basis for a tachycardia is either reentry or accelerated pacemaker activity. Accelerated pacemaker activity most commonly results from enhanced normal or latent pacemaker activity; triggered activity is probably responsible for some clinical arrhythmias but its exact role and importance remain to be elucidated. The clinical distinction between these mechanisms is not always possible.

Chapter 8 gives an overview of tachycardias, and Chapters 9 through 12 outline the specific characteristics of the tachycardias, classified by their atrial, AV junctional, or ventricular sites of origin. This section describes some very general characteristics of tachycardias.

The term *paroxysmal* means a tachycardia with a sudden onset and termination, a characteristic of reentrant arrhythmias. *Nonparoxysmal* refers to tachycardias with a gradual onset and termination, as expected with an increasing or decreasing rate of pacemaker impulse formation. The maximum rates of pacemaker tachycardias tend to be slower than reentrant tachycardias, but considerable overlap exists.

Slower rates for a pacemaker tachycardia occur because progression through the slow diastolic depolarization-repolarization process is required to generate each repetitive response. During reentry, on the other hand, the next impulse can be generated as soon as an area has completed its absolute refractory period. Sinus or other atrial pacemakers may achieve maximum rates of 200 beats per minute, sites in the His bundle may achieve a rate of 150 beats per minute, and sites in the bundle branches may be limited to 120 beats per minute. When sympathetic tone is increased, the rates of all pacemakers accelerate, with the sinus node usually predominating. Pacemaker

tachycardias originating from areas below the sinus node are therefore produced either by local effects such as ischemia and inflammation, or by certain drugs (e.g., digitalis) which may specifically accelerate the rate of pacemaking sites other than the sinus node.

Ladder Diagrams

Figure 1–11 illustrates both supraventricular and ventricular tachycardias using ladder diagrams. There is no separate example of an accelerated pacemaker tachycardia from the His bundle, since this is very similar to the ventricular tachycardia due to accelerated pacemaker activity within the bundle branches. When constructing a ladder diagram, vertical lines are used to indicate each apparent chamber depolarization (the P waves and QRS complexes). Diagonal lines connecting the P waves and QRS complexes indicate AV conduction. Use of this simple system often permits the testing of proper conclusions regarding P and QRS relationships that would otherwise be difficult.

In Figure 1–12, ladder diagrams are used to illustrate one example of why it is important to determine the mechanism of an arrhythmia's generation as well as its location. Two supraventricular tachycardias, one resulting from an abnormality of impulse formation (enhanced automatic-

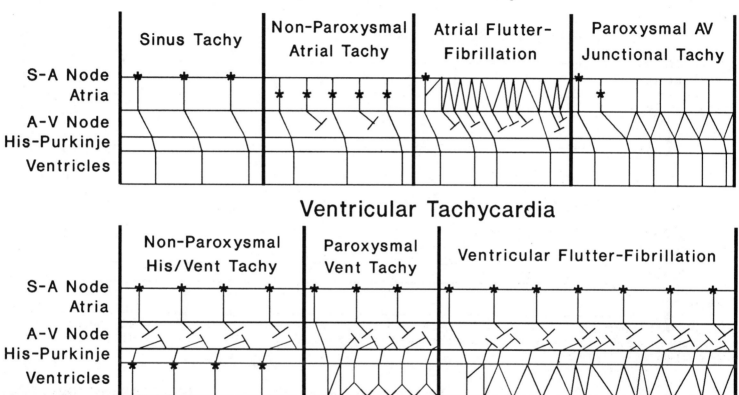

FIGURE 1–11. These ladder diagrams summarize the various tachycardias. The top line represents the sinoatrial (SA) node, and the succeeding spaces represent the atria, the AV node, the His-Purkinje (or bundle branch) system, and the ventricles, respectively. Asterisks indicate pacemaker activity; vertical lines indicate chamber depolarization; slanted lines indicate conduction through a particular area; short perpendicular lines at the end of slanted lines indicate AV block; and zig-zag lines indicate reentry. The rare SA nodal and focal atrial reentry tachycardias are not depicted. Note that premature beats may arise from either reentry (e.g., the first premature beat of the atrial flutter-fibrillation example) or a pacemaker (e.g., the first premature beat of the paroxysmal AV junctional tachycardia example), and that either cause may initiate sustained reentry tachycardias.

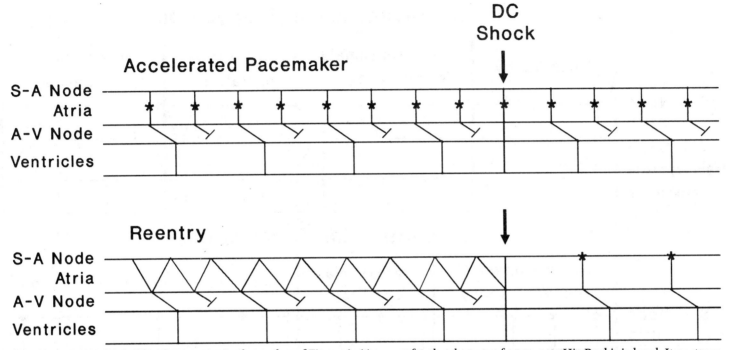

FIGURE 1–12. This ladder diagram is similar to that of Figure 1–11 except for the absence of a separate His-Purkinje level. It portrays the differing responses to DC shock of a tachycardia produced by an accelerated pacemaker and one produced by reentry. Asterisks indicate pacemaker discharge.

ity) and the other from impulse conduction (reentry), are illustrated, as well as why DC shock is effective only when a reentry mechanism is present. Pacemaker arrhythmias persist so long as the precipitating factor is present, whereas reentry arrhythmias result from a transient prob-

lem that produces a self-perpetuating reentry circuit. DC shock stops a reentrant arrhythmia by interrupting the reentry loop, whereas it does not eliminate the factor causing enhanced pacemaker activity. The tachycardia promptly recurs following the shock.

Electrophysiologic Study

Reentrant arrhythmias frequently can be induced in the electrophysiology laboratory using programmed electrical stimulation of the atria and ventricles to reproduce the patient's clinical arrhythmia and to guide or test therapy, or to achieve both objectives. Tachyarrhythmias due to abnormal automaticity sometimes can be induced with β-adrenergic stimulation, whereas programmed electrical stimulation of the heart will not induce such arrhythmias. The arrhythmias thought to be due to early afterdepolarizations may be induced if the rate is slowed, and those due to delayed afterdepolarizations may be induced with acceleration of the atrial or ventricular rates. Programmed electrical stimulation, however, rarely induces these tachyarrhythmias.[8] Chapter 6 discusses the role of electrophysiologic testing in the diagnosis and treatment of arrhythmias.

Basic Principles of Rhythm-Strip Interpretation

The 12-lead ECG typically contains one to three cardiac cycles for each of the leads, and usually suffices for confirmation of normal sinus rhythm but not for diagnosis of an abnormal rhythm. For arrhythmia diagnosis, it is optimal to use a longer rhythm strip of at least 15 seconds. Many diagnoses of simple arrhythmias can be made from a brief rhythm strip of a single lead, whereas more difficult diagnoses may remain impossible even when long strips from multiple leads are observed. The simultaneous recording of two or more ECG leads with different ori-

entations may provide helpful additional information. The interpreter must appreciate the limitations in arrhythmia diagnosis from rhythm strips alone and, at times, include several possibilities in the differential diagnosis even at the conclusion of examination.

Systematic Electrocardiographic Analysis

The approach to the diagnosis of cardiac arrhythmias is discussed through a step-by-step analysis of the rhythm strip (Table 1–2).

ARE SINUS BEATS PRESENT?

The first step in the diagnosis of an arrhythmia is to locate one sinus beat or, ideally, a run of normal sinus beats. The shape of the P, QRS, ST, and T intervals and the PR, QRS, and QT intervals of these beats define what is "normal" for that rhythm and allow comparison with abnormal beats. Sinus beats provide a touchstone for comparison with all other beats and, if two sinus beats are present, the sinus rate also can be determined. When possible, more than one lead should be examined in order to measure the intervals and morphologies of normal beats as precisely as possible (Figs. 1–13 and 1–14).

MEASUREMENT OF THE PR, QRS, AND QT INTERVALS

The PR interval should be measured in three leads and averaged (see Fig. 1–14). Measuring this interval in only one lead may be inaccurate because part of the P wave or QRS complex may be isoelectric in a given lead and the interval will be incorrectly short or long. When three leads are recorded simultaneously, the onset of the P wave can be judged more accurately and the interval from this point to onset of the QRS complex showing the earliest activation, will provide an even more accurate PR measurement. The normal PR interval should be between 0.12 and 0.20 seconds. The longest measured QRS complex should also be recorded. The measurement can be made in any limb or precordial lead as long as the onset and offset of the QRS complex are clearly demarcated. The normal duration of the QRS complex is less than 0.10 seconds. With duration of the QRS complex between 0.10 and 0.12 seconds, a fascicular block or nonspecific conduction delay may be present. With a duration of 0.12 seconds or more, a complete bundle branch block is usually present. The QT interval is measured from the beginning of the QRS complex to the end of the T wave and should also be assessed in several leads. In some cases, the T wave may be broad with a prominent U wave, making it difficult to

Table 1–2. ARRHYTHMIA ANALYSIS

1. Is there a normal sinus beat or run of sinus rhythm?
2. What are the atria doing?
3. What are the ventricles doing?
4. What is the AV relationship?
5. Are there premature beats or pauses?
6. If a tachyarrhythmia is present:
   a. What are the characteristics of onset, termination, or interruption?
   b. What is the response to autonomic maneuvers?
   c. What is the response to pacing or cardioversion?

AV = atrioventricular.

determine when the T wave ends and the U wave begins. In this setting, it is appropriate to note the prominent U wave but not fix a specific number on the QU interval. Since the QT interval has a normal range that varies with rate, the QT interval should be corrected (QT_c) for rate by using either a nomogram relating the observed QT and RR intervals to a corrected QT interval,[9] or by Bazett's formula, wherein

$$QT_c = K \times \sqrt{RR}$$

When the QT and RR interval are measured in seconds, the $K = 0.37 \pm 0.024$ for men and $K = 0.40 \pm 0.04$ for women[10] and the upper normal QT_c is 0.44 seconds. As general rules, the measured QT interval should be less than 0.40 seconds if the rate is between 60 and 100 per minute, or it should be less than half of the RR interval.

WHAT ARE THE ATRIA DOING?

Although it seems natural to focus initial attention on the more prominent QRS complexes, it is more important to discipline oneself first to "find the P waves." This may be difficult, because these smaller waves may be obscured not only by the QRS complexes but also by the ST-T waves. Calipers are, at times, essential for finding the P waves and for determining the atrial rhythm. In this search, it is important to develop suspicions based on solid clinical concepts. For example, because an atrial pause is often caused by a premature P wave that has occurred too early to conduct through the AV conduction system to the ventricles, one should always search in the T wave prior to a pause for a missing P wave. This may require observation of several different ECG leads. Also, when a long PR interval is present in the setting of a supraventricular tachycardia, the P wave or waves are likely obscured by the preceding QRS and ST-T waves. When suspected, a bedside maneuver aimed at slowing the atrial rate or AV conduction through altering parasympathetic tone, may result in correct rhythm interpretation (see Chapters 4, 9, and 10).

ABNORMAL P WAVES

The P wave morphology is altered when its origin is remote from the sinus node area. Determining the location of an ectopic P wave site requires more than one lead. The normal sinus P wave comes from the high right atrium and is generated first by right atrial and then by left atrial depolarization with a vector that is leftward and inferior (between 0° and 90°). The first portion of the P wave is directed anteriorly and the terminal portion

A

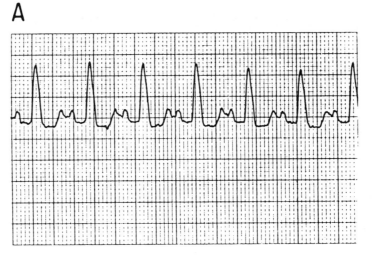

$$Rate = \frac{60{,}000}{R-R \ (msec)}$$

$$R-R = 520 \ msec$$

$$Rate = 115/min$$

B

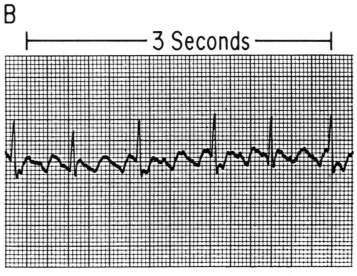

3 Seconds

5 Beats in 3 sec.

$$5 \times 20 = 100/min$$

FIGURE 1–13. The heart rate can be estimated by counting the number of 0.2-second boxes (big boxes) in a single RR interval and dividing this number into 300 (or for rapid heart rates, dividing the number of small boxes between an RR interval into 1500). Either method gives a quick and rough estimate of heart rate. A more precise calculation of rate (*A*) can be made by dividing 60,000 by the RR interval in milliseconds, or when the rate is irregular (*B*), counting the RR intervals during a 3-second sample (or even longer when necessary) and multiplying by 20 or by whatever factor is appropriate to index the heart rate to beats per minute.

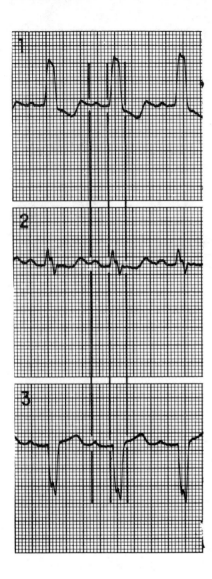

FIGURE 1–14. A simultaneous recording of leads 1, 2, and 3 facilitates accurate measurement of the important ECG intervals. Note that the QRS duration (0.16 seconds) is most accurately reflected in lead 1, and that the PR interval (0.24 seconds) and the QT interval (0.52 seconds) are most accurately assessed in lead 2.

is directed posteriorly (hence in V_1, the P wave is normally diphasic with a terminal negative component). Ectopic or retrograde P waves will have a different P vector; the latter will be directed superiorly, resulting in P wave inversion in leads II, III, and aVF. Ectopic P waves originating in the left atrium will be inverted in I and may be directed either inferiorly or superiorly. Right atrial P waves will have a different morphology from the sinus P but may have the same general vector.

WHAT ARE THE VENTRICLES DOING?

It is important to consider the rate, regularity, and appearance of the QRS complexes. As previously noted, the appearance of the QRS complex may be altered by an abnormality in impulse conduction in one of the bundle branches, or by various other factors that have no relationship to cardiac rhythm. Indeed, bundle branch block is only important in consideration of arrhythmias because, when both bundle branches are involved, second- or third-degree AV block may produce a serious bradycardia (Fig. 1–15). Bundle branch blocks are considered "incomplete" when there is a minor disturbance in the QRS complex, resulting in its prolongation but a total duration of less than 0.12 seconds. Complete right bundle branch block will produce a QRS of at least 0.12 seconds while left bundle branch block typically produces a QRS of at least 0.14 seconds. Consideration of left

bundle branch block is complicated by the presence of relatively separate anterior and posterior divisions (or fascicles) of the left bundle. Therefore, incomplete left bundle branch block is usually due to an abnormality in the left anterior or posterior fascicle, resulting in marked axis deviation (see Chapter 14). When there is a QRS abnormality with an incomplete left bundle branch block pattern but without axis deviation, the most likely cause is left ventricular hypertrophy rather than a primary conduction disturbance.

WHAT IS THE AV RELATIONSHIP?

Once P waves and QRS complexes are identified, it is important to try to determine the relationship between them. This process may be facilitated with ladder diagrams. Location of the P wave may be difficult, because there may be aspects of either the QRS complex or the T wave that mimic P waves in appearance. Therefore, one should attempt to identify the shortest interval between two waves that are definitely P waves. Walking the calipers to either side of this interval will allow determination of whether other "notches" are indeed on-time P waves or just part of the QRS, ST, or T waves (Fig. 1–16A; see Figure 1–15B and C).

When the PR relationship is constant, AV association is presumably present. Sometimes, however, obvious dissociation is present on a later rhythm strip; only

for the short period during which the initial rhythm strip was observed did an "isorhythmic" or constant P-QRS relationship mimic association. Isorhythmia (similar atrial and ventricular rates) occurs during AV dissociation either by coincidence or because an interaction other than an electrical one exists between the atria and ventricles. If one suspects that AV dissociation is present, a prolonged rhythm strip with or without an autonomic intervention may be necessary for confirmation. When isorhythmic AV dissociation is present, one cannot evaluate the status of AV conduction because P waves after the prior T wave and more than 0.2 seconds in front of the QRS complex do not occur. Conclusions regarding AV conduction require observation of the rhythm when isorhythmia is absent.

ALTERED P-QRS RELATIONSHIPS

When the relationship between the P wave and QRS complex is altered, there may be either a persistence of AV association or the development of AV dissociation (Table 1–3). "AV dissociation" means the atria and ventricles are beating independently, but it does not define the pathophysiologic mechanism. AV dissociation may be due to interference in conduction of an antegrade atrial impulse by retrograde conduction into the AV node from either junctional or ventricular activity (Fig. 1–17). Such interference may be the result of either atrial slowing or

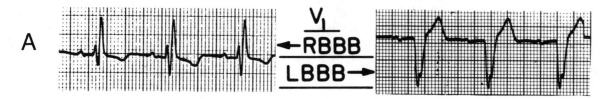

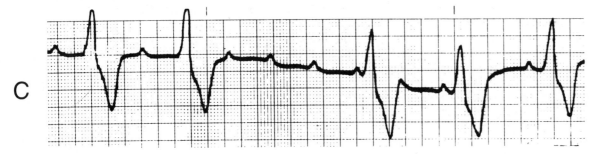

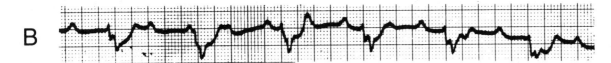

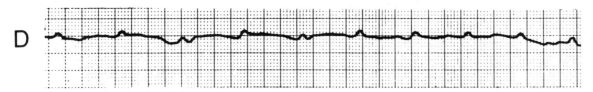

FIGURE 1–15. A typical sequence of progressive intraventricular and atrioventricular conduction abnormalities is illustrated. (*A*) Initially, there are first-degree AV block and right bundle branch block (RBBB), with a long PR interval. Shortly thereafter, complete left bundle branch block (LBBB) appears, also with a long PR interval. (*B*) Complete AV block develops suddenly, within 24 hours. The patient is initially asymptomatic because of an accelerated ventricular pacemaker at a rate of 60 beats per minute. (*C*) This situation does not persist, however, and instability of the ventricular pacemaker results in progressive slowing with pauses. (*D*) The situation finally culminates in complete ventricular asystole, with only P waves manifested on the ECG.

A Variable A-V Block

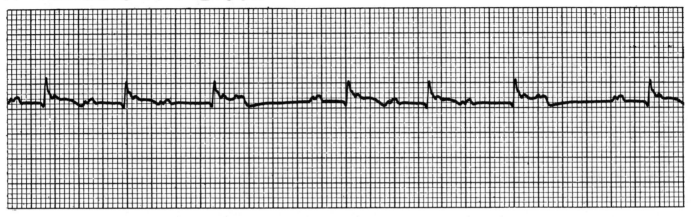

B Complete A-V Block

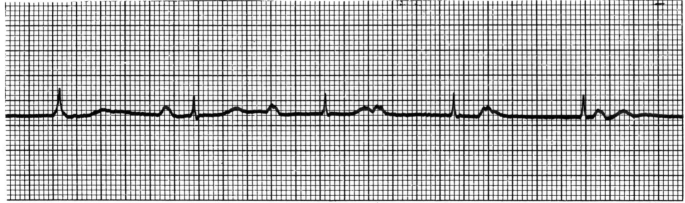

FIGURE 1–16. (*A*) The PR interval is variable, as is the RR interval, with a constant QRS morphology. These features define AV association with varying AV conduction. (*B*) The PR interval varies, but the RR interval is constant. The ventricles, therefore, cannot be under the control of the atria. This defines AV dissociation, which in this case was due to AV block, as confirmed by the numerous P waves that should have conducted but did not.

Table 1–3. CAUSES OF AV DISSOCIATION

MECHANISM	EXAMPLES
Interference:	
Slowing of the atrial pacemaker	Sinus bradycardia with AV junctional rhythm
Speeding of a lower pacemaker	AV junctional or ventricular tachycardia
AV block	Third-degree AV block

AV = atrioventricular.

ventricular speeding. The other cause of AV dissociation is block of the atrial impulse in the AV conduction system. Table 1–3 lists the causes of AV dissociation. More than one process may be present on occasion.

If AV dissociation is due to interference, the ventricular rate should be faster than or the same as (isorhythmic) the atrial rate. In addition to noting the relative atrial and ventricular rates, however, the clinician should carefully assess the absolute atrial and ventricular rates, as they are somewhat predictive of the basic mechanism responsible for the AV dissociation. If the atrial rate is less than 60 beats per minute, atrial slowing is likely to be responsible; if the ventricular rate is more than 60 beats per minute, ventricular speeding is likely to be responsible.

If AV dissociation is due to AV block, the ventricular rate is almost always slower than the atrial rate. The position of nonconducted P waves is key to the diagnosis; if a P wave appears at a time when it would be expected to conduct but fails to do so, AV block is present. That is, a P wave falling after the T wave of a prior beat and preceding the next QRS complex by more than 0.2 seconds should have conducted to the ventricles. If no such P wave occurs on the ECGs available for review, then the status of AV conduction cannot be assessed; either additional rhythm strips must be reviewed or an intervention performed to change the timing of the P waves relative to the QRS complexes. For example, carotid sinus massage could slow the atrial rate and change the P-QRS relationship, causing a P wave to occur at a time that it should conduct, and thus allow an assessment of the status of AV conduction.

Both AV dissociation and AV association with variable AV block result in a variable PR interval. If the PR interval is variable because of variable block, the resulting RR interval should also be vari-able. If the ventricular rhythm is dissociated from the atrial rhythm, on the other hand, the ventricular rate is almost always regular. Thus, in the presence of a variable PR interval, a variable RR interval indicates AV association, whereas a constant RR interval indicates AV dissociation (see Figure 1–16).

ARE THERE PREMATURE BEATS OR PAUSES?

After the basic rhythm has been defined, one should look for premature beats and attempt to identify their origin. Guidelines for this decision are presented in Chapter 7.

An interruption of the basic rhythm may result in a pause reflecting a nonconducted premature beat, AV block, or failure of the primary pacemaker. Determination of the cause of the pause is important in determining the correct diagnosis as well as in selecting the proper therapeutic approach, because both AV

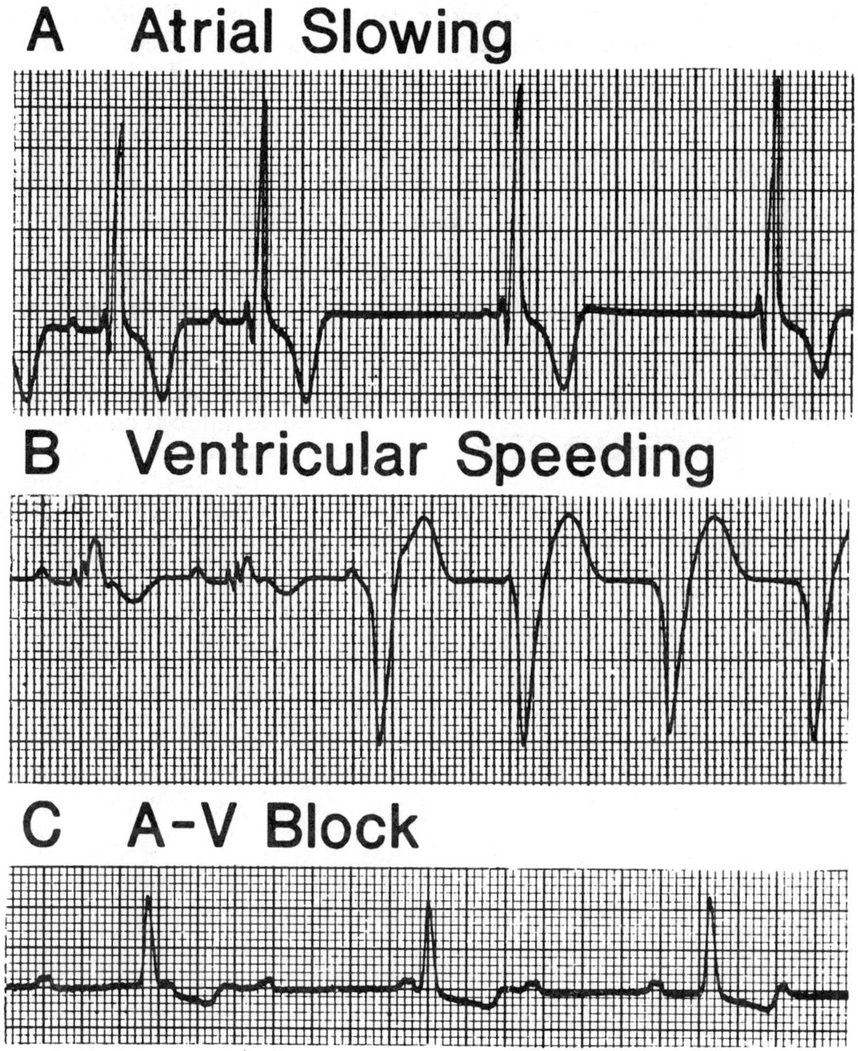

FIGURE 1–17. The three causes of AV dissociation: atrial slowing, ventricular speeding, and AV block. (*A*) The atrial rate slows and the late atrial activity then encounters interference from normally timed junctional escape beats. (*B*) The normally timed atrial activity (third P wave) encounters interference from early ventricular activation. (*C*) There is no interference (i.e., there is no atrial slowing or ventricular speeding). Therefore, AV block must be present as the cause of the AV dissociation. The presence of AV block is confirmed by the numerous P waves that should have conducted but did not.

block and sinus arrest or exit block can lead to serious bradyarrhythmias.

TACHYARRHYTHMIAS: ONSET, OFFSET, CHANGE

Additional steps to be followed when a tachyarrhythmia is present can be found in Chapter 8. New questions should be considered at this point, including the characteristics of onset, offset, or interruption, and the response of the arrhythmia to autonomic interventions or other maneuvers such as pacing.

REFERENCES

1. Wit AL: Cellular electrophysiologic mechanisms of cardiac arrhythmias. Ann NY Acad Sci 432:1–17, 1985.
2. Zipes DP: Genesis of cardiac arrhythmias: Electrophysiologic considerations. In Braunwald E (ed): Heart Disease. WB Saunders, Philadelphia, 1988, pp 581–620.
3. Akhtar M, Tchou PJ, and Jazayeri M: Mechanisms of clinical tachycardias. Am J Cardiol 61(Suppl 1)61:9A–19A, 1988.
4. Cranefield PF: Action potentials, afterpotentials and arrhythmias. Circ Res 41:415–423, 1977.
5. Belhassen B, Shapira I, Pelleg A, Copperman I, Kauli N, and Laniado S: Idiopathic recurrent ventricular tachycardia responsive to verapamil: An ECG-electrophysiologic entity. Am Heart J 108:1034–1035, 1984.
6. Gomes JA and El-Sherif N: Atrioventricular block: Mechanism, clinical presentation, and therapy. Med Clin North Am 68:955–967, 1984.
7. Packer DL and Prystowsky EN: Wolff-Parkinson-White syndrome: Further progress in evaluation and treatment. Prog Cardiol 1:147–187, 1988.
8. Sung R, Keung EC, Nguyen NX, and Huycke EC: Effects of β-adrenergic blockade on verapamil-responsive and verapamil-irresponsive sustained ventricular tachycardias. J Clin Invest 81:688–699, 1988.
9. Kissin M, Schwarzchild MM, and Bakst H: A nomogram for rate correction of the Q-T interval in the electrocardiogram. Am Heart J 35:990–992, 1948.
10. Bazett HC: An analysis of the time-relations of the electrocardiogram. Heart 7:353–370, 1920.

The Patient History

BARRY W. RAMO, MD

Outline

Many people have experienced symptomatic arrhythmias at some time during their lives; these arrhythmias are usually due to isolated premature beats or sinus tachycardia and have no prognostic significance. Most patients ignore these infrequent episodes of more rapid or irregular heart action, but at times, treatment may be required if only because the patient is made uncomfortable by the symptoms. In other patients with presyncope or syncope, angina, unexplained confusion, fatigue, or heart failure, a carefully recorded history may suggest a significant underlying arrhythmia wherein appropriate treatment may prevent death or severe disability. Further complicating diagnosis are those patients who may have relatively minimal or even no symptoms and yet who have an arrhythmia with the potential for disastrous hemodynamic or electrical consequences.

Figure 2–1 is a Venn diagram illustrating four populations of patients with ar-

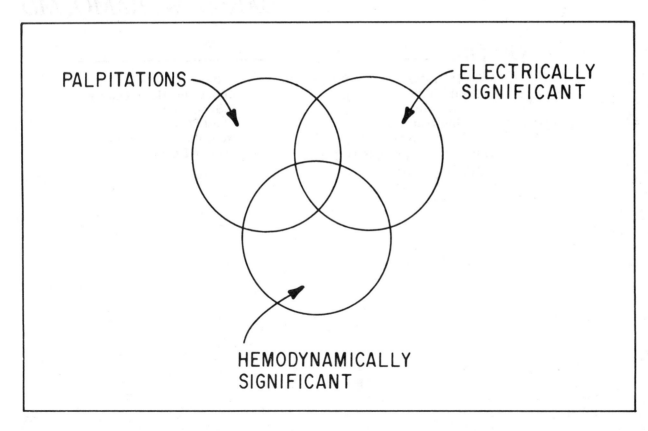

FIGURE 2–1. Four populations of patients with arrhythmias. The *palpitations* subgroup includes patients who are able to sense changes in heartbeat rhythm either spontaneously or by palpating the pulse (i.e., they have symptoms specifically related to the change in rhythm and therefore are aware of their heartbeat patterns). In the *electrically significant* subgroup are those whose arrhythmia has the potential for leading to death from asystole or ventricular fibrillation. The *hemodynamically significant* subgroup includes those whose arrhythmias significantly decrease blood pressure and cardiac output, or increase myocardial oxygen demands, or both. Note that any two or all three subgroups may overlap. Those outside all three circles have asymptomatic arrhythmias with no clinical significance.

PALPITATIONS

ELECTRICALLY SIGNIFICANT

HEMODYNAMICALLY SIGNIFICANT

rhythmias. Also illustrated is the potential for overlap among the three symptomatic or significant subgroups. For example, in a patient with a normal cardiovascular system and palpitations due to sinus tachycardia or premature ventricular complexes (PVCs), neither arrhythmia has electrical or hemodynamic significance, and the patient would be categorized in the nonoverlapping portion of the "palpitations" circle or subgroup. On the other hand, in a patient with palpitations due to paroxysmal atrial fibrillation who also has syncope, the arrhythmia is likely hemodynamically significant, with hypotension due to either a rapid rate or a post-tachycardia pause. Such a patient would reside in the area of overlap between the "palpitations" and "hemodynamically significant" subgroups. If this patient also had antidromic ventricular preexcitation, then an "electrically significant" arrhythmia (e.g., atrial fibrillation leading to ventricular fibrillation) would also be possible, and such a patient would reside in the area of overlap of all three subgroups.

It is the clinician's task to determine whether a known or suspected arrhythmia is (1) benign with no significance; (2) electrically significant with a risk of asystole or ventricular fibrillation; or (3) hemodynamically significant as defined by a significant reduction in blood pressure and cardiac output or an increase in myocardial oxygen consumption, or both. The first step in this process is the patient history.

This chapter discusses the use of the patient history in the diagnosis of arrhythmias due to abnormalities of impulse formation and conduction that result in tachycardias, bradycardias, or premature beats, or in any combination of these cardiac-rhythm disturbances.

MECHANISMS RESPONSIBLE FOR SYMPTOMS

The symptoms of a cardiac-rhythm disturbance are determined by a variety of factors depending on the arrhythmia itself and the patient. Arrhythmia-related factors include, most importantly, the arrhythmia's rate and regularity and the presence or absence of atrioventricular (AV) dissociation, and, to a lesser degree, the arrhythmia's site. Patient-related factors of equal or even greater importance include the severity and type of underlying heart disease, the vascular tone, and the blood volume.

The final hemodynamic significance is determined by how these factors interact to produce a fall in cardiac output, a fall in blood pressure, an increase in myocardial oxygen demands, or any combination of these responses (Figs. 2–2 and 2–3). Factors that can contribute to the severity or chronicity of the resulting hypotension and inadequate cardiac output include:

- A baroreceptor reflex inadequate to maintain appropriate peripheral vascular resistance
- Diminished intravascular volume
- Left ventricular dysfunction that limits the stroke volume or cardiac output response to an arrhythmia

Similarly, the development of myocardial ischemia depends on the extent of coronary artery disease and the degree of ventricular hypertrophy, as well as the patient's ability to maintain an adequate coronary perfusion pressure.

The variability in these factors explains why patients with markedly different symptoms may have identical arrhythmias or, conversely, identical symptoms yet different arrhythmias. Similarly, arrhythmias due to abnormalities of either impulse formation or impulse conduction may result in clinical syndromes that are indistinguishable on the basis of their mechanism. In some instances, however, the mechanism of the arrhythmia contributes specific clinical features that are described in the following sections dealing with the symptomatic correlates of premature beats, bradycardias, and tachycardias.

Premature Beats

Premature beats, regardless of basic mechanism, are often just a nuisance in that they are symptomatic but have no prognostic significance. Even when oc-

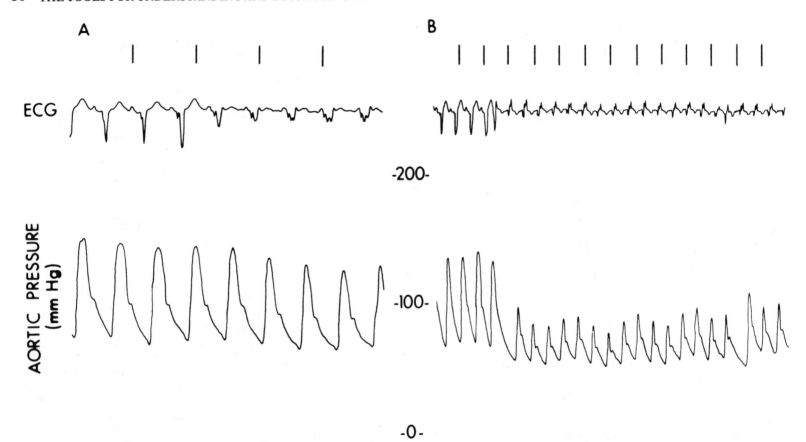

FIGURE 2–2. (*A*) Sinus rhythm is interrupted by an accelerated ventricular rhythm causing transient atrioventricular (AV) dissociation with a progressively shorter PR interval. As the contribution of atrial systole to stroke volume lessens, aortic pressure gradually falls. (*B*) A premature ventricular complex (PVC) causes abrupt AV dissociation that continues during a subsequent long run of accelerated ventricular rhythm. Aortic pressure also falls abruptly to less than 100 mmHg and, as compensatory mechanisms come into play, subsequently rises slowly but variably to greater than 100 mmHg. This variability in pressure reflects the variable contribution of atrial systole to stroke volume and is also due to the AV dissociation. Time lines represent intervals of 1.0 second.

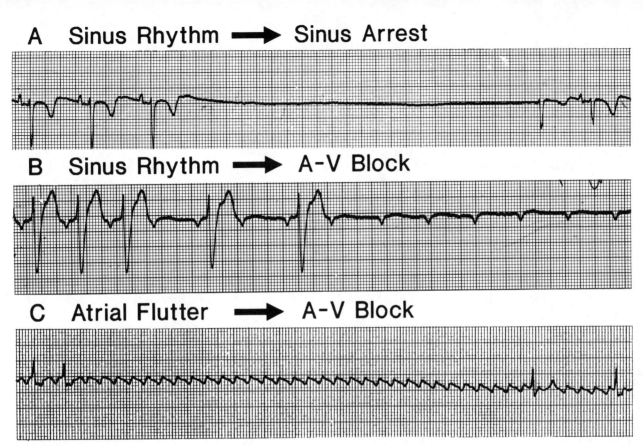

A Sinus Rhythm ➤ Sinus Arrest

B Sinus Rhythm ➤ A-V Block

C Atrial Flutter ➤ A-V Block

FIGURE 2–3. Three different bradyarrhythmias with the potential for causing syncope. (*A*) Sudden failure of the sinus as well as all escape pacemakers produces a 5.2-second pause that is terminated by a junctional escape beat. Enhanced parasympathetic tone is the likely cause of this failure of impulse formation. (*B*) This bradyarrhythmia occurs during sinus rhythm and is due to the combination of a failure of AV conduction and a failure of all escape pacing. The constant PR interval (0.18 seconds), even after the pauses due to dropped P waves, indicates type II, second-degree AV block (i.e., the RP interval varies but the PR interval remains constant). The QRS complex is also wide, and in combination with the failure of an escape pacemaker to emerge from the bundles distal to the site of block, it demonstrates features typical of distal conduction-system disease. (*C*) This bradyarrhythmia occurs during atrial flutter with rapid AV conduction (150 beats per minute) and results from a sudden increase in AV block plus a failure of escape pacing. It produces a 6-second pause. The QRS complex is narrow, and it is likely that the AV node is the site of block and that both the block and inhibition of escape pacing are due to enhanced parasympathetic tone.

curring frequently, they are rarely of hemodynamic significance, but they commonly produce feelings of fullness in the throat or chest, a sudden need to cough, or an irregular sensation within the chest. The beats are sensed for four reasons. First, premature ventricular beats may occur in synchrony with atrial contraction and produce cannon A waves in the neck and pulmonary veins that are sensed (Fig. 2–4; see also Figs. 3–2 and 3–3). Second, premature beats can open the aortic valve and eject blood, and this process or the early beat itself may be sensed or appreciated by the patient in some way independent of any cannon A waves (Figs. 2–4 and 2–5). Third, premature beats are frequently followed by a pause, and this too may be sensed. A common description is "I feel a fluttering in my chest and then my heart stops" (see Fig. 2–5). Fourth, the large stroke volume of the beat following the premature beat generates a large pulmonary and systemic arterial pulse that may be felt as a sense of fullness or a "thumping sensation."

Activity does not necessarily decrease the frequency of premature beats but it distracts patients. Patients most often complain of premature beats when they are inactive and resting.

No matter how frequently single premature beats occur, they usually do not produce symptoms of inadequate cerebral blood flow. The one exception occurs when a patient with a slow resting heart rate and limited cardiac reserve develops a bigeminal rhythm. The resulting marked decrease in the effective heart rate may cause an impaired blood pressure response to sudden changes in posture or a diminution in cardiac output (Fig. 2–6). On other occasions, premature beats may cause neurologic symptoms by an indirect route when they are sensed and lead to anxiety and hyperventilation with dizziness, paresthesias, and other neurologic features typical of the syndrome.

Bradycardias

When bradycardias cause hypotension with critically decreased cerebral blood flow, the perfusion defect is global and symptoms of cerebrovascular insufficiency occur, such as transient episodes of presyncope or syncope depending on chronicity or severity on both factors. The cause of a bradycardia may be slowing of either the primary pacemaker or AV block, but a severe bradyarrhythmia can only ensue if there is also concomitant failure of escape pacemakers to function appropriately (see also Chapter 13, pages 304 to 310, and Chapter 14, pages 339 to 340). The corresponding clinical syndrome reflects both the rapidity with which the bradycardia progresses and its severity. Both pacemaker failure and AV block can produce abrupt hypotension with correspondingly precipitous presyncope or syncope, or both.

An inadequate heart rate response to activity, as well as the loss of atrial contraction with any concomitant AV dissociation, can limit the cardiac output and may cause exercise intolerance with exertional dyspnea and fatigue. Bradycardias may also contribute to congestive heart failure because an inadequate cardiac output activates the renin-angiotensin system, with resulting salt and water retention. With the combination of depressed ventricular function and bradycardia, exercise may also result in a fall in blood pressure and neurologic symptoms.

Tachycardias

Tachycardias may produce an awareness of a rapid heart action (a variety of palpitations) or more serious symptoms of hemodynamic impairment either by increasing myocardial oxygen demands, with anginal syndromes and impaired ventricular function; by producing hypotension, with resulting neurologic symptoms; or by limiting the cardiac output, with heart failure symptoms. Some tachycardias due to reentrant or, more rarely, triggered mechanisms may lead to syncope and sudden death. Arrhythmias due to enhanced pacemaker activity, such as sinus tachycardia, nonparoxysmal AV junctional tachycardia, or accelerated

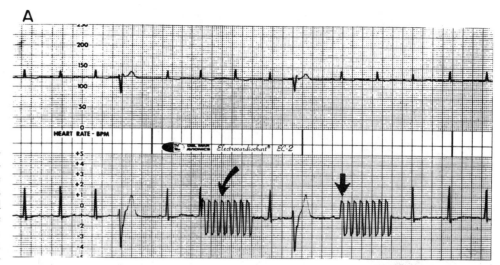

FIGURE 2–4. This dual-channel ambulatory electro-cardiogram (ECG) is from a physician who was experiencing palpitations. (*A*) After a "flip-flop" sensation, he pressed the symptom-marker button (curved arrow) as quickly as possible. Shortly thereafter, he experienced a second flip-flop sensation and was able to activate the marker button even more quickly (straight arrow). After the first premature ventricular complex (PVC), an intervening sinus return beat occurs before the symptom marker, and it is possible that the flip-flop sensation could have come from either the premature beat itself or the postpremature sinus beat. After the second PVC, however, the symptom-marker button was activated before the returning sinus beat, isolating the symptom to the premature beat itself. (*B* and *C*) With practice, the physician became quite adept at rapidly activating the symptom-marker button after each palpitation. Note that the symptom markers occur simultaneously with or slightly before the returning sinus beat following each PVC. Given a cellular electromechanical coupling interval of 40 to 60 milliseconds plus the inevitable additional delay between the symptom and reflex activation of the marker button, however, the symptoms obviously preceded any mechanical component associated with the return cycle. Given these observations and the flip-flop character of the sensations, the symptoms obviously arose from either the PVC itself or, more likely, the resulting cannon A waves in the systemic and pulmonary veins.

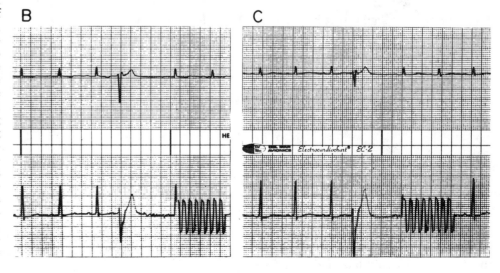

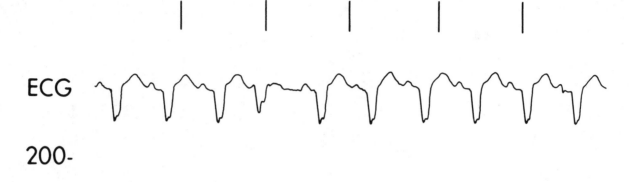

ECG

200-

AORTIC PRESSURE (mm Hg)

100-

0-

FIGURE 2–5. In this recording of aortic root pressure and the ECG, normal sinus rhythm is interrupted by a single PVC. The PVC itself generates enough of a stroke volume to open the aortic valve and create a small, premature pulse wave. After the PVC, there is a pause, resulting in an augmented stroke volume and pulse pressure of the post-PVC beat. Either of these mechanical events may be sensed and may explain some of the "palpitations." Time lines indicate intervals of 1.0 second.

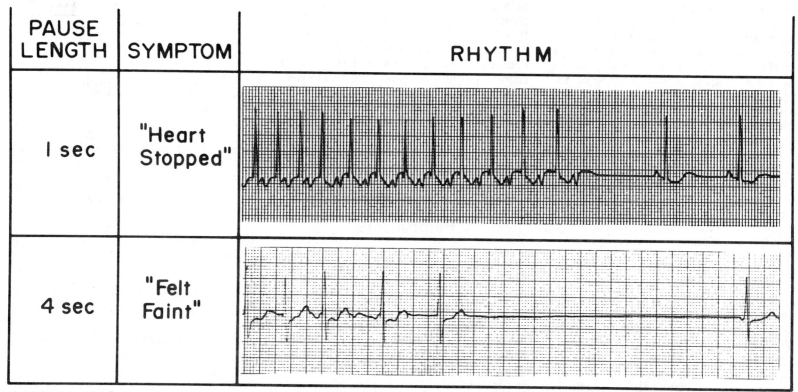

PAUSE LENGTH	SYMPTOM	RHYTHM
I sec	"Heart Stopped"	
4 sec	"Felt Faint"	

FIGURE 2–6. In the top strip, paroxysmal AV junctional tachycardia first slows slightly and then stops abruptly, producing a brief pause that is terminated by prompt sinus escape. Because the patient was aware of a rapid heartbeat rhythm, the sensation of the heart "stopping" occurred when the rhythm terminated. In the bottom strip, atrial flutter-fibrillation stops abruptly with marked suppression of escape pacemaker activity, resulting in a 4-second pause and the symptom of "feeling faint." The pause is terminated by a junctional escape beat.

ventricular rhythms, generally do not reach heart rates that lead to serious hemodynamic consequences.

The rate of the arrhythmia and the patient's overall hemodynamic status determine if symptoms of hemodynamic impairment occur, but in general it is rare for a tachycardia below the rate of 150 beats per minute to produce syncope. One exception occurs when accelerated ventricular rhythms at rates of 60 to 120 beats per minute (usually in association with significant underlying ventricular dysfunction) produce significant hypotension because of the concomitant AV dissociation and loss of atrial contraction (see Fig. 2–2). Supraventricular and ventricular tachycaridas both involve ranges of heart rate that are sufficiently rapid to cause significant hemodynamic impairment.

The clinical presentation of reentrant arrhythmias is characteristic because they usually are initiated by single premature beats and terminate abruptly, whereas pacemaker tachycardias typically begin gradually. Some automatic tachycardias end abruptly owing to exit block, but sinus tachycardia invariably slows gradually. Patient symptoms reflect these electrophysiologic differences in that palpitations due to reentry start and stop suddenly, whereas with sinus tachycardia, for example, the onset and offset are more gradual. Presyncope and syncope in tachycardia settings may also reflect asystole following their termination because

of pathologic "overdrive suppression" of normal escape pacemakers. This phenomenon is particularly common in patients with paroxysmal atrial flutter-fibrillation, one of the most frequent varieties of the "tachycardia-bradycardia" syndrome (see Fig. 2–6). On occasion, rapid regular palpitations may follow the perception of an isolated premature beat when the latter causes anxiety, an outpouring of catecholamines, and sinus tachycardia.

SPECIFIC SYMPTOMS DUE TO ARRHYTHMIAS

Palpitations

Palpitations, defined as an awareness of one's own heartbeat, are the most common cardiac symptoms and may result from one or more factors, including an irregular heartbeat, an increased heart rate, or an increase in myocardial contractility. No symptom is more troublesome and frightening to patients yet so often benign. Palpitations may lead to a cardiac neurosis, particularly when the physician insists on treating them or otherwise implies that they reflect heart disease. The patient with sinus tachycardia who is treated with a β-blocker may become fatigued, depressed, lose hair, or experience nightmares or other side effects that make palpitations seem like a pleasure in comparison. The key to the correct treatment of the patient

Table 2–1. IMPORTANT HISTORICAL DESCRIPTORS IN DIFFERENTIAL DIAGNOSIS OF PALPITATIONS

Are they regular or irregular? What is the rate?	Doctor taps out rhythm on tabletop or has patient tap out rhythm.
How do they start and stop? (sudden vs. gradual)	Ask "Is it there one second and gone the next?" (or vice versa)
What are the inciting and associated factors?	Determine what the patient was doing at the onset and whether any drugs or other potential stimulants were being used.
Are there associated symptoms?	Ask specifically about presyncope, syncope, angina, dyspnea, polyuria

is to diagnose accurately the arrhythmia responsible for the palpitations, a process that begins with the history. Some important historical points in the differential diagnosis of palpitations are listed in Table 2–1.

PALPITATIONS AT NONTACHYCARDIAC HEART RATES

Intermittent isolated palpitations at a nontachycardiac heart rate usually reflect premature beats. Patient thresholds for perceiving premature beats are quite variable, both from patient to patient and within the same patient at different times. Most patients with frequent premature beats are asymptomatic, but sadly, others are aware of almost every single one. Even though premature beats may be seen with equal or increased frequency during periods of activity on ambulatory monitoring and during exercise testing, it is unusual for patients to note an increase in their frequency with activity; they are usually maximally symptomatic at rest. This phenomenon probably reflects the diminution in environmental sensory input during rest or inactivity and the enhanced likelihood that such internal stimuli will be sensed.

Patient descriptions of how premature beats feel are also quite variable. Patients may complain of a sudden need to take a deep breath as the pulmonary and systemic arterial fullness generated by the increased stroke volume of the postpremature beat or the fullness in the jugular and pulmonary veins caused by the cannon A wave creates a transient feeling of dyspnea. Occasionally patients may perceive this brief sensation as a chest discomfort. They may also note a fullness in the throat, a heaviness in the chest, or a feeling of irregularity within the chest. "My heart turned over," "A bird was fluttering in my chest," and "There was a flip-flop sensation" are common descriptions. The physician should determine if the sensations are due to one premature beat, a sequence of premature beats, or a sustained tachycardia. Neither the mechanism nor the site of origin of premature beats can be reliably differentiated by history. On occasion, symptoms may occur in some combination, as when perception of an isolated premature beat causes anxiety and a catecholamine-induced sinus tachycardia, or when the ectopy causes a subsequent reentry tachycardia. Inattention to such details may result in an incorrect diagnosis of paroxysmal tachycardia when the patient is only having intermittent premature beats, or premature beats followed by sinus tachycardia.

Palpitations may also occur secondary to an increased force of contraction with little or no change in heart rate and thus not reflect an arrhythmia. In such instances, patients frequently complain of "hard beats" that are regular and not rapid. Having the patient or a companion count the pulse rate and regularity during an episode of palpitations is very helpful in determining the rate.

RAPID, REGULAR PALPITATIONS

The most common cause for rapid, regular heart action is sinus tachycardia, and the questions outlined in Table 2–1 are helpful in its diagnosis. It is frequently perceived as a sensation of the heart beating hard as well as fast. Sinus tachycardia is often precipitated by physical activity, emotional stress, or the use of stimulants such as coffee, cigarettes, alcohol, and certain drugs (both legal and illegal); a careful history concerning these points is important. Because sinus tachycardia is the result of an increase in automaticity of the sinus node, the tachycardia gradually accelerates and slows. Although it is not uncommon for patients to miss the gradual onset and complain that the palpitations "were suddenly there," they usually describe the resolution as gradual over several minutes.

Patients with symptomatic sinus tachycardia due to anxiety or extraordinary awareness of their heart action frequently experience a similar rapid heart rate when they exercise, and note that when they stop exercising, their heart rate gradually slows. When asked to compare the sensations associated with the exercise-induced tachycardia and its resolution to their spontaneously occurring palpitations, they usually describe them as the same. Another helpful question to ask is whether their symptoms might be similar to what they would likely experience if called upon to give a 5-minute extemporaneous speech in front of a crowd.

A second important historical point concerning sinus tachycardia is the rate. Patients with sinus tachycardia rarely have heart rates greater than 140 beats per minute unless they are exercising or in a state where high adrenergic drive is present, such as shock, the postoperative period, or thyrotoxicosis. Most commonly, sinus tachycardia at rest manifests a heart rate of between 100 and 120 beats per minute. Patients can frequently recognize this characteristic rate, as well as the regularity of sinus tachycardia, by having either the physician or themselves tap out the rhythm. It is often surprising how slow the rate is when the doctor or patient taps out the rhythm on a tabletop or a knee, even though the patient initially described the rate as "fast." When such tapping is unsuccessful, it is often useful to teach the patient or a companion or both to count the pulse rate and regularity during episodes of palpitations. If they report "It was too fast to count," the patient was probably experiencing a tachyarrhythmia other than sinus tachycardia.

As mentioned, patients with paroxysmal tachycardias frequently indicate that "one second it was there and the next it was not" (or vice versa). Examining the onset and termination of the arrhythmia in more detail than just whether it was sudden or gradual may provide additional important clues to the correct diagnosis. Because almost all reentry tachyarrhythmias begin with a premature beat, the patients will often describe a "sudden thump" initiating a sustained tachycardia. Alternatively, they may note that the tachycardias are initiated by a "fullness" in the chest or throat, which likewise reflects a premature beat's cannon A waves. The method by which the arrhythmia terminates may also provide diagnostic clues. Patients with paroxysmal AV junctional tachycardias (both atrioventricular nodal reentry and atrioventricular reciprocating tachycardias using a bypass tract) often note that straining, deep breathing, or gagging terminates the arrhythmia. Young patients may find handstands quite effective in stopping attacks. Patients may also be quite aware of the sensation that occurs at the termination of the tachycardia. In the top part of Figure 2–6, the sudden termination of an AV reciprocating tachycardia with a 1-second pause caused the patient to feel as though "my heart had stopped." In the bottom part of Figure 2–6, following termination of atrial fibrillation with a 4-second pause, the patient "felt faint." If self-initiated maneuvers are successful in terminating an arrhythmia, the patient may not consult a physician.

RAPID, IRREGULAR PALPITATIONS

Patients with paroxysmal atrial fibrillation characteristically complain of the sudden onset of rapid and irregular heart action. This cadence can be reproduced by the knee- or tabletop-tapping technique; the patients can almost immediately recognize this chaotic rhythm. Often patients will notice that lying down reduces the intensity of the palpitations but that the symptoms invariably return on trying to resume normal activity. Even a low level of exercise speeds AV conduction disproportionately and results in a rapid ventricular rate.

Paroxysmal atrial fibrillation, like AV junctional reentry, in addition to beginning abruptly also terminates abruptly. The patient may become symptomatic at termination when pathologic overdrive suppression of the sinus node and other potential escape pacemakers causes a prolonged pause with presyncope or syncope (see Fig. 2–6, bottom). On occasion, the posttachycardia-bradycardia is worsened by the drugs (such as the type Ia and type Ic agents, β-blockers, and calcium antagonists) used to treat the tachycardia; what was previously slight dizziness at termination may progress to overt syncope following the institution of drug therapy. Rarely, a similar posttachycardia depression of the sinus node may occur when paroxysmal ventricular tachycardia and retrograde ventriculoatrial capture cause penetration and capture of the sinus node with resulting pathologic overdrive suppression.

Polyuria

Polyuria during, after, and rarely even before the onset of reentry supraventricular tachycardias is thought to be due to increased levels of atrial natriuretic hormone associated with an increase in atrial pressures or stretch resulting from the tachycardia (both AV junctional reentry and atrial reentry) or premature atrial contractions (in those patients with polyuria prior to their tachycardia), or to any combination of these causes. Polyuria in association with palpitations, therefore, is a clue that patients are having supraventricular tachycardias.

Fatigue

Patients with slow, fixed heart rates due to either AV block or sinus slowing frequently have a decreased exercise tolerance with fatigue as a prominent complaint (Fig. 2–7A). A common clinical example of this phenomenon occurs in patients with fixed-rate ventricular pacemakers and has led to the development of pacemakers that are responsive to activity (see Chapter 16). Patients with atrial fibrillation and an uncontrolled ventricular response to exercise may similarly have a markedly and inappropriately depressed exercise tolerance because they develop a rapid tachycardia at a low level of exertion (Figure 2–7B). The clinical importance of whether an arrhythmia develops during exercise with corresponding symptoms or whether it is present at rest but asymptomatic and becomes clinically manifest only during exercise usually depends on the presence and degree of associated ventricular dysfunction. Fatigue and symptoms from an inadequate cardiac output response to exercise, for example, are more profound in patients with underlying heart disease.

Congestive Heart Failure Symptoms

Protracted tachycardias and bradycardias can cause a decrease in cardiac output that may lead to a compensatory volume overload and signs of congestive heart failure such as dyspnea, orthopnea, paroxysmal nocturnal dyspnea, nocturia, and, with right-heart failure, peripheral edema. When the arrhythmia is accompanied by a loss of appropriately timed atrial systole, the stroke volume and cardiac output may be further compromised.

Chest Pain

Angina pectoris may be an important and unexpected symptom of cardiac arrhythmias. Tachycardias can produce myocardial ischemia not manifest under any other circumstances, as well as worsen preexistent angina. For example, a patient with coronary artery disease may have a normal exercise tolerance with no angina when in sinus rhythm and yet develop typical ischemic pain when a paroxysmal tachyarrhythmia develops.

Even patients with no obstructive coronary artery disease may develop angina and, rarely, even myocardial infarction if the arrhythmia is sufficiently rapid and sustained, because the increased myocardial oxygen demands of a very rapid heart rate, particularly in combination with hypotension, can produce subendocardial ischemia and infarction.

Tachyarrhythmias may give few if any clinical evidence of their presence, or, in addition to angina, they may cause syncope or dyspnea with the patient being unaware of any rapid heart action. In patients with coronary artery disease, dyspnea results when global left ventricular ischemia causes transient heart failure and even pulmonary edema, but tachycardias can worsen left ventricular function regardless of the cause of underlying heart disease. Thus, the clinician must carefully evaluate patients with unexplained angina (as well as dyspnea or syncope) for the possibility of a silent (nonpalpitating) tachyarrhythmia.

Bradyarrhythmias rarely produce angina pectoris, but an occasional patient with coronary artery disease and profound bradyarrhythmias can have rest angina. Presumably, cardiac dilatation increases the left ventricular internal diameter and wall tension, with a resulting increase in myocardial oxygen demands. Such patients have been successfully treated with permanent pacemakers that increase the heart rate. The resulting decrease in left ventricular size and wall tension decreases myocardial oxygen demands despite the increase in heart rate.

Neurologic Symptoms

In adult patients, even with known cerebrovascular disease, seizures or focal neurologic signs are only rarely related to global hypoperfusion due to an arrhythmia. An exception occurs when an arrhythmia (usually a bradycardia) results in a prolonged period of hypotension in the setting of underlying cerebrovascular disease; a focal neurologic deficit may then ensue. Another exception occurs in children, who may present with seizures

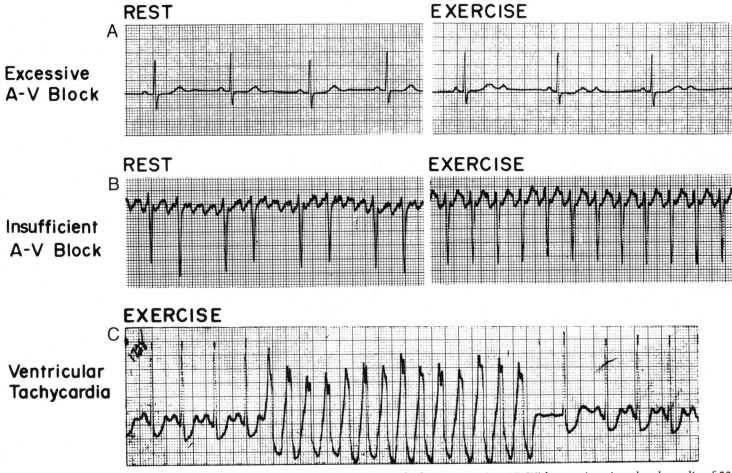

FIGURE 2-7. Three examples of arrhythmias that produce symptoms only during exercise. (*A*) With a resting sinus bradycardia of 52 beats per minute, exercise results in 2:1 AV block and reduces the ventricular rate to 43 beats per minute. (*B*) With atrial flutter, a 6:2 conduction ratio produces an overall resting ventricular rate of 108 beats per minute. With minimal exercise, AV conduction increases to 2:1, and the ventricular rate speeds excessively to 170 beats per minute. (*C*) During exercise, a sinus tachycardia of 140 beats per minute is interrupted by a sudden 14-beat run of ventricular tachycardia with a rate of 210 beats per minute.

Table 2–2. DIFFERENCES IN NEUROLOGIC SYMPTOMS DUE TO ARRHYTHMIC VS. NONARRHYTHMIC MECHANISMS

SYMPTOMS OR SIGNS	MECHANISMS	
	ARRHYTHMIC	NONARRHYTHMIC*
Syncope, presyncope	Yes	Rarely with akinetic seizures, vertebrobasilar artery insufficiency
Confusion, somnolence	Rare and brief	Yes
Focal neurologic signs	Rare†	Yes
Seizures	Rare‡	Yes
Vertigo, nystagmus	No	Yes

*Embolic or hemorrhagic cerebrovascular accident (CVA), reversible ischemic neurologic deficit (RIND), seizures, subclavian steal syndrome.

†Preexisting neurologic deficits (e.g., unilateral weakness from an old CVA) may be exacerbated temporarily.

‡More common in children.

as a manifestation of an arrhythmia. Conversely, primary neurologic processes rarely present as syncope, although it may occur rarely with vertebrobasilar arterial insufficiency. With the onset of syncope due to an arrhythmia or other causes of hypotension, often there may be a few tonic twitches of the face or extremities, which must not be confused with seizure activity. A careful history often reveals that what was being called a "seizure" was actually such twitches and the stertorous breathing caused by global cerebral ischemia. Table 2–2 outlines the differences in neurologic symptoms due to cardiac and noncardiac etiologies.

PRESYNCOPE AND SYNCOPE

Both paroxysmal bradycardias and tachycardias can cause hypotension with cerebral hypoperfusion. A reduction in cardiac output and blood pressure sufficient to cause neurologic symptoms usually results in global cerebral ischemia. The symptoms reflect this, with the two most common being presyncope ("dizziness" and "faintness" are common descriptive terms used by patients) and syncope (see Fig. 2–6, bottom); confusion or somnolence, or both, are much less frequent. The course of the fall in blood pressure with different arrhythmias is variable, so the timing of syncope varies correspondingly. The fall in blood pressure associated with the onset of a sustained tachycardia generally lasts for only 5 to 20 seconds because the baroreceptor reflex causes peripheral vasoconstriction and a return of the blood pressure toward normal (see Fig. 2–2). Brief or less severe hypotension may result in only presyncope, with transient feelings of being lightheaded. Patients commonly report that they "nearly blacked out." These symptoms must be distinguished from the vertigo often seen with vertebrobasilar arterial insufficiency, wherein nausea, diplopia, and dysarthria are common associated symptoms. Patients who claim to be "dizzy" should be carefully questioned to ascertain whether the symptoms are not, in fact, presyncope. On average, it takes the body about 6 to 10 seconds to compensate with arteriolar vasoconstriction following the onset of an arrhythmia; if a blood pressure sufficient to maintain cerebral perfusion is not effected within 10 to 15 seconds, syncope will occur. The time to syncope is even shorter if there is underlying cerebrovascular disease. Some patients with exercise-induced tachycardias become syncopal only with the onset of the tachycardia during the period of exercise (see Fig. 2–7C).

The syncopal episodes caused by cardiac arrhythmias (Morgagni-Adams-Stokes attacks) are associated with characteristic symptoms and should be distinguishable from other causes by examining the "3 Ps" of syncope: Precipitating factors, Prodrome, and the Postsyncopal state with the "s" standing for the syncopal episode itself (Table 2–3).

Precipitating Factors. Cardiac syncope may or may not be accompanied by any precipitating factors. The majority of arrhythmias occur spontaneously and are not associated with any particular activ-

TABLE 2–3. THE "3 Ps" OF CARDIAC SYNCOPE

Precipitating factors:	*Usually none.* More rarely, exercise, alcohol, antiarrhythmic agents, antihypertensive agents, diuretics, hypokalemia, hypomagnesemia.
Prodrome:	*Usually no warning.* If present, less than 30 seconds; include presyncope, dim or darkened vision ("gray outs"), sense of withdrawal from environment, palpitations, and sudden feeling of falling or fading away.
Syncope:	*Duration < 1 min.* No seizures, rare incontinence.
Postsyncope:	*Wide awake in <2 min.* No postictal state or focal neurologic signs.

ity, although exercise can occasionally precipitate tachyarrhythmias (see Fig. 2–7C). Patients may develop rapid paroxysmal atrial fibrillation after overindulging in alcohol (the "holiday heart syndrome"). Medications may also predispose patients to the development of bradyarrhythmias or tachyarrhythmias. The class Ia antiarrhythmic agents (quin-

idine in particular) may produce torsades de pointes (a rapid polymorphic ventricular tachycardia), and both class Ia and Ic agents may increase the frequency or severity, or both, of extant ectopic activity or cause new ventricular arrhythmias. Diuretics may produce hypokalemia and hypomagnesemia (important factors in patients with out-of-hospital sudden death), or cause syncope directly by volume depletion. Syncope in a patient taking antiarrhythmic drugs or agents that can alter serum electrolytes in a proarrhythmic fashion (see Chapter 15) should be ascribed to a drug-related arrhythmia until proved otherwise.

Prodrome. Syncope can occur at the very onset, during, or after a tachyarrhythmia (see Figs. 2–2 and 2–6). Syncopal episodes occurring at the onset of an arrhythmia are typically sudden, with no prodrome or warning; the patient may be unaware of palpitations or of the presence of any arrhythmia. This type of problem is due to the sudden fall in blood pressure and stroke volume associated with the abrupt onset of either a very rapid tachycardia or a profound bradycardia. The faster the heart rate, the less likely are palpitations; likewise, there may be no angina or dyspnea. Being unaware of their hearts' action, patients see a neurologist first because the possibility of a cardiac etiology is never considered.

Syncope may also occur after an arrhythmia is established; this sequence is more likely to be associated with palpitations but is a more unusual presentation and usually reflects a speeding or slowing of the heart rate or worsening left ventricular function, or the presence of both conditions. For example, an increased catecholamine response to hypotension may accelerate the tachycardia's rate and lead to syncope. Patients with an adequate cardiovascular reserve may be able to tolerate heart rates up to 250 beats per minute without significant symptoms. Faster rates (or slower rates with less reserve) are more likely to be associated with presyncope, weakness, or frank syncope.

Finally, as it has been noted, syncope may occur following the termination of tachycardia, because the rapid discharge of all potential pacemakers by the repetitive impulses during the tachycardia causes overdrive suppression and results in a period of asystole following its termination. This phenomenon is made worse by virtually all of the drugs used to treat the tachycardia.

Syncopal Period. With regard to the syncopal episode itself, if it is due to a cardiac arrhythmia, the duration is usually very brief and rarely lasts more than 1 minute. An episode lasting more than 2 minutes is usually not cardiac (unless cardiopulmonary resuscitation [CPR] had to be performed). The patient often describes such brief episodes as "I woke up just as I hit the floor." Patients may twitch and often develop a stertorous, snoring type of breathing and turn ghastly white—"the paleface syndrome"—owing to the absence of blood flow to the brain and upper part of the body. Urinary and bowel incontinence is rare and tongue biting is unusual, although passive traumatic injury to the tongue resulting from a fall may occur. Generalized motor seizures due to an arrhythmia may occur in children but are extremely rare in adults.

Postsyncopal State. There are no postsyncopal symptoms because generalized seizures or focal neurologic deficits rarely occur. The patient with cardiac syncope awakes alert and oriented. Rarely, patients who are unconscious for several minutes (usually owing to a profound bradyarrhythmia) will be a bit confused on awakening, but this symptom clears rapidly.

VASOVAGAL SYNCOPE

The characteristics of cardiac syncope due to tachycardias or sudden bradycardias can be summarized as "up-down-up." An alert patient briefly loses consciousness without warning and then awakens fully alert. In contrast, vasovagal or vasodepressor syncope, although it can be abrupt, usually differs in terms of the "3 Ps" (Fig. 2–8). It is frequently characterized by a protracted prodrome associated with a feeling of intense warmth, nausea, and a feeling of needing fresh air. The episodes may be precipitated by pain or micturition, but classically are associated with anxiety, donating blood, the sight of blood, and by a warm and "closed-in" environment. The Sunday morning "church syncope" that finds matrons fainting in their pews all over the country is well known to emergency department physicians. While sitting in a warm, crowded church, these people experience a sensation of nausea and a desire to leave but are embarrassed to stand for fear of calling attention to themselves. They vasodilate, turn white, and lose consciousness. Vasovagal syncope lasts only until the patient can be placed in a recumbent position and can even be prevented if the patient recognizes the prodromal symptoms and lies down. The postsyncopal state is not associated with confusion, but patients often complain that if they try to reassume the upright position, they feel faint again.

Vasovagal syncope is characterized by a fall in both blood pressure and heart rate. The bradycardia is due to failure of both sinus and lower escape pacemakers as well as the AV nodal block that may be seen during these episodes (see Fig. 2–8). Although the bradycardia contributes significantly to the fall in blood pressure, a concomitant peripheral vascular "vasodepressor" response due to vasodilatation may also contribute importantly to the hypotension. In extreme cases, pacemaker therapy for patients with repetitive profound increases in vagal tone and periods of asystole is sometimes useful as long as

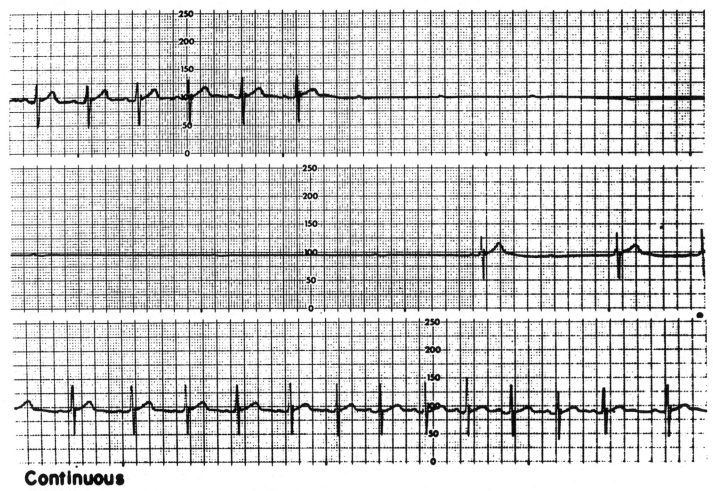

Continuous

FIGURE 2–8. A continuous recording obtained during ambulatory ECG monitoring in a patient with a history of fainting. Symptoms of nausea and malaise were noted before any cardiac arrhythmias occurred. The patient lost consciousness during this period of asystole produced by sudden AV nodal block. Note that the sinus impulse also continues to slow and that no escape pacing activity occurs during the time of failure of AV nodal conduction. This sequence is commonly recorded during fainting episodes due to parasympathetically mediated "vasovagal" syncope.

the peripheral vasodepressor response is not the dominant factor in producing the hypotension (see Chapter 13, pages 318–319). The relative contributions of the peripheral vascular factors versus the bradycardia in causing the syncope must be differentiated before proceeding to pacemaker therapy, to be certain that correcting the bradyarrhythmia will prevent the hypotension and, therefore, the syncope.

DEPRESSED MENTAL FUNCTION

Another variety of cerebral vascular insufficiency resulting primarily from bradyarrhythmias is depressed mental function, with lethargy, confusion, and somnolence. The arrhythmia leads to a reduced cardiac output and blood pressure with decreased cerebral perfusion but without overt loss of consciousness. Patients with intermittent episodes of unexplained confusion may be suffering from intermittent bradyarrhythmias and show a dramatic recovery of their old personalities and energy with implantation of a permanent pacemaker. The physician is urged to be very careful in selecting for pacemaker implantation only those patients with both symptoms and profound, persistent slowing of the heart rate (rates less than 45 beats per minute), because

many older patients have unrelated neurologic symptoms and sinus bradycardia with periods of sinus arrest less than 3 seconds. A trial of temporary pacing may be useful to determine if increasing the rate will effect an improvement in mentation.

It is important to reemphasize what neurologic symptoms arrhythmias do *not* cause. Transient cerebral ischemia from an arrhythmia results in global ischemia; *focal* defects such as hemiparesis, seizures (except in children), or posterior cerebral circulation ischemia (diplopia, dysarthria, and dizziness) are rarely due to arrhythmias. Ambulatory electrocardiogram monitoring and electrophysiologic studies generally have a very low yield in evaluating such problems, and the physician must look elsewhere to determine their cause.

Sudden Death

Patients resuscitated from sudden death can sometimes relate a history that is helpful in diagnosing the cause. Exercise may be a precipitating factor. Angina pectoris or equivalent nonpainful symptoms such as acute dyspnea may incriminate ischemic heart disease. Not uncommonly, patients note a preceding change

in an established anginal syndrome even though angina may not be present at the time of the cardiac arrest. The patient's prodrome may be similar to previous episodes of syncope that did not result in sudden death, and the questions relating to such syncopal spells should be addressed carefully. A loss of consciousness can have a variety of causes, and it is reasonable to ask whether the patient truly "died." Patients with ventricular fibrillation will only very rarely convert to sinus rhythm without defibrillation, so it is key to determine whether the rescue unit performed CPR or defibrillation, or both, and what initial rhythm was recorded. Patients with syncope due to bradyarrhythmias (save for agonal asystole) will usually spontaneously awaken without the need for CPR. The postresuscitation course should also be characterized to determine whether the patient sustained an acute myocardial infarction. Patients who die suddenly usually have coronary artery disease, but at least two thirds have no evidence of acute myocardial infarction. These patients constitute a high-risk subgroup more likely to have a second episode of sudden death. In general, they are candidates for aggressive evaluation, including electrophysiologic testing.

The Physical Examination

ROBERT A. WAUGH, MD

Although conventional electrocardiography is the most widely available tool for arrhythmia diagnosis, an electrocardiograph (ECG) machine is frequently not immediately available in many clinical settings where rhythm disturbances are encountered. A careful bedside examination may provide the diagnosis, and in addition, it is challenging and intellectually rewarding to predict accurately what the electrocardiogram subsequently confirms. Sometimes the bedside examination provides important support for the diagnosis made from the ECG and should be repeated at frequent intervals in unstable patients and in those whose diagnosis and therapeutic plan are still being determined.

The bedside examination may be helpful in diagnosis when arrhythmias present in one of four ways: (1) isolated premature beats, (2) sustained tachycardias, (3) arrhythmias at normal heart rates (60 to 100 beats per minute), and (4) bradycardia. Table 3–1 summarizes the physical findings in patients with premature beats and tachycardias, and Table 3–2 summarizes the findings in patients with normal and bradycardiac heart rates.

USEFUL COMPONENTS OF THE BEDSIDE EXAMINATION

An evaluation of the arterial pulse volume or blood pressure or both, the jugular venous wave form, and cardiac auscultation are most helpful in arrhythmia diagnosis. The assessment of the jugular venous wave form and careful auscultation of the heart have the highest yield of useful information. The arterial pulse examination is of use when, with a regular ventricular rate, a variation in its amplitude or the systolic blood pressure, or in both, suggests that atrioventricular (AV) dissociation is contributing to a variation in stroke volume. Inspection and palpation of the precordium are rarely helpful in arrhythmia diagnosis.

TECHNIQUE AND NORMAL WAVE FORMS

Neck Veins

Elevate the patient's thorax to whatever level maximizes the visibility of the pulsations of the internal jugular veins. The neck should be slightly flexed to relax the neck muscles. The morphology of each of the components of the jugular venous pulse is then analyzed and timed against either the contralateral carotid pulse or an auscultated first heart sound.

The normal venous pulse shows a dominant A wave (due to right atrial systole) followed immediately by an X descent (due mainly to right atrial relaxation). The subsequent V wave and Y descent are usually much smaller. With heart rates less than beats per 60, the A wave may be difficult to discern, and the most prominent feature of the jugular venous pulse is the X descent. This occurs because with slow heart rates the neck veins fill passively during the long diastolic cycle, and the next A wave (a low-pressure event) does little to distend the already filled neck veins, (Fig. 3–1). In such instances, a prominent downward flick (X descent) of the neck vein, synchronous with the carotid pulse, provides a ready visual marker from which to judge the preceding A wave and the following V wave and Y descent. The interval between the observed A wave and the palpated carotid pulse also provides a bedside clue to the PR interval. With practice, one can become proficient at detecting first-degree AV block.

The Arterial Pulse

For arrhythmia diagnosis, besides determining heart rate and regularity, the arterial pulse should be assessed by measuring the beat-to-beat systolic blood pressure and carotid pulse amplitude during held respiration. With a regular rhythm, a beat-to-beat variation in systolic pressure of greater than 10 mmHg is significant and implies marked variation in left ventricular filling, usually due to AV dissociation.

Auscultation

Particular attention should be given to any variation in the intensity and degree

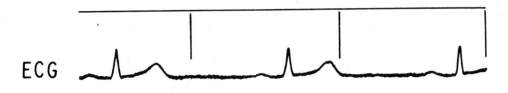

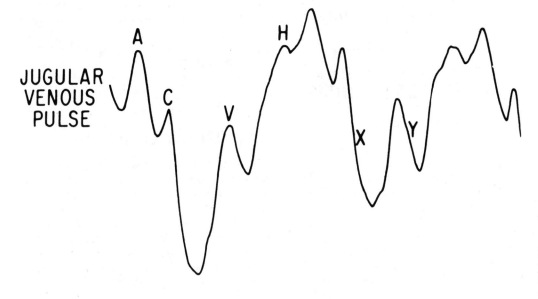

FIGURE 3–1. In this normal jugular venous pulse, the positive waves are labeled on the first complex and the negative waves are labeled on the second complex. At the bedside, the most conspicuous clinical feature of this venous pulse was a prominent downward movement (or collapse) that corresponded to the X descent (see text). A = A wave; C = C wave; H = H wave; V = V wave; Y = Y descent.

Table 3–1. PHYSICAL FINDINGS: PREMATURE BEATS AND TACHYCARDIAS

RHYTHM	VENOUS PULSE	ARTERIAL PULSE	AUSCULTATION
		Premature Beats	
PVC and PJC	Cannon A waves	Augmented pulse amplitude after the pause.	Wide split of S_1 and S_2; S_2 may not occur if very early.
PAC	Variable A waves (cannon if early enough)	No pulse augmentation unless compensatory pause is evident.	Normal split of S_1 and S_2 unless aberration is present.
		Tachycardias	
Paroxysmal AV junctional tachycardia	Constant A wave	Constant pulse amplitude.	Constant S_1; normal split of S_1 and S_2 unless aberration is present.
Atrial flutter	Flutter waves with dominant Y descent	Constant pulse amplitude if AV block is constant.	Constant S_1 unless AV block is variable; normal split of S_1 and S_2.
Atrial fibrillation	Dominant Y descent (fibrillation waves are inapparent)	Pulse amplitude varies directly with prior cycle length.	Variable S_1; normal split of S_1 and S_2 unless aberration is present; any S_3 is difficult to hear during short RR intervals.
AJR and VT with AV dissociation*	Irregular cannon A waves	Variable pulse amplitude	Variable S_1; AJR—normal split of S_1 and S_2 unless aberration is present; VT—split of S_1 and S_2; variable diastolic gallops.
AJR and VT with VA association*	Regular (usually cannon) A waves	Constant pulse amplitude	Constant S_1; AJR—normal split of S_1 and S_2 unless aberration is present; VT—wide split of S_1 and S_2; any gallops are constant.

AJR = accelerated junctional rhythm; AV = atrioventricular; PAC = premature atrial complex; PJC = premature junctional complex; PVC = premature ventricular complex; S_1 = first heart sound; S_2 = second heart sound; S_3 = third heart sound; S_4 = fourth heart sound; VA = ventriculoatrial; VT = ventricular tachycardia.

*Heart rates for both accelerated junctional and idioventricular rhythms may be < 100 beats per minute.

of splitting of the first heart sound (note: the first heart sound is normally narrowly split) as well as the degree and type of respiratory splitting of the second heart sound. Note also any variations in the timing and loudness of diastolic gallops.

PREMATURE BEATS

The Venous Pulse

Whether isolated premature beats introduce abnormalities in the neck veins depends on their prematurity and on whether AV dissociation occurs (Table 3–1). The neck veins are easiest to analyze when the intrinsic rhythm is slow and when the premature beats either are superimposed on a normal venous pulse morphology or are infrequent enough to avoid interfering with the easy identification of the venous waves of the normal beats. When premature beats are ventricular and do not conduct retrograde to the atria, the next "on-time" right atrial depolarization typically occurs while the tricuspid valve is closed, resulting in the quick upward "flick" of an accentuated, reflected A wave in the neck (the "cannon" A wave of AV dissociation). When this occurs in the setting of a normal venous pressure, the resulting cannon A wave may be detected as a strikingly positive but usually brief wave (Fig. 3–2A). When the same events occur with an elevated venous pressure, the cannon A wave may be much less apparent, because full neck veins cannot appreciably distend further. Similarly, when the ventricular extrasystole is late, there may be little or no perturbation in the A wave, because it occurs when the tricuspid valve is open (Fig. 3–2B).

Cannon A waves may occur without AV dissociation and in settings other than with premature ventricular complexes (PVCs) or ventricular tachycardia, and, therefore, cannot be used to identify definitively either that AV dissociation is present or that the origin of the arrhythmia is ventricular. For example, cannon A waves may occur with junctional (or His) depolarizations that either do not conduct retrograde or that conduct retrograde and superimpose atrial contraction on a closed tricuspid valve. The latter phenomenon may also occur with PVCs (Fig. 3–3). "Premature" cannon A waves may also occur when very early premature atrial complexes (PACs) occur during the ventricular systole of the prior beat and are superimposed on a closed tricuspid valve. Depending on the coupling interval or ventriculoatrial (VA) conduction time, premature cannon A waves may occasionally hint of either an atrial origin or retrograde VA capture from a PVC. With PACs, cannon A waves may occur without a ventricular response if such atrial beats are so premature that they do not conduct through the AV node (i.e., physiologic block occurs).

The Arterial Pulse

Palpation of the arterial pulse can be helpful in detecting the occurrence of a premature beat by revealing its premature occurrence (typically with a diminished amplitude), the pause following such a premature beat, or the augmented pulse pressure of the beat ending the pause (Fig. 3–4).

Auscultation

Auscultation is most useful when premature beats produce no detectable changes in the venous pulse or occur so early that perceptible arterial pulsations do not occur. In such instances, one can almost always hear a first heart sound and, depending on whether the stroke volume is sufficient to open the semilunar valves, a second heart sound. When such premature beats are supraventricular and not associated with aberrant conduction, the first and second heart sounds are typically normal. When premature beats are either supraventricular with aberration or ventricular, there may be wide splitting of both the first and second heart sounds due to asynchronous ventricular activation. Such splitting may result from exaggeration in the normally delayed activation of the right ventricle, or may be paradoxical due to a reversed sequence of ventricular activation, with the left-sided heart sounds following the right-sided heart sounds (Fig. 3–5).

SUSTAINED TACHYCARDIAS
The Venous Pulse

The neck vein manifestations of tachycardias are quite variable (see Table 3–1). The clinical findings depend on several aspects of the arrhythmia, including: (1) the site of origin of the tachycardia, (2) the presence or absence of coordinated atrial systole (e.g., ectopic atrial tachycardias versus atrial fibrillation), (3) the timing of the atrial systole relative to ventricular

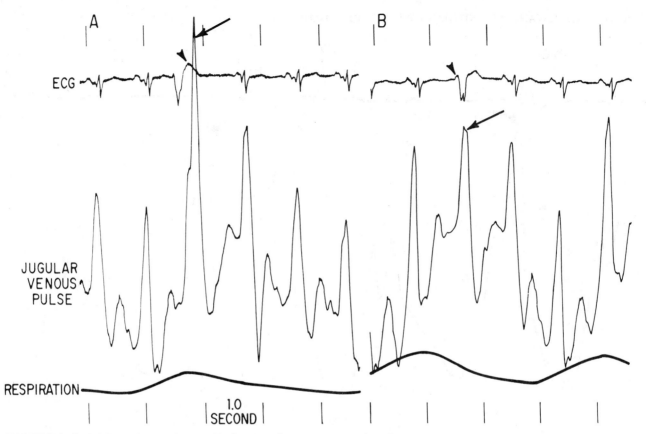

FIGURE 3–2. (*A*) Transient atrioventricular (AV) dissociation results when an on-time P wave (arrowhead) occurs during a premature ventricular complex (PVC) while the tricuspid valve is closed. This phenomenon causes a larger-than-normal right atrial pulse pressure that is reflected in the jugular venous pulse (JVP) as an accentuated but on-time pulsation (cannon A wave: arrow). (*B*) A PVC from the same focus occurs and is also associated with transient AV dissociation but with a normal A wave in the jugular venous pulse (arrow). A cannon A wave does not occur, because the PVC is relatively late (note that the PVC begins after the on-time P wave [arrowhead] and has fusion-beat characteristics). Consequently, right atrial emptying in response to atrial systole is virtually complete by the time the PVC closes the tricuspid valve.

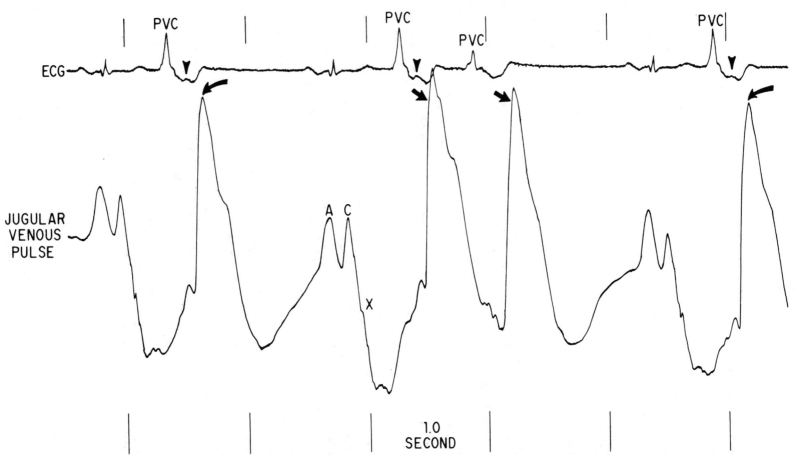

FIGURE 3–3.   In this jugular venous pulse recording, the sinus beats demonstrate a normal morphology with a dominant A-C complex and X descent. The second and last beats are single PVCs that conduct retrograde (note the early P waves following the PVCs [arrowheads]) and produce cannon A waves (curved arrows), which are also early. When two PVCs occur in a row (fourth and fifth beats), back-to-back, coupled cannon A waves (straight arrows) are seen. Cannon A waves also occur in the pulmonary venous circuit, producing venous distention that can be sensed by the patient.

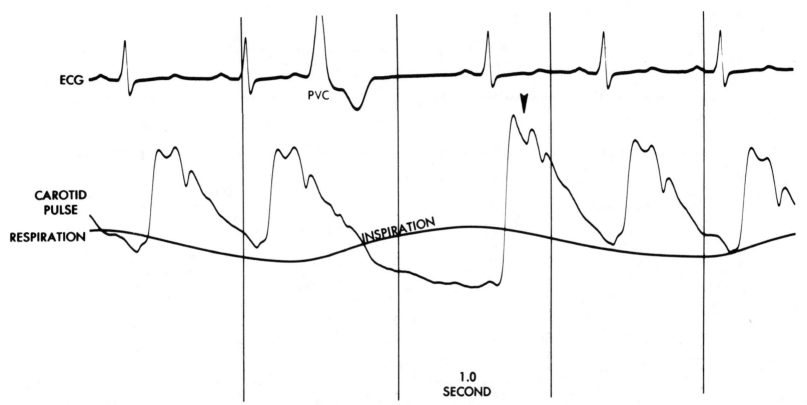

FIGURE 3–4. A single PVC results in transient AV dissociation, making the cycle following the PVC longer than the normal cycle. This long cycle results in augmented ventricular filling that in turn produces a wider pulse pressure for the beat following the PVC (arrowhead). The premature beat itself is so early that the stroke volume is inadequate to open the aortic valve, and no premature arterial pulse occurs.

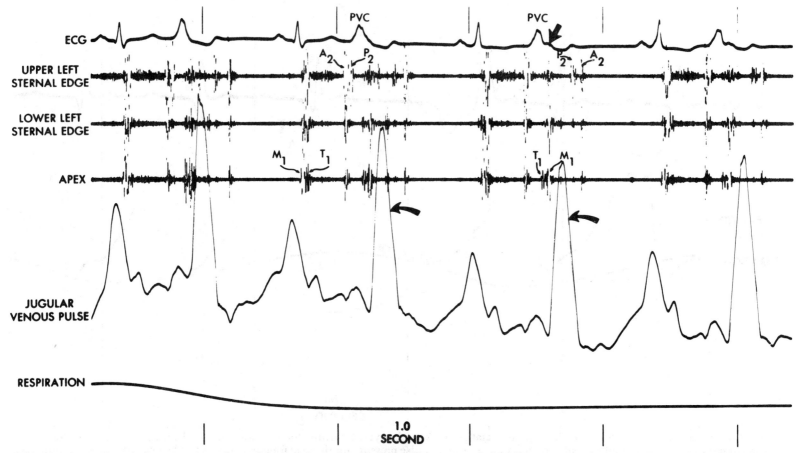

FIGURE 3–5. This simultaneous recording of the jugular venous pulse and heart sounds from a patient in sinus rhythm with ventricular bigeminy shows several features typical of PVCs. AV dissociation occurs (note on-time P wave [straight arrow]), with resulting cannon A waves (curved arrows). These PVCs are from the right ventricle and produce prominent paradoxic splitting of the second heart sound (P₂, A₂) and the first heart sound (T₁, M₁). The first and second heart sounds of the normally conducted beats are narrowly split, but the degree of splitting is accentuated and reversed by the PVCs.

systole, and (4) the presence of AV dissociation.

As the heart rate increases, the ability to discern the various components of the jugular venous pulse becomes more difficult. For example, a sinus tachycardia of 120 beats per minute produces 600 neck vein events per minute (i.e., three positive waves and two negative waves per beat). Fortunately, one can still usually discern the dominant A wave just prior to the carotid pulse.

In the presence of ectopic atrial tachycardia with first-degree AV block, there may still be a dominant A wave, although the associated prolongation of AV conduction time moves this wave farther away from both the first heart sound and the carotid upstroke. If the PR prolongation is sufficient or the heart rate fast enough, or if both conditions are present, atrial systole may either become superimposed on the V wave, producing one prominent diastolic pulsation, or occur immediately before or after the V wave, producing a bifid, predominantly diastolic pulsation. Figure 3–6 shows an example of this phenomenon, although not at a tachycardiac heart rate.

With paroxysmal junctional tachycardia either originating in the AV node or occurring in association with an accessory pathway, the morphology of the jugular venous pulse depends on the timing of atrial systole relative to ventricular systole. With the typical variety of atrioventricular nodal reentry, retrograde conduction from the node to the atrium is usually short (less than 70 milliseconds) and results in "cannon" A waves due to right atrial systole occurring in synchrony with a closed tricuspid valve. If retrograde atrial activation is sufficiently delayed (such delays are occasionally observed with either the "fast-slow" variety or atrioventricular nodal reentry or accessory pathways showing very slow retrograde VA conduction), the A wave can occur just before the next ventricular depolarization and result in a normally positioned jugular venous A wave.

When the tachycardia is due to generalized atrial reentry, the jugular venous morphology depends on the rate and regularity of reentry. When the tachycardia is slower and orderly (i.e., atrial flutter), venous pulsations corresponding to the atrial rate (flutter waves) may be observed. These flutter waves are occasionally quite prominent, particularly with concomitant pulmonary hypertension (Fig. 3–7), but are usually more difficult to see at the bedside because they are relatively low-amplitude and are variably superimposed upon the C, X, V, and Y events that occur as part of each ventricular cycle independent of atrial activity (Fig. 3–8). Whenever the tachycardia rate is regular and in the range of 150 beats per minute, one should search carefully for evidence of flutter waves in the venous pulse because an atrial rate of 300 beats per minute with a 2:1 ventricular response is so typical of atrial flutter.

When generalized atrial reentry is more rapid and irregular (i.e., atrial fibrillation), there is a loss of both coordinated atrial systole and relaxation; the A waves disappear and the X descents become diminutive. Even though low-amplitude fibrillation waves can be easily recorded by phonocardiography, they are usually not visible at the bedside. The most prominent venous pulse feature then becomes a dominant Y descent, occurring immediately after the carotid pulse (Fig. 3–9). In some patients with atrial fibrillation, particularly if the venous pressure is elevated, this aspect of the jugular venous pulse may falsely suggest tricuspid regurgitation. Whenever the cardiac rhythm is irregularly irregular, evidence of atrial fibrillation with a dominant Y descent in the venous pulse is commonly found.

The jugular venous pulse manifestations of ventricular tachycardia depend on the status of VA conduction: when AV dissociation is present, variable cannon A waves are present, reflecting the different atrial and ventricular rates, and they provide important confirmation of the diagnosis. With ventricular tachycardia and 1:1 retrograde conduction, however, "fixed" regular cannon A waves are usual and are not as helpful in the differential diagnosis. A return to the bedside once the rhythm strip has been obtained may be useful in sorting out atrial activity when it

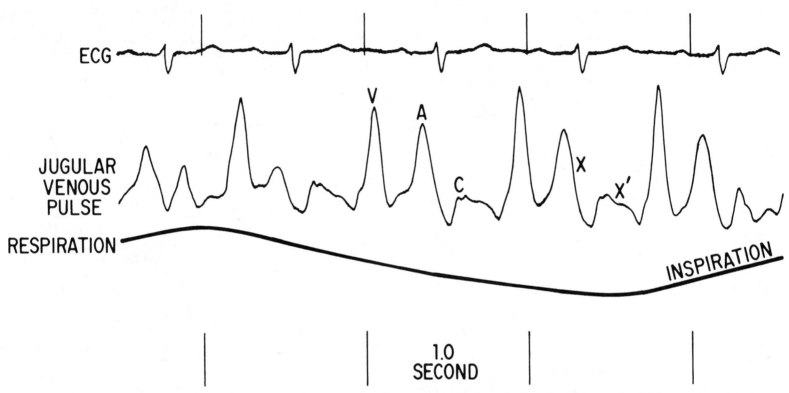

FIGURE 3–6. In this recording of the jugular venous pulse wave taken from a patient in sinus rhythm, the PR interval is 0.26 seconds and the A wave occurs well before the C wave. Atrial relaxation (X descent) also occurs early and is no longer superimposed on the systolic descent of the heart, lessening the X' descent during ventricular systole. At the bedside, the close temporal proximity of the V and A waves and diminutive C wave and X' descent produced a venous pulse in which the most prominent feature was a bifid diastolic wave.

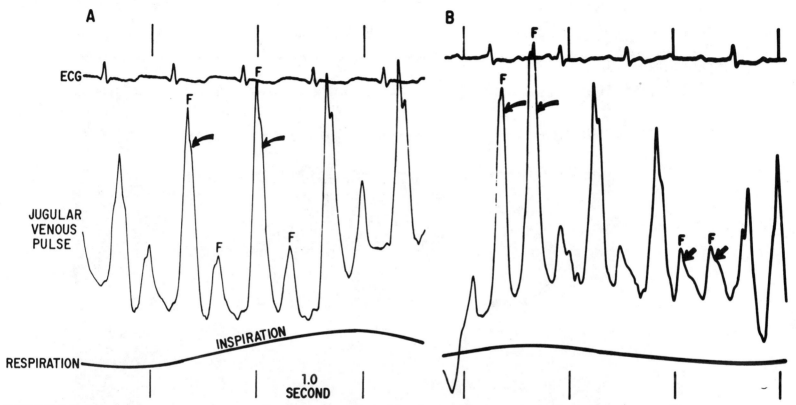

FIGURE 3–7. This jugular venous pulse recording is from a patient with pulmonary hypertension and relatively slow atrial flutter (200 beats per minute) with variable AV conduction. (*A*) Regular 2:1 AV conduction is present, and there are flutter waves (F) (also at 200 beats per minute). Every other flutter wave is accentuated (curved arrows) because it occurs when the tricuspid valve is closed, resulting in an augmented right atrial pressure. (*B*) Variable AV conduction occurs in association with a variable pattern in the accentuation of the flutter waves (F). On the left, coupled cannon A flutter waves (curved arrows) are seen, whereas on the right, unaccentuated flutter waves (straight arrows) result from atrial contractions that occur when the tricuspid valve is open.

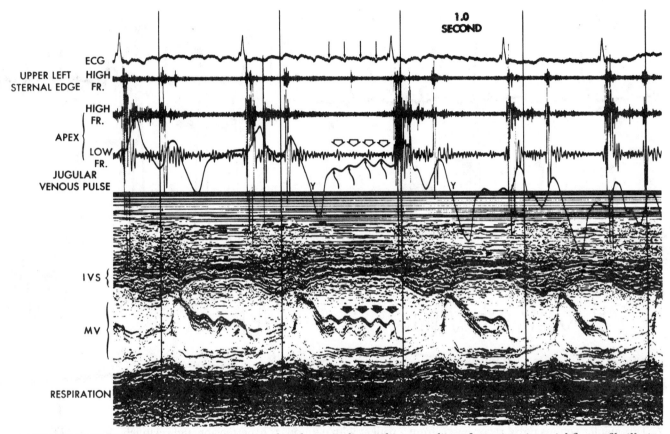

FIGURE 3–8. This simultaneous time-motion echo-phonocardiographic recording of a patient in atrial flutter-fibrillation shows typical flutter waves in the electrocardiogram (ECG) (straight arrows), flutter waves in the jugular venous pulse (curved arrows), and flutter waves in the mitral valve echo (MV) (solid arrowheads). The low-frequency recording at the apex (lower trace) also shows low-frequency "flutter" sounds (open arrowheads), the mechanism for which remains unexplained. Note the common periodicity of the flutter waves in the ECG, jugular venous pulse, mitral valve echo, and the sounds at the apex. In this particular example, the venous flutter waves are diminutive, and the overall morphology of the jugular venous pulse has the clinical appearance of atrial fibrillation with a dominant Y descent. FR = frequency; IVS = interventricular septum.

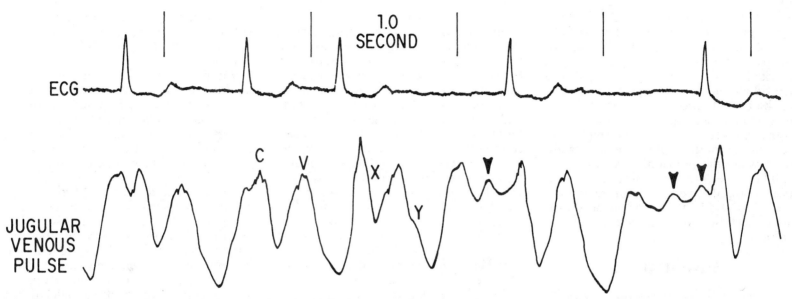

FIGURE 3–9. In this jugular venous pulse recording, atrial fibrillation results in a loss of coordinated right atrial systole and, therefore, the A wave. The C wave (due to tricuspid valve closure), V wave (due to passive venous filling of the right atrium), and Y descent (due to emptying of the right atrium) are unimpaired. A remnant of an X descent persists because the entire heart moves inferiorly during ventricular systole, causing a small drop in venous pressure that is much less than the now-dominant Y descent. During long RR intervals, low-pressure fibrillatory waves (arrowheads) can be recorded but are rarely noted at the bedside.

cannot be clearly discerned on the surface ECG tracing (see Table 8–1).

The Arterial Pulse

The hemodynamic consequences of ventricular tachycardias are usually more severe than those of supraventricular tachycardias. There are, however, numerous exceptions to this rule, because the severity of hemodynamic compromise of any tachycardia depends largely on its rate and the clinical setting in which it occurs. Thus, for example, ventricular tachycardia at a rate of less than 200 beats per minute in an otherwise healthy heart is generally well tolerated, whereas atrial flutter at a rate of 240 to 300 beats per minute with 1:1 conduction, even in an otherwise healthy heart, may be associated with syncope. In general, however, significant arterial hypotension, particularly in association with only a modest increase in heart rate, should always suggest the presence of ventricular tachycardia. With regular ventricular tachycardia and AV dissociation, variation in the carotid pulse amplitude reflects whether an appropriately timed atrial systole has augmented the stroke volume for that particular beat.

Similarly, auscultation of the systolic blood pressure during a held breath will reveal variation in systolic blood pressure of greater than 10 mmHg and also a marked variation in the intensity of the Korotkoff sounds. Once again, going back to the bedside provides important information in answering the question, "What is the atrioventricular relationship?" The recognition of these phenomena is facilitated when the ventricular rate is 120 to 130 beats per minute or slower. In addition, a regular ventricular rate is necessary to eliminate the effect of a variable diastolic filling period on stroke volume.

Auscultation

Palpation of the arterial pulse to determine rhythm regularity and rate may be misleading with heart rates of 150 beats per minute or more. Cardiac auscultation, on the other hand, is a sensitive method for discerning whether the arrhythmia is absolutely regular or even slightly irregular. An absolutely regular tachycardia is suggestive of paroxysmal AV junctional tachycardia (PJT), atrial flutter with fixed AV conduction and, commonly, ventricular tachycardia. A more irregular tachycardia suggests an arrhythmia originating in the atrium, such as atrial fibrillation, multifocal atrial tachycardia, or ectopic atrial tachycardia with variable AV block.

The other auscultatory clues during tachycardia are due to the same variables that influence the jugular venous pulse tracing. When there is a constant relation between atrial and ventricular depolarization, the position of the mitral valve at the onset of ventricular systole is constant, and therefore, the intensity of the first heart sound is constant. The first heart sound varies in intensity, however, whenever there is variable AV or VA conduction because of the resulting variability in mitral valve position at the onset of ventricular systole.[1] A constant-intensity first heart sound is therefore typical of sinus tachycardia, ectopic atrial tachycardia with a fixed AV conduction ratio, paroxysmal junctional tachycardia, generalized atrial reentry with a fixed AV conduction ratio (i.e., atrial flutter with fixed 2:1, 3:1, or 4:1 conduction), and ventricular tachycardia with a fixed retrograde VA conduction. A variable intensity of the first heart sound in the setting of a regular tachycardia, on the other hand, is a classic occurrence with AV dissociation and should always raise the possibility of ventricular tachycardia. Less often, variable loudness of the first heart sound reflects an atrial rate that differs from the ventricular rate due to variable retrograde VA block. With ventricular tachycardia, the variation in loudness of the first heart sound may be phasic, with a gradual crescendo-decrescendo cadence as the dissociated atrial beats "march through" the regularly occurring ventricular cycles and regularly affect the position of the mitral valve at the onset of ventricular systole.

Variable diastolic gallop sounds (including fourth heart sounds and, when atrial systole is superimposed on passive early diastolic ventricular filling, summation gallops) are typical of AV dissociation but may be difficult to detect when there is an increased heart rate because of the abbreviated diastolic cycle. Wide splitting of the first and second heart sounds should suggest that the ventricles are being activated asynchronously either from a ventricular focus or by aberrant conduction. Occasionally, with ventricular tachycardia at relatively slower rates, one may even detect whether or not the second heart sound is physiologically but widely split (i.e., right bundle branch block type of activation) or paradoxically split (i.e., left bundle branch block type of activation).

ARRHYTHMIAS OCCURRING DURING NORMAL HEART RATES

Arrhythmias that occur during normal heart rates (60 to 100 beats per minute) usually involve AV conduction abnormalities or AV dissociation due to speeding of a pacemaker in the His bundle or bundle branches (Table 3–2).

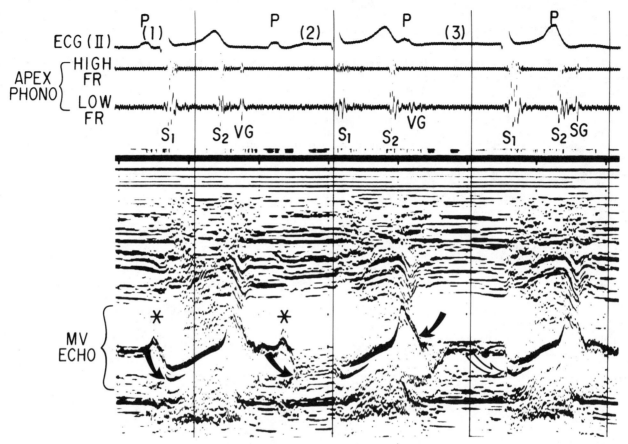

FIGURE 3–10. This echophonocardiogram (simultaneous mitral valve [MV] echocardiogram and apex phonocardiogram) is from a 12-year-old boy with congenital complete heart block. The first PR interval (1) is normal (0.14 seconds) and produces a normal A wave (*) of the anterior mitral valve leaflet with normal closure of the mitral valve (first arrow left) and normal loudness of the first heart sound (S_1). The second PR interval (2) is prolonged (0.46 seconds). The resulting A wave (*) is in mid-diastole with premature closure of the mitral valve (second arrow from left) and softening of the subsequent S_1. With the third PR interval (3), which is markedly prolonged (0.76 seconds), the A wave of the mitral valve is imperceptible because it is superimposed on passive early diastolic left ventricular filling (third arrow from left). This third PR interval is followed by reopening of the mitral valve in mid-diastole, and then reclosure (open arrow) by the subsequent ventricular systole, with resulting augmentation of S_1. The last atrial systole (note the superimposition of the P wave on the last T wave) sums with passive left ventricular filling, producing a summation gallop (SG). Time lines indicate intervals of 1.0 second. FR = frequency; P = P wave, S_2 = second heart sound; VG = third heart sound.

Table 3–2. PHYSICAL FINDINGS: ARRHYTHMIAS WITH NORMAL HEART RATES AND BRADYCARDIAS

RHYTHM	VENOUS PULSE	ARTERIAL PULSE	AUSCULTATION
*Normal Heart Rates**			
Type I second-degree AV block	Increasing jugular A wave—carotid pulse interval and loss of dominant X descent	Increased pulse amplitude following pause	Progressive softening of S_1 after each pause; S_4 common; variable summation gallop may occur.
Atrial flutter or fibrillation	Flutter or fibrillation waves (both frequently inapparent at bedside) with dominant Y descent	Pulse amplitude constant if AV block constant	Constant S_1 if AV block is constant; normal split of S_1 and S_2 unless aberration is present; any S_3 is more constant.
Bradycardias			
Sinus bradycardia	Constant but diminutive A wave; X descent usually most prominent feature	Constant pulse amplitude	Constant S_1; normal split of S_1 and S_2 unless aberration is present; any gallops are constant.
High-degree AV block with coordinated atrial rhythm	Cannon A waves	Variable pulse amplitude	Variable S_1; splitting a function of escape pacer site or aberration; variable gallops.
High-degree AV block with atrial flutter-fibrillation	Dominant Y descent; flutter-fibrillation waves (usually inapparent at bedside)	Constant pulse amplitude	More constant S_1; splitting of S_1 and S_2 is a function of escape pacer site or aberration; any S_3 is constant; no variable summation or atrial gallops.

AV = atrioventricular; S_1 = first heart sound; S_2 = second heart sound; S_3 = third heart sound; S_4 = fourth heart sound.

*For acclerated junctional and idioventricular rhythms at rates < 100 beats per minute, see Table 3–1, Tachycardias.

The Venous Pulse

When an arrhythmia's rate is between 60 and 100 beats per minute, particularly if it is regular, sinus rhythm is usually inferred to be present. Careful scrutiny of the neck veins, however, may reveal either a prolonged interval between the A wave and the carotid pulse (e.g., first-degree AV block; see Fig. 3–6) or two or more A waves for each ventricular beat. The latter suggest the presence of atrial flutter (with either a very slow atrial rate and 2:1 conduction block, or with a more usual atrial flutter rate and higher ratios of AV block) or ectopic atrial tachycardia with block. When an arrhythmia in this rate range is due to an accelerated lower pacemaker (from either the His bundle or the ventricle), one should search for the typical irregular cannon A waves of AV dissociation or the fixed cannon A waves of retrograde VA conduction. When such a regular, accelerated lower pacer is superimposed upon atrial fibrillation with AV block, or when the rhythm is irregularly irregular and due to atrial fibrillation with a well-controlled ventricular response, the neck vein morphology is that of atrial fibrillation with a dominant Y descent. When the rhythm is regularly irregular, it may be due to recurring ectopic beats, sinus rhythm with second-degree AV block, or, rarely, atrial flutter with variable 2:1 and 4:1 conduction. With type I second-degree AV block, the intervals between the jugular venous A wave and the carotid pulse progressively increase, with a progressive diminution in the X descent prior to the dropped p wave (or pause). With type II second-degree AV block, the intervals between the jugular A wave and the carotid pulse remain constant both before and after the blocked atrial beat (or pause). Remarkably, Wenckebach's observations of these two varieties of block predated the clinical use of the string galvanometer and were made using carotid and jugular venous pulse tracings.[2]

The Arterial Pulse

Arrhythmias in this rate range typically are not associated with significant hemodynamic deterioration. When there is AV dissociation and a regular ventricular rate, variable carotid pulse amplitude and systolic blood pressure may provide clues that AV dissociation is present and contributing to variability in left ventricular stroke volume.

Auscultation

With atrial fibrillation, the loudness of the first heart sound varies inversely with the length of the prior RR interval. This variation is usually more pronounced and easier to recognize than the similar variation that occurs with atrial fibrillation and a rapid ventricular response. With type I second-degree AV block, progressive lengthening of the PR interval is associated with increasing degrees of premature closure of the mitral valve and progressive softening of the first heart sound until the blocked atrial beat occurs, when the cycle repeats. During the long PR intervals, atrial gallops may also be more easily heard. With marked PR interval prolongation (to 0.5 seconds or more) due to first-, second-, or third-degree AV block (or with AV dissociation from other causes), the first heart sound intensity may increase again (see Fig. 3–10). This occurs because with very long PR intervals, the effects of atrial systole on AV valve position are effectively lost. That is, atrial systole is superimposed either on the opening of the AV valves that occurs with passive early diastolic ventricular filling or is so early that it occurs during ventricular systole at a time when the AV valves are closed. During the long subsequent diastolic cycle, the AV valves passively reopen and remain opened until the next ventricular systole, with a secondary augmentation of the first heart sound's loudness.[1]

Auscultation may also reveal the presence of bundle branch block with wide splitting of the first heart sound and wide, but physiologic splitting of the second heart sound typical of right bundle branch block. With left bundle branch block, the first heart sound may be widely (and "paradoxically") split, but much more frequently the first heart sound is single, and paradoxic splitting of the second heart sound is the accoustic hallmark. The acoustic findings of ventricular arrhythmias in this rate range are usually more dramatic, particularly when there is AV dissociation. In addition to the variable loudness of the first heart sound and, depending on the site of the accelerated pacemaker, normal or abnormal splitting of the first and second heart sounds, variable diastolic gallops occur as atrial systoles march through the diastoles of successive cycles. These variable gallops are much more likely to be detected in this setting (as compared with tachycardia settings) because of the longer diastolic "listening" periods.

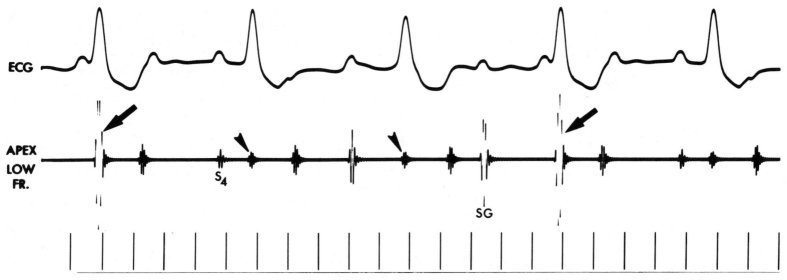

FIGURE 3–11. In this example of AV dissociation due to heart block, note the variation in loudness of the first heart sound (soft with long PR intervals [arrowheads] and loud with short PR intervals [arrows]) and the diastolic gallops that vary in timing from presystolic (S_4) to early diastolic (summation gallop [SG]) as the independent P waves progress through the diastolic cycle of the ventricular escape rhythm. FR. = frequency.

BRADYCARDIAS

Heart rates of less than 60 beats per minute may be due to sinus bradycardia (with or without AV dissociation), default of the sinus pacemaker (i.e., sinus arrest) with escape junctional or ventricular rhythms, or AV block (see Table 3–2). The last two mechanisms also typically produce AV dissociation.

The Venous Pulse

With sinus bradycardia, the jugular venous pulse is typically normal with a small A wave and dominant X descent (see Fig. 3–1), unless AV dissociation due to the sinus rate slowing below that of an escape His pacemaker produces variable cannon A waves. With sinus arrest and loss of coordinated atrial contraction and relax-

ation, the venous pulse approximates that of atrial fibrillation with a dominant Y descent. When high-degree AV block occurs during atrial fibrillation, the venous pulse morphology is also that of atrial fibrillation, with a dominant Y descent. For the remaining arrhythmias, the venous pulse findings depend upon whether AV dissociation is present. In the special instance of isorhythmic AV dissociation, the atrial and ventricular rates are very closely at-tuned, and the jugular venous pulse A wave may vary from "on-time" and nor-mal in amplitude to later and "cannon" in amplitude. When there is a sinus atrial mechanism and high-degree AV block, variable cannon A waves are present.

The Arterial Pulse

While systolic hypotension may be pres-ent with high-degree AV block and very slow ventricular escape rates, the blood pressure may be very well maintained even with heart rates as low as 30 beats per minute. With isorhythmic AV dissoci-ation, a phasic and slow variation in the arterial pulse amplitude and measured systolic pressure may occur that is diffi-cult to recognize at the bedside because the beat-to-beat effects of a variation in the timing of atrial systole on the stroke vol-ume are small and gradual. When there is retrograde VA block from either the His or ventricular escape pacer site and, therefore, AV dissociation, variable am-plitude in the carotid pulse and systolic blood pressure are usually present.

Auscultation

With isorhythmic AV dissociation the intensity of the first heart sound may differ very little from beat to beat. Over time, the loudness of the first heart sound may vary slowly and phasically, but if very gradual, the change may be quite difficult to appre-ciate at the bedside. When the bradycar-dia is due to AV block with a junctional es-cape pacemaker, auscultation may show only variable loudness of an otherwise normal first heart sound (as atrial systole variably affects mitral valve position at the onset of ventricular systole),[1] a normal second heart sound, and variable diastolic gallops. When the bradycardia is due to high-degree AV block with a ventricular escape pacemaker, the same phenomena ensue (Fig. 3–11), but there also may be wide splitting of the first and second heart sounds, with the respiratory behavior of the latter dependent upon whether the es-cape pacemaker resides in the left ventri-cle (right bundle branch block type of ac-tivation) or the right ventricle (left bundle branch block type of activation). The aus-cultatory events of high-degree AV block in the setting of atrial fibrillation differ from those of sinus rhythm only in that variability of the first heart sound is mini-mal and summation and atrial-gallop sounds do not occur.

REFERENCES

1. Burggraf GW and Craige E: The first heart sound in complete heart block: Phono-echocardiographic cor-relations. Circulation 50:17–24, 1974.
2. Wenckebach KF: Beiträge zur Kennt-nis der menschlichen Herztätigkeit. Archiv Anat Physiol: Physiologiche Ab-teilung. 1906, pp 297–354.

CHAPTER 4

Autonomic Maneuvers

MENASHE B. WAXMAN, MD
ROBERT W. WALD, MD

In many instances, one may either suspect or be certain that a cardiac arrhythmia or conduction disturbance is present, but neither the physical examination nor the rhythm strip contains sufficient information to permit a precise diagnosis. No P waves may be apparent, or some may be visible and others obscured by either QRS complexes or T waves. Alternatively, all of the P waves may be clearly visible, but their "association" or "dissociation" with the QRS complexes may not be certain. Because the processes of impulse formation and conduction are both influenced by the two parts of the autonomic nervous system (sympathetic and parasympathetic), an alteration of this balance may cause a change in the rhythm sufficient to permit a diagnosis. At times, this change may actually terminate the arrhythmia. The autonomic condition produced by sympathetic and parasympathetic input may be called *autonomic tone*. Autonomic tone can be manipulated by maneuvers and agents that alter baroreceptor activity, such as carotid sinus massage; intravenous (IV) drugs such as atropine, isoproterenol, and phenylephrine; the Valsalva maneuver; amyl nitrite inhalation; and exercise.

Maneuvers that change autonomic tone, particularly vagal tone, have been extensively used in arrhythmia diagnosis and have become part of the clinician's standard repertoire. In this chapter, we describe the use of modifications of autonomic tone in a wide range of arrhythmias to provide a general approach to the analysis and treatment of rhythm disturbances that can supplement and expand other techniques.[7]

CAROTID SINUS MASSAGE

Physiology

Baroreceptors capable of sensing arterial blood pressure are widely distributed in the common carotid arteries, the aortic arch, and the subclavian arteries. The best-known concentration of baroreceptors is in a small swelling at the bifurcation of the common carotid artery, known as the *carotid sinus*, located beneath the angle of the jaw.[8] A branch of the ninth cranial nerve (the nerve of Hering) arises from this sinus and courses up to the vasomotor center of the medulla. A rise in blood pressure excites pressure-sensitive receptors in the carotid sinus that send impulses up the nerve of Hering in proportion to the pressure increase. This process results in a subsequent increase in efferent vagal nerve traffic to the heart and to the body. The sinus node, the atrioventricular (AV) node, the His bundle, and any other structure innervated by the vagus nerve are affected. The rate of impulse formation, both in the sinus node and in other supraventricular sites with pacemaker capability, is decreased, and conduction through the AV node is impaired. Carotid sinus massage can deform the pressure-sensitive receptors in a manner similar to that of an intraluminal rise in blood pressure. Concomitant with the increase in vagal efferent activity is a reciprocal reduction in sympathetic efferent traffic, resulting in an additive action on the receptor sites in question (Fig. 4–1). A reduction in perfusion pressure, such as occurs following amyl nitrite inhalation, reduces baroreceptor firing and leads to vagal tone withdrawal and sympathetic tone increase. The interrelationship between sympathetic and vagal tones during carotid sinus massage is illustrated in Figure 4–2.

Technique for Proper Execution

The patient should be supine with the head maintained midline in a hyperextended posture. An electrocardiographic strip-chart recorder should be continuously running in full view of the physician applying the carotid sinus massage. The area of the carotid sinus can be identified by gentle palpation. Use of the thumb is particularly advantageous in view of its favorable surface area relative to that of the carotid sinus. The intensity and duration of the pressure should be varied according to the clinical needs.[9,10] Under no circumstances should carotid sinus massage

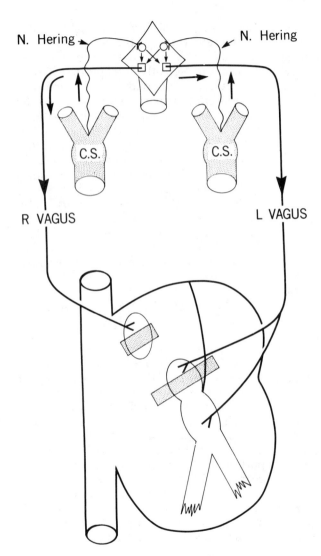

N. Hering

N. Hering

C.S.

C.S.

R VAGUS

L VAGUS

FIGURE 4–1. The major central interconnections of the carotid sinus baroreceptors (C.S.) and the cardiac efferent vagus nerve distribution. The nerves (N.) of Hering provide afferent connections from the carotid sinuses to the vasomotor center in the medulla. The vagus nerves, in turn, course from the vasomotor center to provide parasympathetic innervation for the sinus and atrioventricular (AV) nodes as well as for the His bundle.

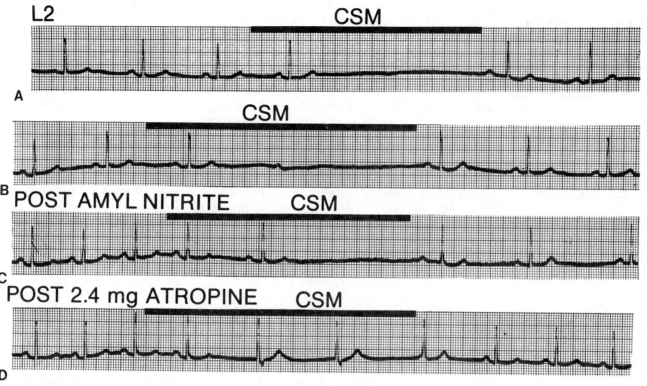

FIGURE 4–2. The first two applications of carotid sinus massage (CSM) result in substantial pauses. In (*A*), the pause is due to sinus slowing, and in (*B*), it is due to both sinus slowing and AV block. In (*C*), massage produces a shorter pause because amyl nitrite has heightened background sympathetic tone, which opposes the enhanced vagal tone. In (*D*), despite administration of 2.4 mg of atropine, massage still causes substantial sinus node slowing, and His bundle escape beats emerge. As the effects of vagal tone have been blocked by atropine, the slowing induced by the carotid sinus massage is likely due to a concomitant withdrawal of sympathetic tone. His bundle escape beats do not emerge during the longer pauses in (*A*), (*B*), and (*C*), because increased vagal tone depresses His bundle automaticity. When vagal tone is blocked by atropine (*D*), however, His bundle escape beats emerge.

be performed bilaterally. Great care should be taken to exclude patients with cerebrovascular disease. Many clinicians rhythmically massage the carotid sinus. Although massage is often more effective than firm compression of the carotid sinus, we find that the latter approach produces more controlled and reproducible results. The duration of steady compression should not exceed 5 seconds.

Techniques for Enhancing Effectiveness

Four major techniques enhance the effectiveness of carotid sinus massage.[1–3,5–7,10] (Each technique is capable of elevating vagal tone sufficiently to perturb the rhythm without superimposed carotid sinus massage.)

1. *Pretreatment with the anticholinesterase drug edrophonium chloride (Tensilon), in a dose of 5 to 10 mg intravenously.* Within 30 to 40 seconds, the patient experiences many of the nicotinic and muscarinic actions of this agent (e.g., lacrimation, salivation, abdominal cramps, nausea, sweating, and muscle twitching), and carotid sinus massage should be performed at that time. The enhanced effect of carotid sinus massage is directly traceable to an inhibition of acetylcholine hydrolysis by the edrophonium chloride.

2. *Compression of the carotid sinus 5 to 10 seconds after the release of a strong Valsalva maneuver.* At this time, the blood pressure is considerably above control levels.

3. *An increase in blood pressure by means of an α-agonist such as phenylephrine hydrochloride (Neo-Synephrine).* Carotid sinus massage should be applied 30 to 60 seconds after administration of an IV bolus of the phenylephrine, when the blood pressure has climbed substantially above control levels. In all patients, the amount of drug administered should be titrated by IV bolus to a blood pressure not exceeding 180 mmHg. The initial IV bolus should be 0.05 mg. A second bolus of 0.1 or 0.15 mg can be given after allowing a sufficient time for the blood pressure to return to control levels (1 to 3 minutes). Additional boluses may be given in this way, each increased by 0.05 or 0.1 mg over the preceding dose, until the arrhythmia reverts, a blood pressure of 180 mmHg is obtained, or the patient complains of headache. Phenylephrine is contraindicated if the resting systolic blood pressure exceeds 160 mmHg, and it should not be used in patients with suspected intracranial vascular malformations, ischemic heart disease, or heart failure. Also, it should be used with great care in persons over age 60.

4. *An increase in tidal volume produced by a deep breath.* This technique results in a rise in systemic blood pressure during the mid-to-late phase of inspiration, which reaches its maximum during the expiratory phase.[11] A Trendelenburg body position (head downward) can have a similar effect. Both maneuvers produce exaggerated responses in patients with paroxymal junctional tachycardia.

Quantitative Aspects

Deformity of the baroreceptors by extrinsic pressure can produce graded responses depending on the extent and duration of compression, because both afferent traffic up the nerve of Hering and efferent vagal tone are directly related to the degree of blood pressure elevation. The quantitative aspects of carotid sinus massage are extremely important in seeking a sufficient, but avoiding an excessive, increase in vagal tone. In Figure 4–3, six consecutive applications of right-sided carotid sinus massage are shown, each of approximately the same intensity but of increasing duration; the sinus pauses that result are appropriately lengthened. If one bears this technique in mind, excessive sinus pauses, as seen in Figure 4–3 (bottom: 5.6-second asystolic period), or prolonged AV block can be avoided. This is particularly important because the complications from carotid sinus massage, whether of a hemiplegic or an arrhythmic variety, are often related to the induction of excessively prolonged periods of cardiac asystole.[10]

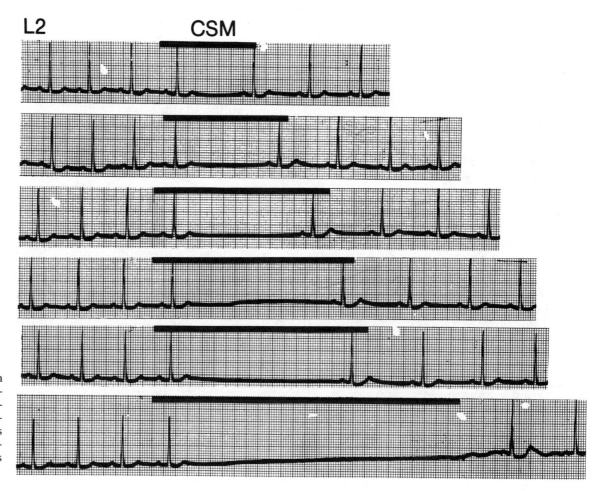

FIGURE 4–3. These six rhythm strips from the same patient are consecutive but not continuous. They illustrate the quantitative aspects of carotid sinus massage (CSM), as progressively longer applications produce progressively longer sinus pauses.

V1 Control

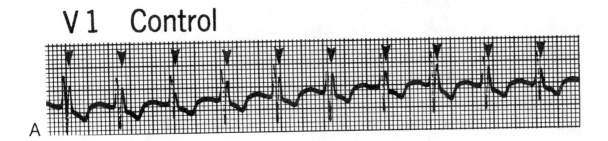

A

CSM

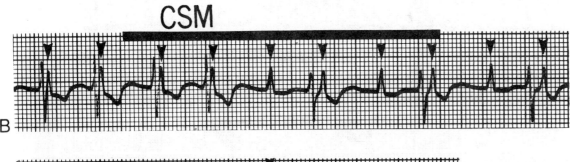

B

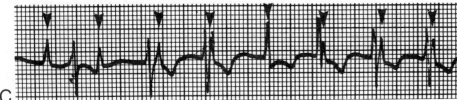

C

FIGURE 4–4. (*A*) Apparent RSR′ complexes occur at a regular frequency of 100 beats per minute. The P waves are not readily seen. In this case of sinus tachycardia with a long PR interval, the P waves (arrowheads) are masquerading as R′ waves. (*B*) Carotid sinus massage (CSM) induces second-degree AV block and exposes the true position of the P wave, clearly indicating that the R′ waves of the RSR′ complexes in (*A*) are indeed P waves. (*C*) As the effects of carotid sinus massage wane, the record returns to its original configuration (last two complexes).

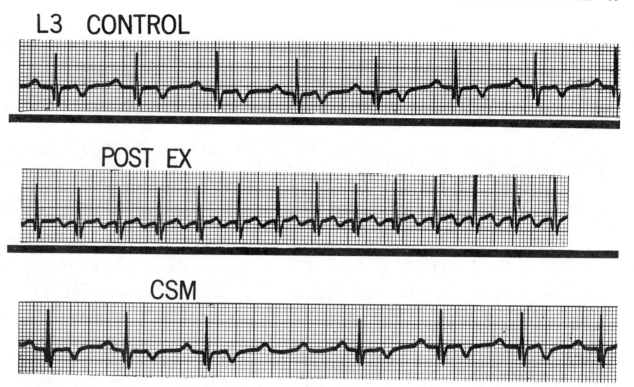

L3 CONTROL

POST EX

CSM

FIGURE 4–5. The top panel shows what appears to be sinus rhythm at a rate of 65 beats per minute with a PR interval of 0.24 second. Enhancement of the AV nodal conductivity by exercise (POST EX) results in precise doubling of the ventricular rate. This finding suggests that the top panel really shows an atrial tachycardia at a rate of 130 beats per minute with 2:1 AV conduction. This situation is further clarified in the last panel: Once the rhythm has returned to that shown in the top panel, an application of carotid sinus massage (CSM) depresses AV nodal conduction and exposes the atrial rate of 130 beats per minute.

CLINICAL USES OF AUTONOMIC INTERVENTION

Defining Atrial Activity

Autonomic maneuvers may affect the atrial frequency and AV conduction time and thereby alter the timing relationship between the P wave and the QRS complex. As a result, P waves hidden within the various electrocardiogram (ECG) wave forms can be readily exposed (Fig. 4–4). Even in cases where the location of a P wave is self-evident, one should always question whether all the P waves are visible. Simple manipulations of autonomic tone may readily answer this question (Fig. 4–5). Atrial flutter, conducting with a 2:1 AV ratio, and especially when ac-companied by abnormal ST and T waves, almost always has obscured atrial activity (Fig. 4–6).

Evaluating Escape Pacemakers

Slowing of the rate through depression either of the sinus node pacemaker or of AV conduction should lead to the emer-

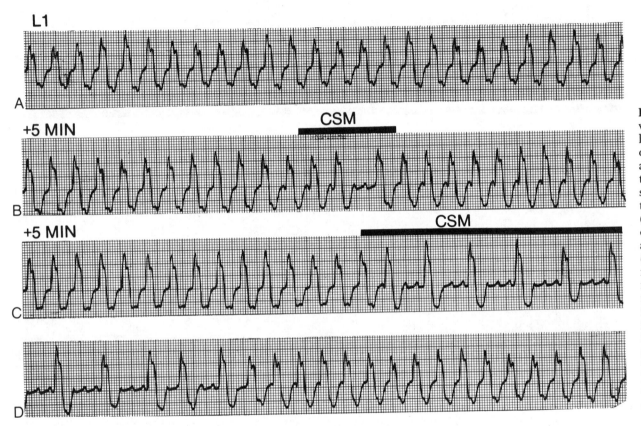

FIGURE 4–6. (*A*) A regular, wide-QRS tachycardia with left bundle branch morphology and no clearly visible atrial activity. (*B*) The situation depicted in (*A*) remains stable until a brief application of carotid sinus massage (CSM) depresses AV nodal conduction and exposes atrial flutter waves. (*C*) and (*D*) A longer application of massage further retards AV nodal conduction, and even more clearly exposes atrial flutter waves that are a perfect multiple of the basic RR interval of (*A*), defining the rhythm in (*A*) as atrial flutter with 2:1 AV conduction and left bundle branch block aberration. Note C and D are continuous.

gence of subsidiary escape pacemakers. Depending on the mechanism of cardiac slowing, a variety of escape pacemakers at different levels within the heart can be exposed. As shown previously (see Fig. 4–2), carotid sinus massage can even depress automaticity of the His bundle pace-

maker. This depressant effect may explain why no escape beats occur during some vagally induced pauses.

Creation of pauses in the heart action may expose escape pacemakers at other sites in the heart (Fig. 4–7). It is not known why depression of AV nodal conduction at

times results in the emergence of ventricular escape beats rather than AV junctional escape beats. Because the His bundle is under vagal control, the increase in vagal tone may depress its spontaneous frequency, thereby allowing the emergence of a subsidiary ventricular pace-

FIGURE 4–7. In this continuous rhythm strip from a patient in atrial fibrillation, carotid sinus massage (CSM) causes slowing of AV conduction with the emergence of ventricular escape beats (dots). After cessation of carotid massage and waning of the vagal effects, AV conduction improves and resumes control of the heart rate.

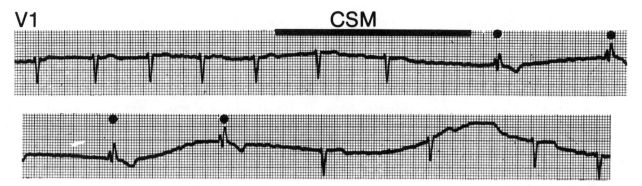

maker. Transient depression of spontaneous frequency is useful in exposing the presence and proper functioning of demand artificial pacemakers at either the atrial or the ventricular level (Fig. 4–8).

Evaluating Tachycardia (Phase-3)–Dependent Bundle Branch Block

Following excitation of a cardiac cell, there is a recovery period, known as the refractory period, during which the cell cannot be reactivated (see Chapter 1, page 4, and Fig. 1–1). Once the refractory period ends, the cell can again be excited. Conduction disturbances within various regions of the heart, especially within the

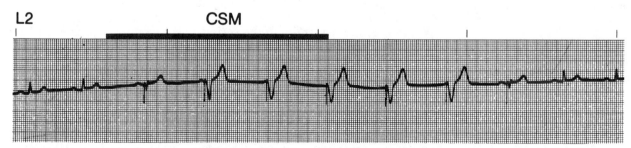

FIGURE 4–8. In this rhythm strip, carotid sinus massage (CSM) results in slowing of the sinus rate with the emergence of demand ventricular escape beats. (In this case, the escape beats are due to an artificial ventricular pacemaker functioning in a VVI mode [see Chapter 16].) Note that the beat following the first pacemaker spike is a fusion beat resulting from activation of the ventricles, which occurs partially through conduction over the normal AV pathways and partially through conduction from the site of ventricular stimulation by the artificial pacemaker. After carotid massage, the sinus node gradually speeds and resumes control of the heart.

bundle branch system, occur whenever the rate of impulses exceeds the refractory period of a group of cells within the circuit. When the refractory period of bundle branch cells is normal (250 to 400 milliseconds), a conduction disturbance may occur only when the supraventricular impulse rate is high (more than 150 beats per minute). When the refractory period of bundle branch cells is prolonged (more than 500 milliseconds), however, conduction disturbances may occur at relatively slow heart rates (less than 120 beats per minute).

The physiology of tachycardia-dependent block[12] is illustrated in Figure 4–9. Alterations in heart rate through manipulations of autonomic tone are particularly effective in eliminating or inducing tachycardia-dependent intraventricular conduction disturbances within the bundle branch system (Figs. 4–10 and 4–11).

Evaluating Bradycardia (Phase-4)–Dependent Bundle Branch Block

Slowing of the primary cardiac frequency may result in intraventricular conduction delays, a process referred to as *bradycardia-dependent bundle branch block*, or phase-4–dependent bundle branch block. The physiology underlying this process[12,13] is illustrated in Figure 4–12. This type of conduction block depends on enhanced phase-4 diastolic depolarization. Bradycardia-dependent block rarely exists by itself and almost always coexists with tachycardia-dependent block within the same bundle. By contrast, tachycardia-dependent block frequently exists without bradycardia-dependent block. Figure 4–13 demonstrates coexistence of both forms of block in the same person. Awareness of the presence of bradycardia- and tachycardia-dependent bundle branch block is especially important when attempting to normalize intraventricular conduction.

Determining the Site of AV Block

The responses of AV conduction and escape pacemaker frequency to manipulations of autonomic tone in the setting of AV block can help in localizing the site of AV block and in determining the seriousness of the conduction disturbance.

PROXIMAL AV BLOCK

Block at the level of the AV node (proximal AV block) is characterized by normal QRS complexes and type I periodicities; the Wenckebach pattern is the classic example. On many occasions, however, there are prolonged periods of fixed 2:1 (or 3:1, 4:1, and so forth) AV conduction with no variation in the PR intervals, and the block cannot be further "typed." Variations of these intervals can be easily evoked by maneuvers that enhance AV nodal conduction by reducing vagal tone or by enhancing sympathetic tone (Figs. 4–14 and 4–15). Congenital AV block is characterized by the failure of development of the AV node or of the fusion of the AV node with the His bundle. Either defect results in the presence of a His bundle escape pacemaker. Because of the rich vagal and sympathetic innervation of this structure, predictable responses in escape beat frequency can be seen with autonomic manipulations, as illustrated in Figure 4–16.

DISTAL AV BLOCK

Block at the level of the bundle branch system (distal or infranodal AV block) also responds fairly predictably to manipulation of autonomic tone. The ECG pattern of distal heart block is characterized by type II patterns of AV conduction (see Chapter 1, pages 13 to 15, and Chapter 14, page 327–329), and it is almost always accompanied by intraventricular conduction disturbances.[1–3,6,7]

As might be expected from the discussion of tachycardia-dependent bundle branch block, rate acceleration is a good method of evoking high-degree distal AV block. Figure 4–17 is an example of sinus rhythm with fixed right bundle branch block and tachycardia (phase-3)–dependent block within the left bundle branch. Second-degree AV block developed when

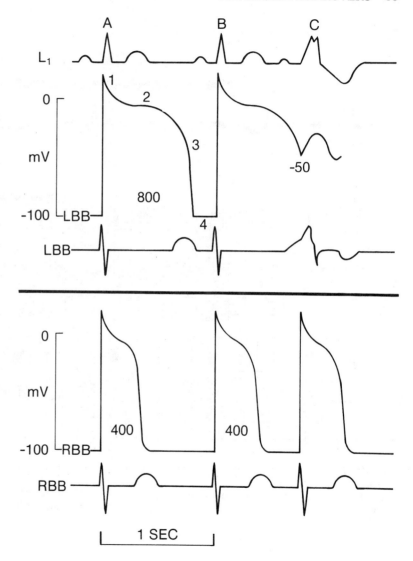

FIGURE 4–9. In this diagram, the recordings (top to bottom) are surface ECG lead 1 (L$_1$), a transmembrane action potential from a Purkinje fiber in the left bundle branch (LBB), an accompanying LBB electrogram, a transmembrane action potential from a fiber in the right bundle branch (RBB), and an RBB electrogram. When an action potential is activated by an oncoming sinus impulse, rapid depolarization (phase 0) ensues, and this depolarization corresponds with activation of the local electrograms and the surface QRS complexes. Action potential repolarization is divided into phases 1, 2, and 3, and recovery is complete by phase 4. The refractory period is essentially equal to the duration of the action potential of the cell. In this example, the duration of the action potential of the LBB cell (800 milliseconds) is longer than that of the RBB cell. The third beat (C) occurs at a faster rate and therefore falls during phase 3 of the LBB cell, when its membrane potential is only −50 mV. A slow, small-amplitude depolarization results, and the LBB electrogram shows aberration. Because these RBB cells have an action potential with a shorter duration (400 milliseconds), they are fully recovered when the early impulse occurs, and their depolarization and the RBB electrogram are normal. The accompanying surface ECG lead 1 shows a pattern of left bundle branch block. Because the early impulse occurs during phase 3 of the LBB action potential, this type of conduction disturbance is called phase-3–dependent (or tachycardia-dependent) block. (Adapted from Singer et al.[12])

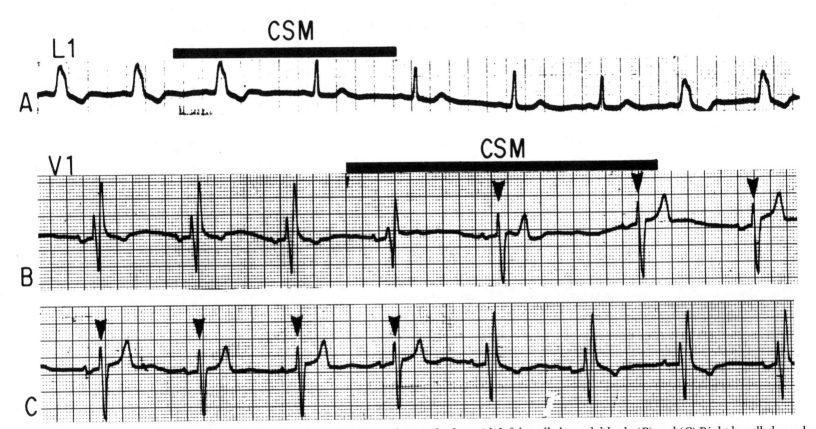

FIGURE 4–10. Rhythm strips from two different patients. (*A*) Normal sinus rhythm with left bundle branch block. (*B*) and (*C*) Right bundle branch block. In each patient, transient sinus slowing due to carotid sinus massage (CSM) normalizes the QRS complexes (A-beats 4-7; B and C arrowheads), identifying tachycardia-dependent (or phase-3–dependent) aberration. Several seconds later, as the enhanced vagal tone wanes, the sinus rates return toward their original values, causing the respective bundle branch blocks to reappear. (*B*) and (*C*) are continuous recordings.

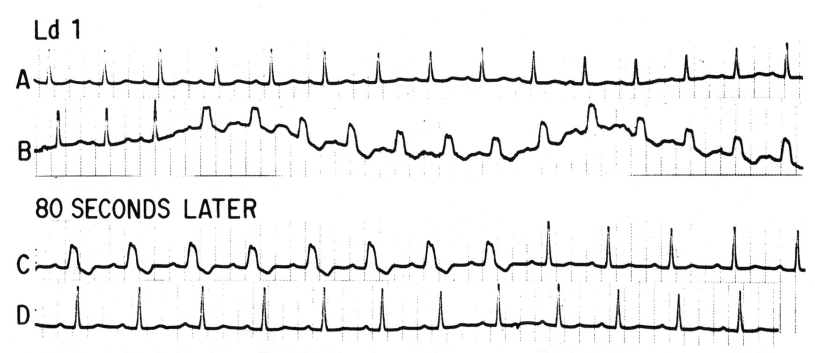

FIGURE 4–11. Tachycardia-dependent (or phase-3–dependent) aberration. (A) Normal sinus rhythm with first-degree AV block and normal intraventricular conduction. (B) Amyl nitrite inhalation lowers the arterial blood pressure, reflexively increasing sympathetic tone and withdrawing vagal tone. These changes result in acceleration of the sinus node, and left bundle branch block emerges once the heart rate reaches a critical value. (C) and (D) Eighty seconds later, the rate slows sufficiently to allow return of normal intraventricular conduction.

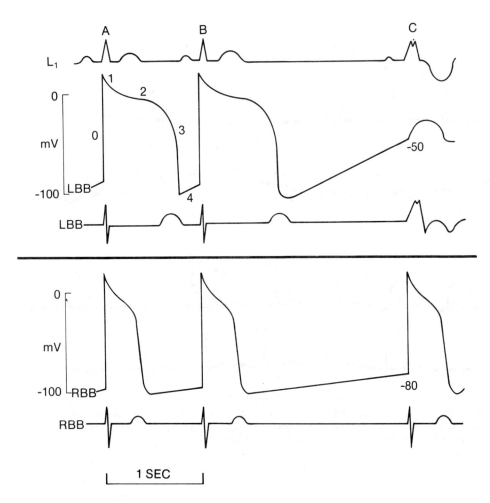

FIGURE 4–12. Surface ECG lead 1 (L₁), transmembrane action potentials, and local electrograms from left bundle branch (LBB) and right bundle branch (RBB) cells are recorded. The LBB cells have been injured and show enhanced spontaneous phase-4 (diastolic) depolarization. Beats A and B are normal. The third beat (C) follows a slowing of the rate that allows the LBB cell to depolarize substantially (to −50 mV). This cell does not discharge spontaneously, as the threshold potential has probably shifted to a less negative value. Therefore, when the sinus-originated impulse invades these cells, a slow, small-amplitude depolarization ensues, and the local electrogram shows aberration. The RBB cells have a normal slope of diastolic depolarization; thus, when activated by the sinus impulse, they depolarize fully, and the RBB electrogram is normal. The ventricles are therefore activated mainly by the normally conducting RBB, and a pattern of left bundle branch block results. Because the late impulse occurred during phase 4 of the LBB action potential, this type of conduction disturbance is called phase-4–dependent bundle branch block (or bradycardia-dependent bundle branch block). (Adapted from Singer et al,[12] and Rosenbaum et al.[13])

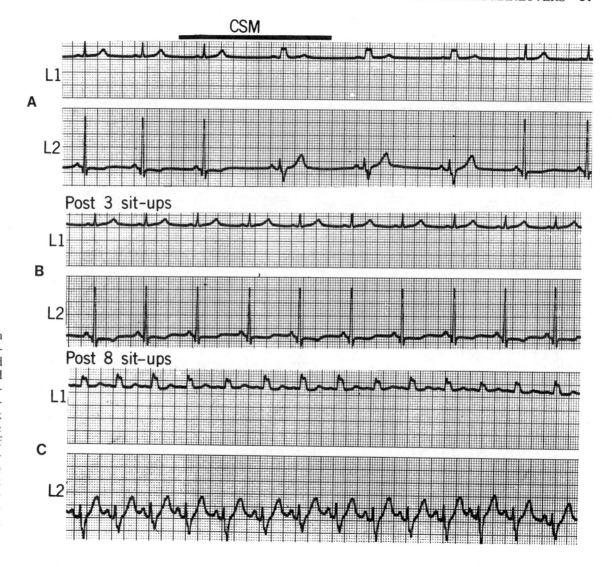

FIGURE 4–13. (*A*) Sinus rhythm with normal intraventricular conduction is seen initially. The background sinus rate is slightly slowed by carotid sinus massage (CSM), and bradycardia-dependent (or phase-4–dependent) left bundle branch block emerges transiently. (*B*) The cardiac rate has been accelerated by means of three sit-ups, and normal intraventricular conduction is present. (*C*) Following additional sit-ups, the heart rate has increased further, and tachycardia-dependent (or phase-3–dependent) left bundle branch block emerges.

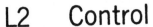

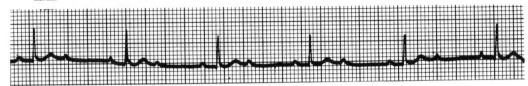

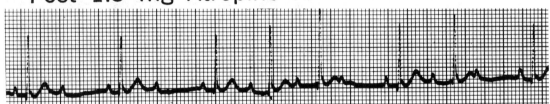

FIGURE 4–14. *(Top)* The control record shows second-degree AV block with a fixed 2:1 AV conduction ratio and normal QRS complexes. Because the RP intervals are constant, the PR intervals are also consistent and the block cannot be typed. *(Bottom)* After IV administration of 1.8 mg atropine, the sinus rate has accelerated somewhat, and AV conduction is augmented, so that the conduction ratios now vary. Note the reciprocal variability in the RP and PR intervals, which is typical of type I second-degree AV block.

the faster sinus rate encroached upon the prolonged refractory properties of the left bundle branch.

THE RESPONSE OF TACHYCARDIAS TO VAGAL TONE

Table 4–1 summarizes the response of common tachycardias to maneuvers that increase vagal tone, such as carotid sinus massage.[1–3,6,7]

Sinus Tachycardia

Sinus tachycardia should transiently slow in response to the increased vagal tone of carotid sinus massage and then reaccelerate gradually as vagal tone wanes with the cessation of massage. With rate slowing, concealed P waves are thereby more readily exposed. In the presence of sinus tachycardia and a high sympathetic tone, however, it is often difficult to obtain gradual slowing in response to carotid sinus massage, and vigorous pressure may be required. This pressure may

result in an abrupt reduction in heart rate that can simulate the termination of a paroxysmal AV junctional tachycardia. Figure 4–18 presents an example of the response of sinus tachycardia in the setting of an acute inferior wall myocardial infarction.

Paroxysmal AV Junctional Tachycardia

Paroxysmal AV junctional tachycardia (paroxysmal AV nodal reentrant tachycar-

L₁ Control

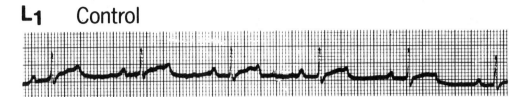

Immediately Post Exercise

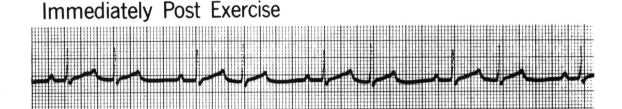

30 secs later

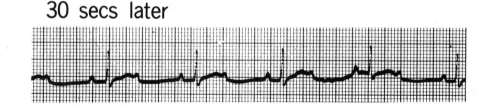

FIGURE 4–15. *(Top)* The control record shows sinus rhythm with second-degree AV block, a 2:1 AV conduction ratio, and normal QRS complexes. Because the RP intervals are constant, the PR intervals are also constant and the block cannot be typed. *(Middle)* After exercise, typical 3:2 AV Wenckebach periods are produced (i.e., there is type I second-degree AV block). *(Bottom)* Thirty seconds later, this augmentation of AV conduction has waned, and AV conduction has returned to its control ratio of 2:1.

dia and paroxysmal atrioventricular reentrant tachycardia [see Chapter 11]) usually terminates in response to an increase in vagal tone if it is of sufficient degree.[10,11,14–16] As well, in some cases spontaneous increases in vagal tone may automatically terminate the tachycardia.[17]

This effect applies equally to episodes confined to the AV node (paroxysmal AV nodal reentrant tachycardia) and to those that incorporate an overt or concealed accessory pathway (paroxysmal atrioventricular reentrant tachycardia). In Figure 4–19, the success of a fixed vagal stimulation protocol in terminating 68 consecutive cases of paroxysmal junctional tachycardia is illustrated.[6]

Although the termination of paroxysmal junctional tachycardia in response to enhanced vagal tone is abrupt, some slowing usually occurs before termination. In

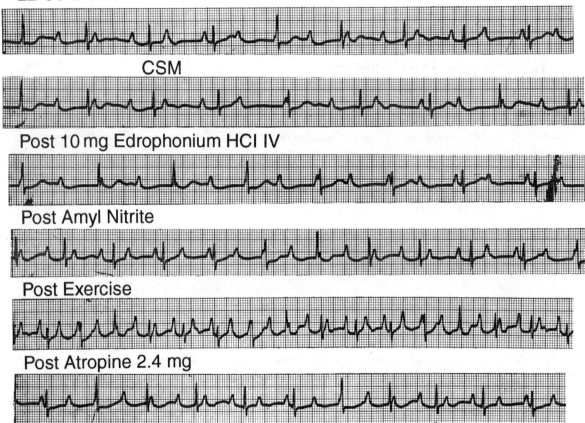

L2 Control

CSM

Post 10 mg Edrophonium HCl IV

Post Amyl Nitrite

Post Exercise

Post Atropine 2.4 mg

FIGURE 4–16. The control record, shown in the top panel, shows AV dissociation due to complete AV block, with a His bundle escape mechanism (note the narrow QRS complex) of 60 beats per minute. In the succeeding panels, manipulations of autonomic tone change both the atrial and His pacemaker rates (sometimes dramatically), but AV dissociation due to AV block persists throughout. Carotid sinus massage (CSM) slows both the P-wave frequency and the His bundle escape rate. Edrophonium chloride (Tensilon), an anticholinesterase drug, has a similar effect. Amyl nitrite elicits a sympathetic response, resulting in acceleration of both the sinus mechanism and the escape pacemaker. Exercise causes the sinus node and His bundle escape pacemakers to accelerate to 170 and 120 beats per minute, respectively. Finally, withdrawal of vagal tone by means of atropine accelerates the sinus rate and His bundle escape rate to 140 and 100 beats per minute, respectively.

V1

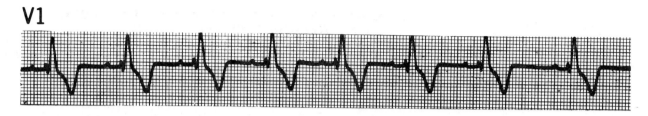

Post Amyl Nitrite

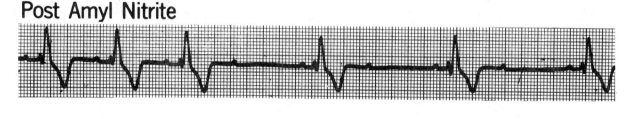

+35 secs

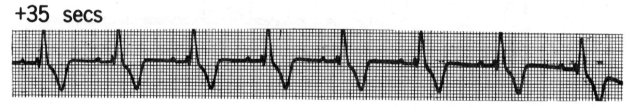

FIGURE 4–17. The top strip shows sinus rhythm with first-degree AV block and right bundle branch block. After the inhalation of amyl nitrite, the sinus rate accelerates slightly, provoking 2:1 AV conduction without the antecedent prolongation of the PR interval. This is typical of type II AV block. When the sinus rate has slowed to control values 35 seconds later, 1:1 AV conduction resumes.

Figure 4–20, four episodes were terminated by means of carotid sinus massage. In each example, the last few RR cycles are prolonged over the control values.

It is important to emphasize that the response of arrhythmias to carotid sinus massage is graded. This response pattern is illustrated in Figure 4–21, wherein an ECG lead V_6 and beat-to-beat heart rate were recorded simultaneously during an episode of paroxysmal junctional tachycardia. Four applications of carotid sinus massage are shown. The first three were applied in a gentle fashion to slow the rhythm reversibly without effecting termination. Stopping after the first three applications of carotid sinus massage might have led to the wrong conclusion that this was a case of sinus tachycardia with transient slowing. The fourth application of carotid sinus massage converted the rhythm to normal sinus rhythm, proving the diagnosis of paroxysmal junctional tachycardia. Rate slowing prior to termi-

**Table 4–1. RESPONSE OF COMMON TACHYCARDIAS
TO INCREASED VAGAL TONE**

ARRHYTHMIA	RESPONSE TO INCREASED VAGAL TONE
Sinus tachycardia	Slowing and reacceleration
Paroxysmal AV junctional tachycardia	1. Slowing and reacceleration 2. Slowing and termination
Atrial flutter	1. Increased degree of AV block 2. Rare conversion to atrial fibrillation
Atrial fibrillation	Increased degree of AV block
Ventricular tachycardia	1. Selective atrial slowing 2. Rare termination

AV = atrioventricular.

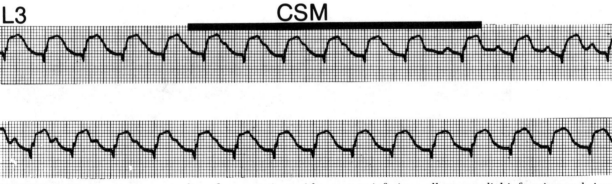

FIGURE 4–18. Continuous recordings from a patient with an acute inferior wall myocardial infarction and sinus tachycardia. *(Top)* The P waves are initially concealed within the T waves. Carotid sinus massage (CSM) slows the atrial rate, and the P waves move away from the T waves, allowing their clear identification. Whereas the initial portion of the response is somewhat gradual, the major slowing is rather abrupt, thereby simulating the termination of paroxysmal junctional tachycardia. *(Bottom)* As the effect of carotid sinus massage wanes, reacceleration is gradual, as is expected for sinus tachycardia. Once the rate has returned to its former value, the P waves are once again hidden within the T waves.

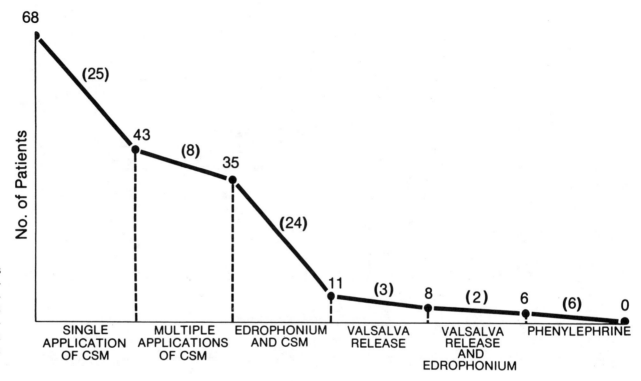

FIGURE 4–19. The success rates (numbers in parentheses) of various vagotonic maneuvers in terminating 68 cases of paroxysmal junctional tachycardia. (From Waxman et al,[10] p. 657, with permission.)

nation is particularly useful in cases that are accompanied by tachycardia-dependent bundle branch block, wherein, if slowing prior to termination is sufficient, normalization of the tachycardia-dependent conduction disturbances may occur. Many vagotonic maneuvers such as head dependency, deep inspiration, phase 4 of the valsalva maneuver, and the administration of phenylephrine act by elevating arterial blood pressure and thereby increasing vagal tone via the baroreceptors.[1–7,11,17]

Atrial Flutter

As shown in Figure 4–6, retardation of AV nodal conduction is an effective means of exposing atrial flutter waves. Carotid sinus massage is equally effective in cases of atrial flutter with tachycardia-dependent bundle branch block. Rarely, atrial flutter may "change" (reentry speeds) to atrial fibrillation during or after carotid sinus massage. Carotid sinus massage applied during sinus rhythm may also rarely induce atrial fibrillation.

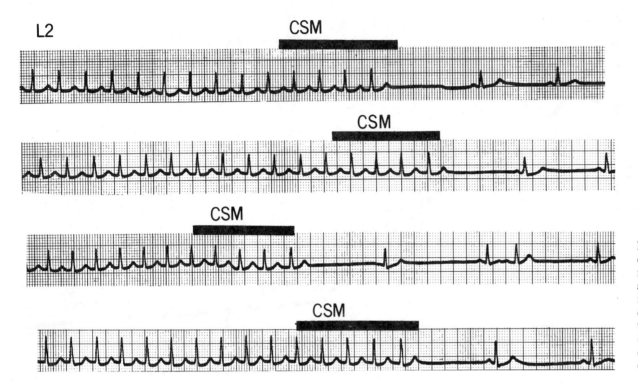

FIGURE 4–20. These four panels from the same patient show reproducible slowing, and then abrupt termination, of paroxysmal junctional tachycardia, induced by the enhanced vagal tone of carotid sinus massage (CSM). These recordings are consecutive but not continuous.

Atrial Fibrillation

In the presence of atrial fibrillation, carotid sinus massage ordinarily depresses AV nodal conduction and reduces the ventricular response. Atrial fibrillation with a rapid ventricular response can result in tachycardia-dependent intraventricular conduction disturbances. In such cases, carotid sinus massage may slow the ventricular response sufficiently to produce brief normalization of phase-3–dependent block, proving aberration as opposed to ventricular ectopy (Fig. 4–22).

On the other hand, atrial flutter-fibrillation with conduction over an accessory AV connection (i.e., ventricular preexcitation) typically results in a rapid ventricular response and a broad, aberrant QRS complex. Because accessory pathways are not responsive to vagal tone alterations, carotid sinus massage and other vagal maneuvers do not slow the ventricular rate or consequently shorten the QRS duration. The fact that carotid sinus massage slows and normalizes the ventricular response in Figure 4–22 rules out the pos-

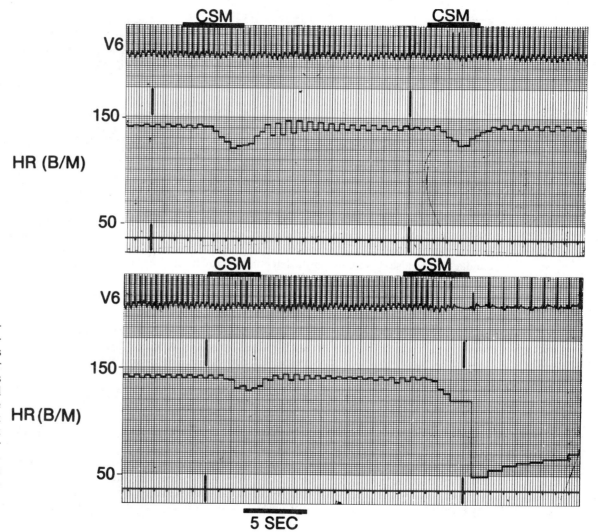

FIGURE 4–21. This continuous recording, from a patient with paroxysmal junctional tachycardia, illustrates the graded slowing of the ventricular rate in response to four applications of carotid sinus massage (CSM). Lead V_6 and beat-to-beat heart rate (HR) are recorded simultaneously. The first three applications of massage result in transient slowing of the ventricular rate without termination of the tachycardia. The fourth application causes initial slowing followed by abrupt termination. B/M = beats per minute. (From Waxman et al,[10] p. 660, with permission.)

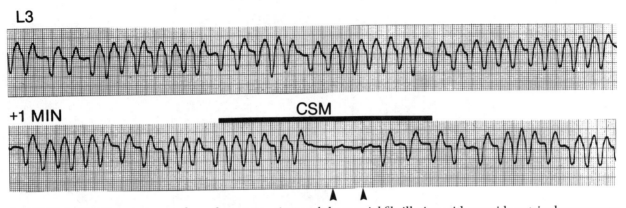

FIGURE 4–22. These strips are from the same patient and show atrial fibrillation with a rapid ventricular response of 160 beats per minute accompanied by tachycardia-dependent left bundle branch block. Carotid sinus massage (CSM) transiently slows the ventricular responses and eliminates the left bundle branch block for two beats (arrowheads). This vagally induced depression of AV nodal conduction and the slowing of the ventricular rate allow the conducted impulses to encounter the left bundle branch cells after phase 3 of recovery (i.e., beyond the refractory period); thus, normal intraventricular conduction is briefly restored.

sibility of rapid conduction over an accessory AV connection.

Ventricular Tachycardia

During ventricular tachycardia, atrial activity is dissociated in approximately 50% to 70% of cases and is associated in the remainder. In Figure 4–23, ventricular tachycardia is associated with 1:1 retrograde ventriculoatrial conduction, and a small consistent notch is seen in every ST segment. Thirty seconds following administration of edrophonium chloride, carotid sinus massage was applied, producing 2:1 retrograde block so that only every alternate ST segment contained a deformity. This proved that there was indeed a concealed P wave in the first instance and shows that the ventricular tachycardia rate remains uninfluenced by this maneuver. Selective slowing of the atrial rate without change in the ventricular rate proves that the rhythm is indeed ventricular tachycardia rather than supraventricular tachycardia with aberrant ventricular conduction. As well, observing selective atrial slowing is a good indicator that carotid sinus massage was properly applied during a case of ventricular tachycardia.

In many instances of ventricular tachycardia, when P waves cannot be identified in the surface recordings, accelerating the dissociated atrial activity may facilitate the diagnosis. The sequence in Figure 4–24 convincingly proves the diagnosis of ventricular tachycardia by (1) providing evidence of AV dissociation during a

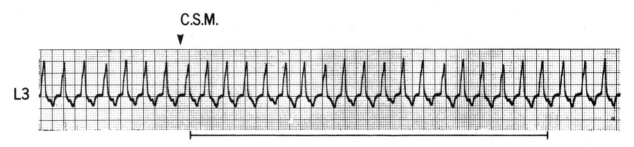

30 SEC POST   EDROPHONIUM HCl

C.S.M.

L3

FIGURE 4-23. Use of carotid sinus massage (CSM) in a patient with a wide-QRS tachycardia produces 2:1 ventriculoatrial block and identifies the ventricular origin of the tachycardia. See text for further discussion. (From Waxman et al,[18] p. 660, with permission.)

tachycardia, (2) demonstrating fusion beats, and (3) demonstrating normal capture beats in the presence of a higher rate than that of the original tachycardia. Normal capture beats appearing at a rate above that of the original tachycardia rule out the possibility of a supraventricular tachycardia with aberrant conduction. A limited number of cases have been published where carotid sinus massage and other vagotonic maneuvers terminated episodes of ventricular tachycardia[5,18-21] or affected the rate of the ventricular arrhythmia.[22] The frequency with which all cases of ventricular tachycardia might be expected to slow and terminate following an increase in vagal tone is unknown, but must be extremely low. Furthermore, the majority of patients in ventricular tachycardia with serious hemodynamic compromise would not be candidates for such interventions. Therefore, attempting termination of a wide-QRS tachycardia by a vagotonic maneuver is applicable only to stable patients. When successful, most cases will prove to be paroxysmal junctional tachycardia with aberrant conduction.[10]

Atrial Fibrillation with Wide QRS Complexes

In the presence of atrial flutter-fibrillation, intermittent wide QRS complexes pose a particular diagnostic problem. The elimination of such wide complexes by means of vagotonic maneuvers strongly favors aberrant ventricular conduction as the pathophysiologic mechanism rather than premature ventricular beats. In Figure 4-25, carotid sinus massage produces AV nodal block, thereby reducing the number of fibrillatory impulses reaching the bundle branches and allowing them to recover their excitability and conduct normally. Thus, aberrant conduction in this case is tachycardia dependent. Once the ventricular rate during atrial fibrillation is controlled by digitalis treatment, aberrant ventricular conduction can be reinvoked by maneuvers that reaccelerate the ventricular response.

Wolff-Parkinson-White Syndrome

The Wolff-Parkinson-White (WPW) syndrome (or ventricular preexcitation) is uniquely amenable to manipulations of autonomic tone. Paroxysmal supraventricular tachycardia involving an AV ac-

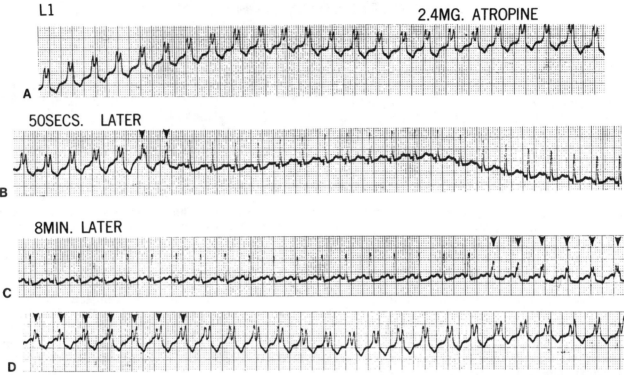

FIGURE 4–24.   (*A*) A wide-QRS tachycardia with no apparent atrial activity. (*B*) When 2.4 mg of atropine is administered 50 seconds later, the atrial rate speeds above the rate of the wide-QRS tachycardia and completely captures the ventricles. During the transition from the wide to the narrow QRS complex, there are convincing fusion beats that are virtually pathognomonic of competition between an atrial and a ventricular focus (arrowheads). The narrowing of the QRS complex at a faster rate than the wide-QRS tachycardia excludes aberration, for all practical purposes, as a cause of the wide-QRS arrhythmia. (*C*) Eight minutes later, when the atrial rate slows to the level of the ventricular tachycardia rate, a series of fusion beats (arrowheads) with incrementally greater contributions by the ventricular tachycardia is seen. (*D*) This process of incremental fusion with the ventricular tachycardia continues for the next seven complexes (arrowheads). Thereafter, the atrial rate falls below the ventricular tachycardia rate, the process of fusion ends, and the QRS configuration returns to the control condition of ventricular tachycardia. (From Waxman et al,[18] p. 659, with permission.)

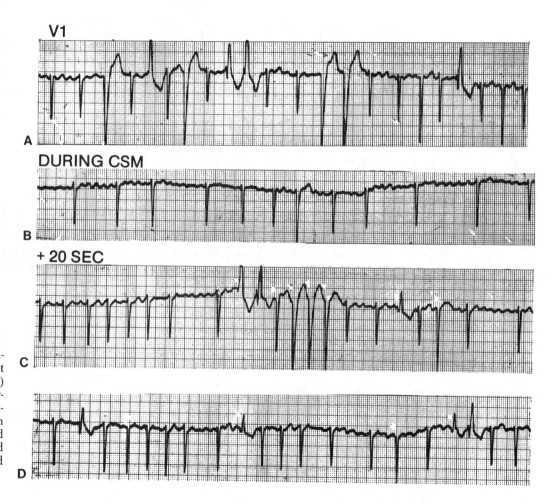

FIGURE 4–25. (*A*) Atrial fibrillation with numerous wide QRS complexes having both right and left bundle branch block configurations. (*B*) During carotid sinus massage (CSM), these aberrantly conducted beats totally disappear—a response highly suggestive of aberrant conduction rather than premature ventricular beats. (*C*) and (*D*) After dissipation of the effects of carotid sinus massage, the ventricular rate speeds, and aberrant conduction returns.

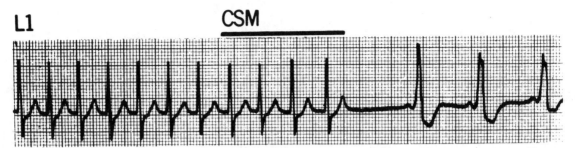

FIGURE 4–26. In this patient with a paroxysmal narrow QRS complex tachycardia, carotid sinus massage (CSM) results in transient slight slowing of the heart rate followed by abrupt termination of the tachycardia (typical paroxysmal atrioventricular reentrant tachycardia). After a brief pause, sinus rhythm resumes, but with a wide QRS complex. At first glance, this sequence might suggest the possibility of bradycardia-dependent aberration to explain the wide QRS complex during the slower sinus rhythm. A closer inspection, however, shows that the PR interval is very short (about 0.08 second) and that the onset of the QRS complex is slurred by a delta wave. These changes are typical of ventricular preexcitation. The QRS complex is narrow during the tachycardia because the accessory pathway is used only in a retrograde (or orthodromic) direction. During sinus rhythm in this particular patient, antegrade conduction over the accessory pathway occurs, resulting in anomalous activation of the ventricles, which produces a delta wave and widening of the QRS complex.

cessory pathway bypass tract (paroxysmal atrioventricular reentrant tachycardia) is readily converted to sinus rhythm with a vagotonic maneuver[10,11,14–16] (see Chapter 11). Such tachycardias involve reciprocation between atria and ventricles, usually using the normal AV node and His-Purkinje system for antegrade conduction to the ventricles, and the accessory connection for retrograde conduction to the atria. A vagotonic maneuver interrupts the tachycardia by blocking conduction within the AV node. Because of the direction of the tachycardia, the QRS com-

plexes are normal during the tachycardia (unless rate-related aberration occurs), and signs of ventricular preexcitation are seen only after sinus rhythm is restored (Figure 4–26). In the presence of aberrant conduction due to ventricular preexcitation, normalization of the QRS complex can be accomplished by evoking His bundle escape beats following sinus node suppression by increased vagal tone. In Figure 4–27, such normalization is accomplished by means of carotid sinus massage. "WPW conduction" may come and go as a function of background heart

rate and autonomic balance in the AV node. If an accessory pathway has a long refractory period, conduction over it may cease when the rate exceeds its recovery time.[23] Conversely, expression of conduction over a bypass tract may require slowing of the cardiac rate to overcome phase-3–dependent block in this structure (Fig. 4–28).

Because the degree of preexcitation depends on the relative velocities of conduction over the bypass tract and the normal AV connections, manipulations of AV nodal conduction time may alter the de-

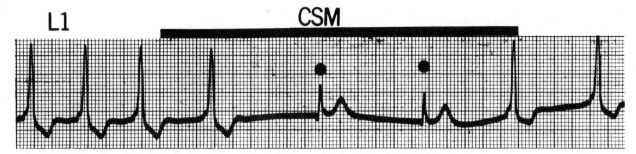

FIGURE 4–27. This strip begins with sinus rhythm and ventricular preexcitation. During carotid sinus massage (CSM), the sinus rate slows and allows an escape junctional (or His bundle) pacemaker (dots) to appear. When the effect of carotid sinus massage wanes, the sinus node regains capture of the ventricles, and ventricular preexcitation resumes.

gree of ventricular preexcitation conduction (Fig. 4–29).

SUMMARY

Autonomic interventions should be viewed as diagnostic and therapeutic tools that occupy an important place in the spectrum of arrhythmia analysis, which ranges from a critical review of long strips of the surface ECG to complex and technologically sophisticated intracardiac recordings, stimulation techniques, and pharmacologic interventions. Each step in this process is characterized by specific advantages and limitations. Whether one is analyzing a rhythm strip with calipers or localizing a His bundle potential with a bipolar electrode, the

maximum information available for interpretation frequently depends on dynamic changes in rhythm.[1–7]

A monotonously repetitive rhythm, no matter how it is analyzed, may remain relatively unyielding; variations in the rhythm are ultimately more informative. Autonomic interventions are so valuable because they provide a simple, usually temporary, perturbation of an otherwise monotonous sequence. The resulting insights are often enormously helpful irrespective of the means of analysis. Some methods can increase the power of rhythm-strip analysis sufficiently to preclude the need for invasive investigations.

Although the range of their potential applications is remarkably broad, practical considerations limit the use of some or many of these interventions. Patients with

cerebrovascular disease should not be subjected to vigorous carotid sinus massage. Individual sensitivity to this maneuver and to most of the other techniques described is highly variable and must be carefully considered or tested at the outset. For example, patients with significant ischemic heart disease or poor left ventricular function should not be given pressor agents; edrophonium has reportedly caused asystolic arrest; atropine can occasionally induce ventricular tachycardia or fibrillation and may exacerbate AV block; isoproterenol or amyl nitrite may be contraindicated in some patients with dynamic left ventricular outflow tract obstruction; patients with unstable angina should not be exercised; and so on. Clearly, deployment of each maneuver requires careful consideration of the pa-

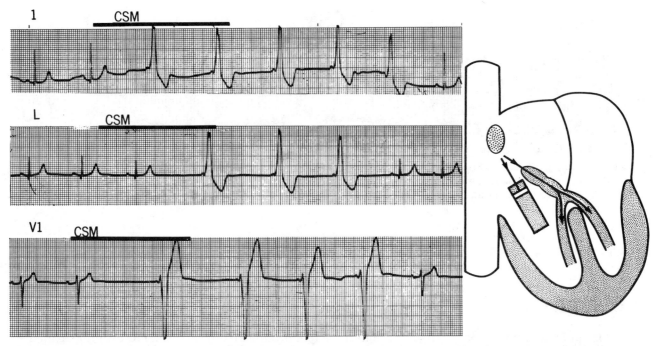

FIGURE 4–28. Ventricular preexcitation is initially absent under control conditions during these three separate recordings. After carotid sinus massage (CSM), however, the sinus node slows, and ventricular preexcitation is evoked for several beats in each strip. In this particular patient with phase-3–dependent block in a right-sided accessory pathway (diagram), conduction over this pathway can occur only when impulses arrive after the completion of phase 3 of the action potential.

tient's underlying condition and clinical status.

We have not listed comprehensively the possible adverse reactions that might ensue from injudiciously applied autonomic interventions. At the same time, other methods of arrhythmia study or termination, including antiarrhythmic drugs or invasive electrophysiologic recording and stimulation techniques, are not entirely free of risk. Moreover, serious hemodynamic or ischemic compromise during an arrhythmia may limit one's ability to deploy any maneuvers other than emergency measures such as electrical cardioversion or pacemaker insertion. Clearly, the choice of approach has to remain a matter of individual clinical judgment. Notwithstanding these caveats, the simple autonomic tools outlined in this chapter should, if extrapolated in imagi-

FIGURE 4–29. In this patient, global preexcitation is evoked during carotid sinus massage (CSM). The enhanced vagal tone selectively slows AV nodal transmission, allowing increased ventricular excitation via the bypass tract, which results in more preexcitation of the ventricles. Note that the fifth beat is wider and different from all other preexcited beats, suggesting that it is displaying the greatest degree of preexcitation. As the sinus node then speeds slightly in concert with the waning of the vagal effects, the degree of preexcitation, though continuing, lessens slightly. The last three QRS complexes like the first four QRS complexes are fusion beats resulting from simultaneous activation of the ventricles, partially via the accessory pathway and partially via the normal routes of intraventricular conduction.

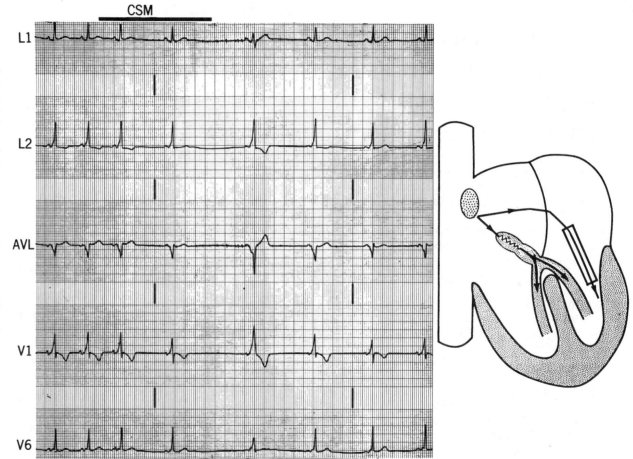

native ways, find numerous and fruitful applications in arrhythmia analysis.

REFERENCES

1. Wald RW and Waxman MB: Clinical approach to cardiac arrhythmias. In: Emergency Management of the Critically Ill. Aberman A and Logan A (eds): Symposia specialists. Miami, 1980, pp 101–124.
2. Waxman MB, Wald RW, and Cameron DA: Interactions between the autonomic nervous system and tachycardias in man. Cardiol Clin, Saunders, Philadelphia, 1983, pp 143–185.
3. Waxman MB and Wald RW: Influences of the autonomic nervous system on tachycardia. In: Tachycardias. Surawicz B (ed) Martinus and Nihoff, Boston, 1984, pp 67–102.
4. Waxman MB and Cameron DA: The reflex effects of tachycardias on autonomic tone. Ann NY Acad Sci 601:378–393, 1990.
5. Waxman MB, Cameron DA, and Wald RW: The effects of vagal tone on ventricular tachyarrhythmias. In: Vagal Control of the Heart: M. Levy and P. Schwartz (eds). Futura Publications, Mt Kisco, NY. In press, 1993.
6. Waxman MB, Wald RW, and Cameron DA: Interaction between the autonomic nervous system and supra-ventricular tachycardias in humans. In: Cardiac Electrophysiology ed 2. Saunders, Philadelphia. In press, 1993.
7. Waxman MB: Supraventricular tachycardias: modulation by autonomic tone. In: Atrial Arrhythmias. DiMarco JP and Prystowsky EN (eds). Futura Publishing, Mt. Kisco, New York. In Press, 1993.
8. Eckberg DL and Sleight P: Human baroreflexes in health and disease, Oxford University Press, Oxford, 1992.
9. Lown B and Levine SA: The carotid sinus: Clinical value of its stimulation. Circulation 23:766–789, 1961.
10. Waxman MB, Wald RW, Sharma AD, Huerta F, and Cameron DA: Vagal techniques for termination of paroxysmal supraventricular tachycardia. Am J Cardiol 46:655–664, 1980.
11. Waxman MB, Bonet JF, Finley JP, and Wald RW: Effects of respiration and posture on paroxysmal supraventricular tachycardia. Circulation 62:1011–1020, 1980.
12. Singer DH, Lazzara R, and Hoffman BF: Interrelationships between automaticity and conduction in Purkinje fibers. Circ Res 21:537–558, 1967.
13. Rosenbaum MB, Elizari MV, Lazzari JO, Halpern MS, Gerardo J, Nau and Levi RJ: The mechanism of intermittent bundle branch block: Relationship to prolonged recovery, hypopolarization and spontaneous diastolic depolarization. Chest 63:666–677, 1973.
14. Waxman MB and Wald RW: Recurrent paroxysmal atrial tachycardia: A complication of ventricular pacing in a patient with occult Wolff-Parkinson-White syndrome. J of Electrocardiology 10:291–298, 1977.
15. Waxman MB, Wald RW, Bonet JF, and Finley JP: Carotid sinus massage-induced elimination of rate-related bundle branch block during paroxysmal atrial tachycardia: A simple method of proving bypass tract participation in the tachycardia. J of Electrocardiol 12:371–376, 1979.
16. Waxman MB and Cupps CL: Spontaneous termination of paroxysmal supraventricular tachycardia following disappearance of bundle branch block ipsilateral to a concealed atrioventricular accessory pathway: The role of autonomic tone in tachycardia diagnosis. PACE 9:26–35, 1986.
17. Waxman MB, Sharma AD, Cameron DA, Huerta F, and Wald RW: Reflex mechanisms responsible for early spontaneous termination of paroxysmal supraventricular tachycardia. Am J of Cardiol 49:259–272, 1982.
18. Waxman MB, Downar E, Berman ND, and Felderhoff CH: Phenylephrine

(neosynephrine) terminated ventricular tachycardia. Circulation 50:656–664, 1974.

19. Waxman MB and Wald RW: Termination of ventricular tachycardia by an increase in cardiac vagal drive. Circulation 56:385–391, 1977.

20. Waxman MB, Staniloff H, and Wald RW: Respiratory and vagal modulation of ventricular tachycardia. J Electrocardiol 14:83–90, 1981.

21. Hess DS, Hanlon T, Scheinman M, Budge R, and Sesai J: Termination of ventricular tachycardia by carotid sinus massage. Circulation 65:627–633, 1982.

22. Waxman MB, Cupps CL, and Cameron DA: Modulation of an idioventricular rhythm by vagal tone. J Am Coll Cardiol 11:1052–1060, 1988.

23. Waxman MB, Wald RW, and Cameron DA: Coexistence of tachycardia dependent (phase 3) left bundle branch block and Wolff-Parkinson-White conduction. PACE 5:100–105, 1982.

CHAPTER 5

Electrocardiographic Monitoring

ROBERT A. WAUGH, MD, and
GALEN S. WAGNER, MD

OUTLINE

The ability to monitor the electrical activity of the heart has changed markedly in recent years as both the variety and the sophistication of monitoring technology have increased. Miniaturization of components, in addition to allowing more sophisticated signal processing at a lower cost, has also increased patient comfort by reducing the size and weight of the telemetry and monitoring devices.

With real-time monitoring (as typified by in-hospital telemetry surveillance systems), radio-frequency transmission of the electrocardiogram (ECG) signal has unshackled the patient from hard-wired systems, while memory loops and "alarm" algorithms have improved the detection and documentation of significant arrhythmias.

Ambulatory ECG monitoring was first introduced by Holter in 1961.[1] Since then, improvements in the portable recorders have allowed longer periods of monitoring using smaller batteries. With the use of simpler recorders and cassette tapes, most patients can handle battery and tape changing, further increasing the utility of long-term ambulatory ECG monitoring remote from the office or laboratory. Modems allow telephone transmission of the ECG signal, making it feasible to monitor patients in their usual environment. Sophisticated signal-processing equipment now allows reasonably accurate detection and quantitation of heart rate, pauses, and arrhythmias.

This increasing complexity and variety of monitoring methods and equipment, however, have also complicated the clinical decisions necessary to apply them in the most cost-effective manner. Some have taken an entrepreneurial approach to ambulatory ECG monitoring and have made inflated or undocumented claims as to the sensitivity, specificity, and predictive accuracy of a given device or system.

A detailed treatise on technologic approaches to ECG monitoring, including the strengths and weaknesses of particular systems, is beyond the scope of this book, and the reader is referred elsewhere.[2] This chapter, however, reviews some of the important technical aspects of ECG monitoring, including the electrodes and lead systems, and some clinical aspects unique to ambulatory monitoring, including symptomatic correlations and artifacts that must be differentiated from clinically significant events.

CLINICAL USE OF MONITORING SYSTEMS

On occasion, particularly in the hospital, the patient first learns that monitoring will be performed when a hospital employee shows up to attach the device. In such instances, patients (and family members or friends) should be reassured that the procedure does not necessarily indicate underlying heart disease, and they should be educated as to why monitoring is being undertaken, how the electrodes are going to be placed on the chest, and what can be done to facilitate the success of the test.

Application of Electrodes

Proper preparation of the skin is an initial critical step in obtaining a high-quality ECG signal. Even if no hair is apparent, the electrode sites should be shaved. Additional preparation includes cleansing the sites and removing the superficial keratinized skin layer to diminish electrical impedance. Removal of this skin layer is accomplished by light abrasion, using a special abrasive paste and gauze pad with vigorous rubbing. Extra fine sandpaper or a specially designed rotating drill with a disposable abrasive pad can be used. (Drawing blood at the prepared site is to be discouraged, however.) The site should then be wiped thoroughly with a clean gauze pad to remove debrided cells and abrasive material. These procedures ensure excellent electrical contact and proper electrode adherence, and they minimize skin irritation. The use of alcohol as an additional cleansing agent is frequently painful, and there is no convincing evidence of an improved ECG signal.

Pregelled disposable electrodes should be removed from their sealed, foil-wrapped package and applied to the designated area with as little finger contact with the adhesive surface as possible. With multiple-electrode packs, the unused electrodes are now individually sealed and will not dry out. The electrodes should be placed on the proper chest or abdominal location, with pressure applied initially at the central pregelled pad and then progressing outward in a circular motion over the entire adhesive area. Particularly for ambulatory ECG monitoring, the electrical impedance between electrodes should be measured. If it is inappropriately high, the offending electrode, or electrodes, should be removed, the skin site prepared again, new electrodes applied, and the impedance remeasured. Next, the ECG leads are applied to the appropriate electrodes by fitting the snap of the lead contact onto the electrode nipple. The resulting ECG signal should be checked to ensure optimal gain and morphology. For telemetry systems, the appropriate alarm rate limits should be set and tested.

For telemetry, the electrodes should be changed as frequently as necessary to obtain an artifact-free ECG signal. For ambulatory monitoring, the electrodes should be changed every 24 hours if possible. Adequate recordings, however, may be obtained from the same set of electrodes for up to 72 hours, depending on how much the patient perspires. Going this long without a shower or bath may prove objectionable to some patients, or to those in their immediate environment.

The skin should be properly prepared each time the electrodes are changed.

Lead Systems

MODIFIED STANDARD LEADS USING PRECORDIAL ELECTRODE POSITIONS

Various lead placements can be obtained by placing the electrodes on different areas on the chest (Fig. 5–1). The two most commonly employed are modified leads II and V_1 (MCL_1). Although not identical to the analogous standard scalar ECG leads, they are sufficiently similar to allow the ECG signal to be related to the morphologic aspects of leads II and V_1 that are used in arrhythmia analysis. For example, like its standard counterpart, modified lead II usually displays maximal P-wave and QRS amplitude. MCI_1, like lead V_1, also displays atrial activity well, but in addition, it allows differentiation of right versus left bundle branch block.

As a practical matter in the intensive care unit, modified lead II involves placing electrodes in areas that may hinder care. The upper right sternal edge and apical precordial areas are frequently valuable auscultatory sites and are also where cardioverter or defibrillator paddles are applied. To obviate the latter problem, specially designed precordial "patches" have been developed that can be used both as ECG monitoring electrodes with peripherally located snap fittings and as

low-impedance sites for paddle electrode placement in delivery of transthoracic countershock. Use of the infraclavicular areas for electrode placement can create skin irritation and a nidus for infection that may prevent these favored sites from being used for subsequent temporary or permanent pacemaker placement.

USE OF ADDITIONAL LEAD SYSTEMS

Standard and Modified Surface Leads. Attachment of electrodes to the arms and the left leg permits recording of standard ECG leads I, II, and III; the right leg electrode serves as a ground lead. When the various arm and leg electrodes are connected in certain configurations, the resulting "mean electrode" can function as a reference point for unipolar recording from an exploring electrode. When the exploring electrode is the right arm, left arm, or left leg electrode versus the "mean electrode," formed by combining the other two limb electrodes, standard leads aVR, aVL, or aVF, respectively, result. When the right arm, left arm, and left leg electrodes are added together and the exploring electrode is a precordial electrode positioned at standard chest wall sites, the standard chest leads V_1 through V_6 result. Lead V_1 is usually an adequate standard lead for identifying P waves. At times, however, P waves are more prominent when the exploring electrode is moved even farther to the right of the sternum and additional interspaces

LEAD	POSITION	R. ARM	L. ARM	R. LEG (Ground)
II	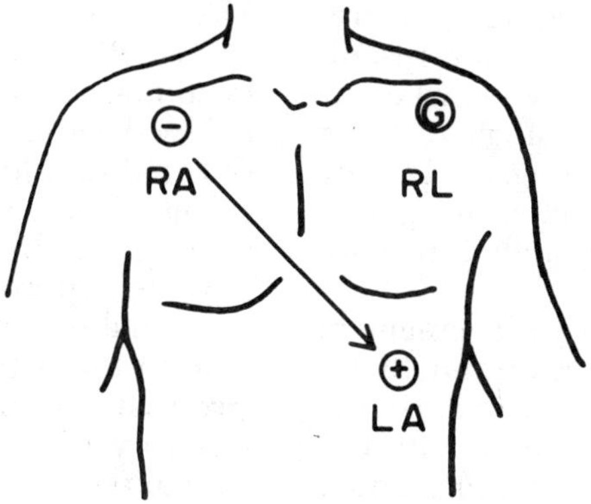	R. Sub Mid-Clavicle	L. Lower Rib Margin	L. Sub Mid-Clavicle
V_1 (MCL$_1$)	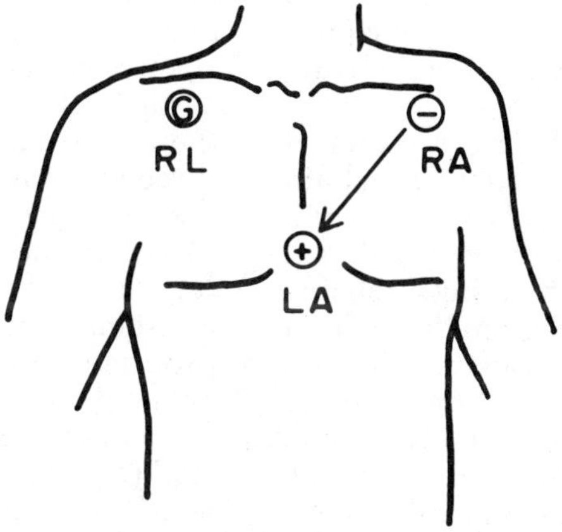	L. Sub Mid-Clavicle	Mid Sternum 4th Inter-Costal Space	R. Sub Mid-Clavicle

FIGURE 5–1. The electrode positions for modified leads II and V_1 (MCL$_1$) are depicted. They offer several advantages for rhythm detection. Lead MCL$_1$, in particular, interferes minimally with the cardiac physical examination, or with paddle placement, should cardioversion or defibrillation be necessary. A = arm; G = ground; L = left; R = right. RA = right arm; RL = right leg; LA = left arm.

are explored. Connection of the right and left arm leads to precordial electrodes positioned at the second and fourth right intercostal spaces, respectively, while the ECG recorder is set to lead I (a Lewis lead) frequently results in a tracing that defines atrial activity more optimally than any of the standard leads.

In addition to detecting atrial activity accurately, the morphologic features of that activity in a given monitoring lead may also be important in arrhythmia diagnosis. This point is illustrated by consideration of the differential diagnosis of atrial tachycardias with 2:1 atrioventricular (AV) block whose atrial rate is in the range of 200 to 220 beats per minute. At this rate, the distinction between atrial flutter and other supraventricular tachycardias may be difficult. Whereas a "sawtooth" configuration of atrial activity establishes the diagnosis of atrial flutter, the right precordial leads, even when flutter is present, often demonstrate P waves that appear discrete. Standard ECG leads II, III, and aVF are most likely to show the sawtooth configuration (Fig. 5-2, *left*). When atrial activity is in the rapid fibrillation end of the flutter-fibrillation spectrum, the standard limb leads may falsely suggest asystole, while lead V_1 usually clearly reveals atrial fibrillation (Fig. 5-2, *right*).

Multiple leads are also helpful in identifying whether premature wide QRS complexes are associated with premature P waves, and in determining whether atrial pauses are due to blocked premature atrial complexes (PACs) (Fig. 5-3). It is also surprising how frequently a premature beat in a single lead closely resembles that patient's normal beats, whereas in a second lead the morphologic features are obviously different (Fig. 5-4). For these and other reasons, monitoring with two or more leads increasingly is becoming the minimum standard.

Esophageal Lead. The placement of an esophageal electrode is minimally invasive (see Chapter 17, particularly for discussion of therapeutic uses). Its use does not require extensive training, and it is so widely available and useful in arrhythmia diagnosis that it is discussed here rather than in the next chapter, which concerns electrophysiologic studies.

When used with ambulatory monitoring, an electrode enclosed in a gelatin capsule with a thin, pliable wire (a "pill electrode") is easily swallowed and well tolerated by patients. Obtaining a reliable esophageal atrial electrogram throughout the monitoring period can be difficult, however, as electrode position tends to drift, causing loss of an adequate signal. For monitoring of inpatients or for monitoring on a short-term basis, stiffer electrodes such as temporary transvenous pacemaker leads, used permanent transvenous pacemaker leads, or electrode-tipped Lehman catheters may be used.

The esophageal atrial electrogram produces a monophasic negative potential as the area of the left atrium is approached. The potential is biphasic when the electrode is directly behind the left atrium and becomes positive as the electrode moves below the area of the left atrium. The site selected should provide a maximal atrial complex that is clearly not a part of the QRS deflection.

Once appropriately positioned, the proximal electrode wire is taped in position to the patient's cheek, and with appropriate connections to either the ambulatory recorder or an ECG machine, one of the leads becomes the esophageal electrogram. When the proximal end of the electrode is connected to the V_3 lead of a three-channel ECG machine, V_1 and V_2 must be affixed to the chest as well. The V_1 through V_3 lead selection switch can then be used to record a simultaneous three-lead rhythm strip of V_1 and V_2, with the esophageal electrogram being displayed in the V_3 channel. (Fig. 5-5). Another type of interface that can be helpful is a signal-splitting device, which with appropriate connections to a standard three-channel machine provides a simultaneous esophageal electrogram, a hybrid lead (e.g., standard lead II and the esophageal electrogram blended together), and the selected standard lead of the surface ECG (Fig. 5-6). Alternatively, a single-channel ECG machine can be used to record an isolated esophageal electrogram,

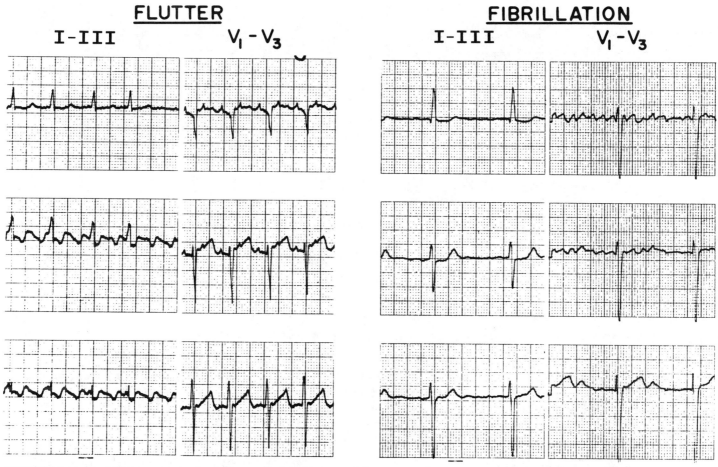

FLUTTER

I-III   V₁ - V₃

FIBRILLATION

I-III   V₁ - V₃

FIGURE 5–2. *(Left)* Supraventricular tachycardia in which atrial flutter is well seen in leads II and III, and in leads V₁ and V₂. In the precordial leads, atrial activation appears discrete, with an isoelectric interval between the P waves. The inferior limb leads, however, show the typical sawtooth configuration of atrial flutter. *(Right)* Supraventricular tachycardia in which fibrillation waves are relatively inapparent in leads II and III but are well seen in precordial leads V₁ and V₂.

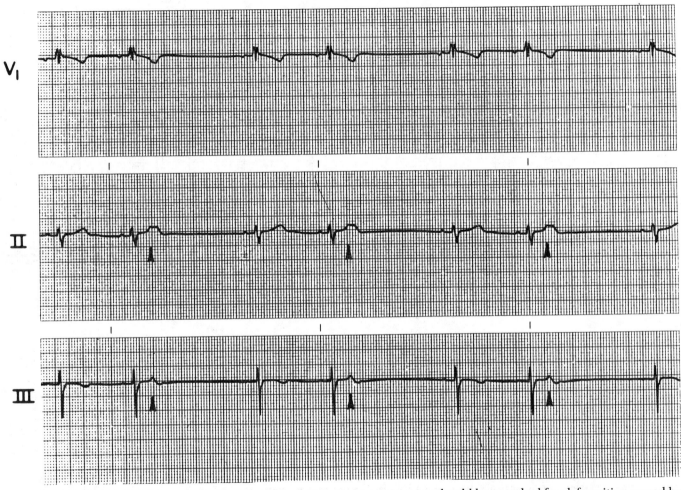

FIGURE 5–3. With atrial pauses, the T waves of the beats prior to any pauses should be searched for deformities caused by premature P waves. In this example of atrial pauses, lead V_1 shows no evidence of ectopic atrial activity, but leads II and III clearly show the ectopic atrial activity (arrowheads), identifying blocked premature atrial complexes (PACs) as the cause for these pauses.

MCL₁

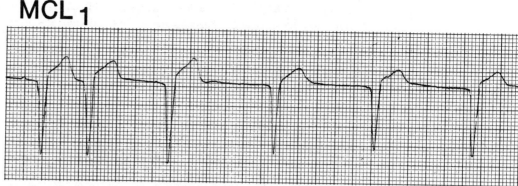

Modified Lead II

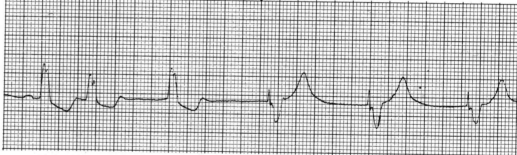

SIMULTANEOUS TRACINGS

FIGURE 5–4. Some of the advantages of monitoring more than one lead are exemplified in this ambulatory electrocardiogram (ECG) from a patient with a VVI pacemaker programmed for a rate of 55 beats per minute. Note that in the anterior precordial lead (MCL₁), the QRS complexes are all remarkably similar to each other, and pacemaker artifact is not clearly identified. In the inferior lead (modified lead II), however, both the pacing spike and the marked change in QRS morphology of the paced beats are easily recognized.

but this method is less satisfactory, as no simultaneous standard surface lead is available for comparison with the patient's clinical arrhythmia.

The esophageal ECG is particularly useful in identifying atrial activity either when it is not apparent on the body surface recordings or when more than the readily apparent atrial activity is suspected (see Fig. 5–6). One must never assume that the AV relationship is 1:1 unless additional atrial activity hidden within the QRS complex (see Fig. 5–5, initial portion of strip) can be excluded. Even when a 1:1 ratio is identified, it is not possible to determine whether the sequence is AV or ventriculoatrial (VA) unless AV block either occurs spontaneously or can be induced (see Fig. 5–5, middle portion of strip). The esophageal electrode is most helpful when it demonstrates that atrial

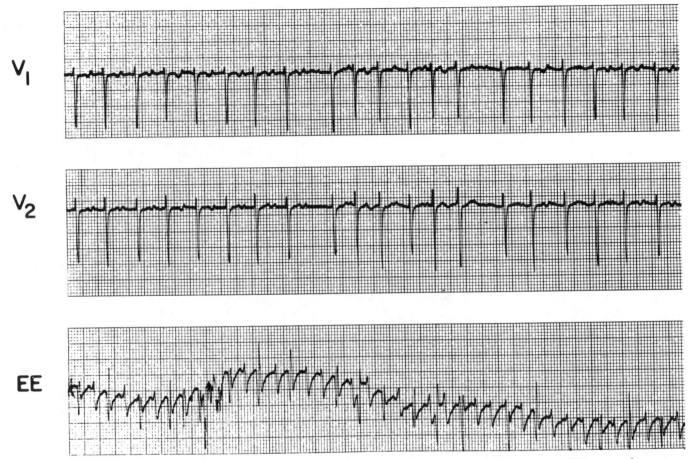

FIGURE 5–5. Initially in this simultaneous recording of leads V_1, V_2, and an esophageal electrogram (EE), a regular supraventricular tachycardia at 150 beats per minute with a 1:1 atrioventricular (AV) relationship is suggested. The EE recording readily proves that there is at least one P wave for each QRS complex but neither defines the sequence of activation (AV versus ventriculoatrial [VA]) nor entirely rules out a second P wave obscured within the QRS complex. In the middle of the tracing, during spontaneous slowing of the ventricular rate, atrial activity is not clearly identifiable in the surface ECG leads V_1 and V_2. The EE lead, on the other hand, readily identifies atrial activity at 300 beats per minute, proving the diagnosis of atrial flutter with 2:1 AV conduction.

Lead II

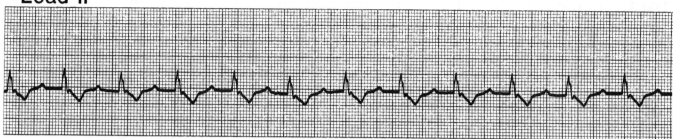

Combined Lead II and Esophageal Electrogram

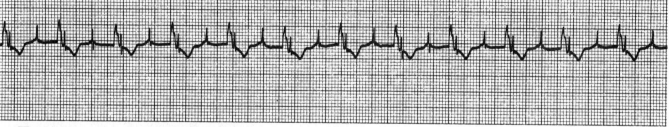

Esophageal Electrogram

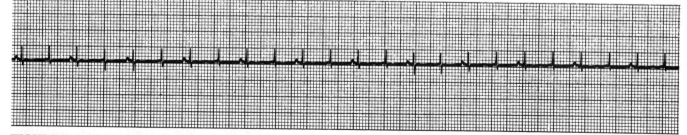

FIGURE 5–6. Using a signal mixing device, separate simultaneous recordings of a standard lead (in this case lead II [*top*]), an esophageal electrode *(bottom)*, and a combination of the two *(middle)* can be obtained. In this case, the suspicion of an atrial tachycardia at 160 beats per minute with 2:1 AV block was confirmed.

activity and ventricular activity are dissociated or that one is a multiple of the other. If such a precise identification of the cardiac rhythm is not possible from an esophageal study, a transvenous intraatrial recording can be obtained.

INTERPRETATION OF RECORDED ECG DATA

The interpretation of the recorded ECG signal is the same regardless of whether it is obtained from telemetry, an ambulatory tape recorder, telephone transmission, or a standard ECG machine, and the guidelines cited throughout this book may be applied. The prognostic aspects of qualitative and quantitative ventricular rhythm analysis are discussed in Chapter 7 (pages 156 to 162) and Chapter 12 (pages 282 to 289, and 291 to 298).

Rhythm-Symptom Correlations

The classic and time-tested indication for long-term ambulatory ECG monitoring is the evaluation of symptoms that suggest an arrhythmic origin, such as palpitations, dizziness, or syncope. It can establish a causal relationship (or lack thereof) between symptoms and underlying rhythm status. Although the history can be quite suggestive of a particular arrhythmia, it may also be misleading. Before initiating antiarrhythmic therapy, particularly with the more expensive and toxic agents, documentation of the arrhythmia is a necessary minimum procedure.

Patients must understand that the diary is a crucial part of the ambulatory monitoring procedure and that they should carefully document the times and types of activities that occur throughout the day, such as taking medications, exercising, eating meals, performing bodily excretory functions, and other types of potentially stressful activities (even without concomitant symptoms). Any symptoms should be similarly documented as to character, time, and corresponding activity. The patient should be discreetly questioned about illiteracy; when this problem or other problems (such as neuromuscular disabilities) prevent the patient from making diary entries, the aid of a literate family member or friend may be enlisted. An alternative and less satisfactory technique is to question the patient when the recorder is returned, with diary entries made retrospectively. In addition to using the diary, patients should be urged also to activate the recorder's symptom marker. Despite aggressive attempts to ensure patient cooperation, up to one third of monitors may be returned with blank or inadequate diaries.

When arrhythmias correspond closely to symptom markers and diary entries, a cause-effect relationship is easy to ascertain (Fig. 5–7). When symptomatic arrhythmias are frequent, however, patients may rapidly lose enthusiasm for documenting each event. This problem results in a recording in which some arrhythmias are associated with use of the symptom marker and diary entries, but many are not, raising the possibility of a "true-true and unrelated" scenario. Education of the patient when the unit is placed, or retrospective inquiry (via the telephone if necessary), or both, offer potential solutions to this problem.

Even evaluation of the symptom "palpitations" can be misleading, because the term has different meanings to different patients (and sometimes, physicians). The most common cause of palpitations is a sympathetically mediated increase in heart rate and inotropic state. When palpitations are associated with obvious sinus tachycardia, the relationship between the symptom and rhythm is also equally obvious. However, in patients with concomitant enhanced parasympathetic tone or chronotropic incompetence, or both, the degree of increase in the heart rate may be more modest and the relationship between palpitations and borderline sinus tachycardia missed.

Another correlative difficulty arises when patients make diary entries and use the symptom marker for every symptom experienced during the recording period. Thus, entries not likely to be related to arrhythmias, such as headache, leg pain, and diarrhea, are intermixed with symptoms such as palpitations and dizziness, for which assessing a cause-effect rela-

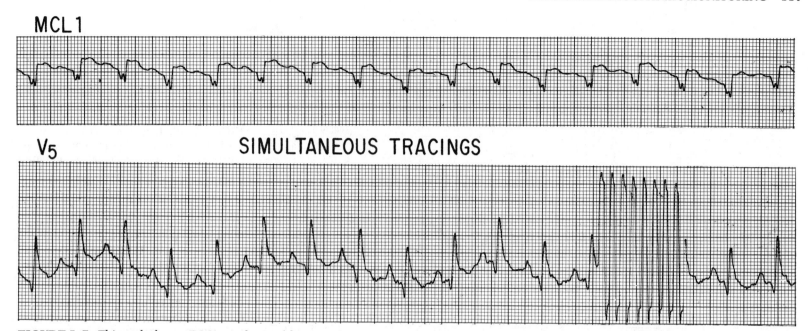

FIGURE 5–7. This ambulatory ECG was obtained from a patient 3 months after myocardial infarction. The use of the symptom marker (toward the end of the bottom strip) was accompanied by the diary entry, "Rapid hard beating of my heart." The onset and offset of this tachycardia were documented to be gradual, and the P-wave morphology was unchanged from the patient's sinus rhythm—all typical features of sinus tachycardia.

tionship to rhythm status is key; therefore, the symptom-rhythm assessment in this situation requires a qualitative judgment made only after careful review and correlation of diary and rhythm.

Another potential confounding variable is the use of the symptom marker; patients frequently use it to indicate non–symptom-related events such as activity status (e.g., "bowel movement"). This is not a problem so long as the diary is accurately kept and carefully reviewed. Children are likely to "play" with the event marker, particularly with recorders whose light-emitting diode clock either illuminates or turns on with event marker use. Despite these difficulties, the correlation among symptoms, activity, and rhythm status is a most important aspect of long-term ambulatory ECG monitoring that should not assume any less importance despite the more sophisticated capabilities of the newer systems.

Evaluation of Pacemaker Function

With the increasing sophistication of today's pacemakers, including their programming and interrogation capabilities,

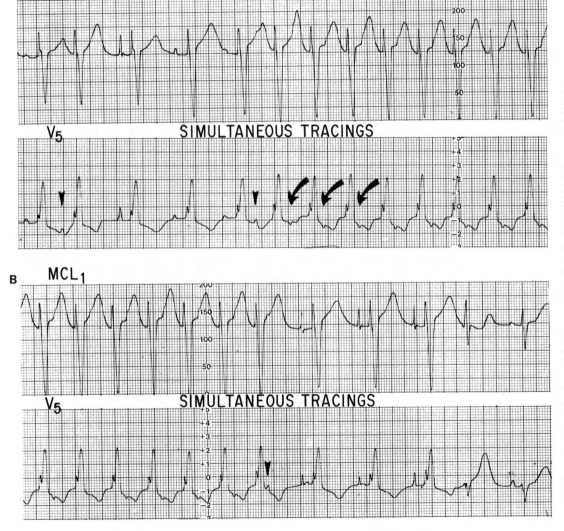

FIGURE 5–8. One month after insertion of a DDD pacemaker, this patient developed paroxysms of rapid heartbeat. Pacer parameters were as follows: rate limits were 70 to 110 beats per minute; AV delay was 0.17 second; post–ventricular atrial refractory period (PVARP) was 0.20 second. An initial PAC (first arrowhead in [A], lower tracing) follows the prior ventricular pacing spike by 0.36 second. Because it follows the PVARP, it is both sensed and tracked (note the ventricular pacing spike approximately 0.17 second later). One beat of AV sequential pacing is followed by two sinus P waves that are also normally tracked. A second PAC (second arrowhead in lower tracing) initiates ventricular pacing at 110 beats per minute. The retrograde P waves following each paced beat (curved arrows) follow the PVARP and are therefore sensed with appropriate ventricular tracking. Consequently, a pacemaker-mediated tachycardia (PMT) occurs and continues until a third blocked PAC (arrowhead in [B], lower tracing) occurs within the PVARP (approximately 0.16 second after the prior pacing spike). It is not sensed, it prevents retrograde VA capture, and it leads to abrupt termination of the PMT. Note the critical role of the retrograde P wave in PMT: The initial ventricular tracking of a PAC (A) has no retrograde VA capture; therefore, no PMT is induced.

as well as the widespread availability of telephone telemetry for pacemaker follow-up, pacemaker and lead malfunctions (including alterations in myocardial pacing thresholds) have become increasingly easier to detect. Nevertheless, the recognition of intermittent problems (such as a lead fracture with intermittent function) and certain pacemaker-induced "malfunctions" such as pacemaker-mediated tachycardia (PMT), pacemaker-induced ventricular arrhythmias, and other "pace-

maker syndromes" may still warrant ambulatory ECG monitoring (see Chapter 16, pages 404 to 408).

This point is illustrated by the case of a patient who underwent DDD pacemaker insertion for sinus node dysfunction with syncope. The post–ventricular atrial refractory period (PVARP) was programmed to 0.20 second, and the upper rate limit was set at 110 beats per minute. Approximately 1 month later, the patient began to notice paroxysms of rapid regu-

lar heart beating lasting from a few seconds to minutes and terminating either spontaneously or following a Valsalva maneuver. Pacer interrogation showed normal parameters, and ambulatory monitoring was undertaken. This monitoring showed typical PMT with retrograde VA capture by the paced ventricular beats and a tachycardia rate of 110 beats per minute (Fig. 5–8). The PMT was corrected by reprogramming the PVARP to encompass the retrograde RP interval. Pace-

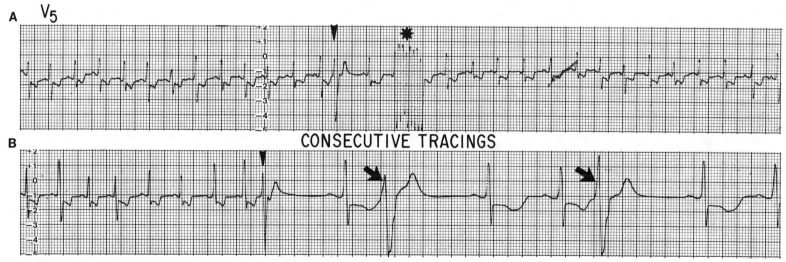

FIGURE 5–9. (*A*) An apparent narrow-complex tachycardia. The PR interval, the width of the QRS complex, and the QT intervals, however, also show marked narrowing. Furthermore, a symptomatic premature beat (arrowhead) led to use of the symptom marker (asterisk), and it, too, was narrowed. (Compare this symptom-marker artifact to that of Fig. 5–7.) These changes are typical of slowed tape recording, which when played back at normal speed produces a "pseudotachycardia." (*B*) A few seconds later, a return to normal recording speed was documented. Compare the premature ventricular complex (PVC) width occurring during tape slowing (arrowhead) to those PVC widths occurring during normal tape speed (arrows). This artifact is most common at the end of a recording period, when battery strength is nearing depletion.

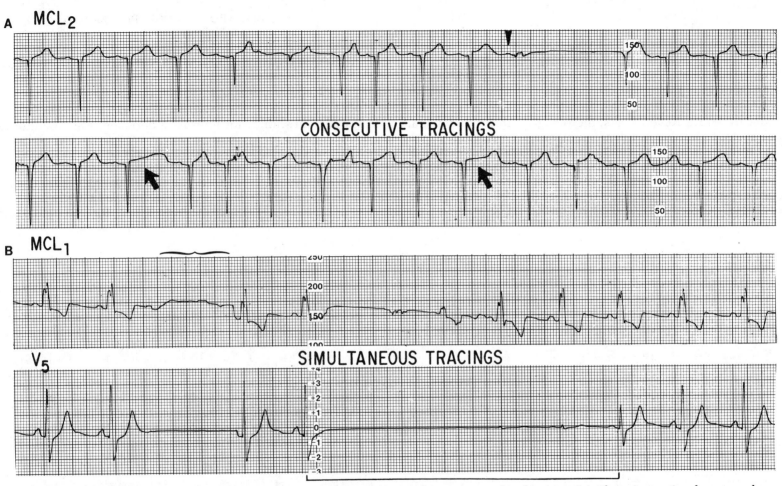

FIGURE 5-10. (*A*) Note the variable QRS configuration and apparent dropped P wave (arrowhead in top strip). Closer inspection, however, shows that the increase in the PR interval is a "pseudopause" due to tape binding followed by release and more rapid movement of tape across the recording head. Note the absence of a P wave immediately in front of the subsequent QRS complex. A short time later (bottom strip), the same thing occurs just after the inscription of a QRS complex, leading to a prolongation in the QT interval (arrows). (*B*) Note the initial pseudopause, which is due to tape binding and then speeding between the inscription of a P wave and the subsequent QRS complex (curved bracket in top strip). The pseudopause is followed by a period of abnormal contact between the tape and recording heads, producing distorted and missing QRS complexes in the upper panel and a 4.4-second pseudopause in the lower panel (square bracket).

maker-mediated tachycardia is analogous to the reentry tachycardia model of preexcitation, in which the pacing wire conducts the impulse antegrade (like the normal conduction system of most AV reciprocating tachycardias) and the His-Purkinje system conducts the impulse retrograde (like the accessory pathway—Chapter 11, pages 240 to 243). Clues to the diagnosis of PMT include retrograde atrial capture outside the PVARP and a tachycardia rate that closely parallels the upper rate limits set for that DDD pacemaker (see Chapter 16).

In addition, pacemaker patients may be at risk for other tachyarrhythmias related to underlying heart disease and may therefore be candidates for ambulatory monitoring for reasons other than evaluation of pacemaker function.

Artifacts Related to Ambulatory ECG Monitoring

A variety of artifacts can occur during the recording and playing back of a tape-recorded analogue ECG signal. These include tape slowing, usually in association with battery failure, leading to a "pseudotachycardia" (Fig. 5–9); tape binding and then speeding, leading to "pseudopauses" or "pseudobradycardias," or to both artifacts (Fig. 5–10A); tape stretch, leading to minor variability in heart rate or regularity; and inconstant contact between the tape and the recording head, causing voltage and morphologic changes in the QRS complex (Fig. 5–10B). Reused recording tape can also create perplexing artifacts when the prior recording is incompletely erased and a second ECG recording is superimposed on the first. Reversal of the recording direction or inversion of the tape when making the second recording further compounds the complexity of the artifact.

REFERENCES

1. Holter NJ: New method for heart studies: Continuous electrocardiography of active subjects over long periods is now practical. Science 134:1214–1220, 1961.
2. David D, Michelson EL, and Dreifus LS (eds): Ambulatory Monitoring of the Cardiac Patient. FA Davis, Philadelphia, 1988.

CHAPTER 6

Electrophysiologic Studies in the Diagnosis of Cardiac Arrhythmias

BARRY W. RAMO, MD, and
MARCEL GILBERT, MD

Electrophysiologic study (EPS) of the heart is a valuable tool used to define the diagnosis, mechanism, prognosis, or treatment of known or suspected bradyarrhythmias and tachyarrhythmias. It is particularly useful for evaluating the effects of drugs on arrhythmias and for evaluating patients who are potential candidates for catheter ablation or for the insertion of devices to control tachyarrhythmias.

In the 1960s, observations made during invasive evaluations of the electrical function of the human heart paved the way for the evolution of modern-day EPS. Two observations were particularly important: (1) clinically relevant arrhythmias could be induced using pacing techniques, and (2) electrical activity could be recorded from the His bundle. Although cardiac pacing had been available as a mode of therapy for several years, it was first used to study arrhythmias by Durrer and coworkers[1] and Coumel and associates in 1967.[2] These investigators and others used programmed atrial and ventricular electrical stimulation in the laboratory to induce arrhythmias that were identical to the patients' spontaneously occurring clinical arrhythmias. Besides the ability to record the His bundle potential,[3] programmed electrical stimulation (PES) of the heart was further developed and used to evaluate the functional characteristics of the sinus node, the atrioventricular (AV) node, and the infranodal His-Purkinje system, as well as accessory pathways. Narrow- and wide-QRS tachyarrhythmias could also be induced with PES. The ability to induce clinically relevant arrhythmias provided a basis for testing pharmacologic therapy that allowed a more precise determination of its effects. This testing was particularly helpful in patients who had very infrequent occurrences of a spontaneous arrhythmia. More recently, EPS has been used in patients who are being considered for an antitachycardia pacemaker device or for an automatic implantable defibrillator,[4] and it is a necessary prerequisite to catheter ablation in the control of various tachyarrhythmias. Table 6–1 outlines the possible indications for EPS in the diagnosis and treatment of arrhythmias.

Patients who have life-threatening arrhythmias or arrhythmias refractory to therapy, or who have accessory pathways and are candidates for radio-frequency catheter ablation, constitute the majority of patients undergoing EPS. Indeed, in patients with recurrent ventricular tachycardia, aborted sudden death in the absence of myocardial infarction, or accessory-pathway–related tachyarrhythmias, EPS is used to guide therapy. In patients with ventricular arrhythmias, empiric therapy carries dual, potentially dangerous burdens: It may be ineffective or worsen the underlying arrhythmia, and it may induce new ventricular arrhythmias (proarrhythmic effect). This chapter discusses the role of EPS in determining arrhythmia diagnosis and prognosis. The role of EPS in guiding therapy is addressed in subsequent chapters that discuss the individual arrhythmias.

TECHNIQUES OF ELECTROPHYSIOLOGIC STUDY

Catheter Sites and Recordings

The individual techniques and protocols for EPS differ from laboratory to laboratory, but in general, a standard format is followed for recording the electrical activity of the heart. The variations in stimulation protocols are based on differing rates and strengths of stimulation, the number of extrastimuli introduced, and the number of sites of stimulation. The numbers of catheters, their location, and where records are made depend on the purpose of the study. For example, a complete study in a patient with syncope or supraventricular tachycardia might require extensive exploration of sinus function and AV conduction as well as stimulation of the atrium and ventricle. The following discussion outlines a generally accepted approach to recording from and stimulating the heart during EPS. Variations in this standard stimulation protocol are determined by the arrhythmias being stud-

**Table 6–1. INDICATIONS FOR
ELECTROPHYSIOLOGIC STUDIES**

Diagnosis*

1. To resolve the differential diagnosis of narrow- and wide-QRS tachycardias, including distinguishing AVNR from AVRT
2. To evaluate cardiac pacemaker function and AV conduction in patients with suspected symptomatic bradyarrhythmias
3. To evaluate syncope of undetermined origin
4. To evaluate patients at risk for sudden death

Therapy*

1. To guide therapy as necessary in patients from categories 1–4 above.
2. To guide therapy of patients with recurrent, sustained ventricular tachycardia, with fibrillation, or with both.
3. To interrupt accessory atrioventricular, AV nodal, or His pathways as well as other supraventricular or ventricular tachyarrhythmias using radio-frequency ablation

AV = atrioventricular; AVNR = atrioventricular nodal reentry; AVRT = atrioventricular reciprocating tachycardia.

*Electrophysiologic study is not to be used when simpler, less invasive, and less expensive methods are more appropriate.

---

ied and are discussed in detail later in this chapter.

Catheters with variable numbers of electrodes are positioned in the atria, His region, coronary sinus, and ventricles and can be used both to record local electrical activity and to stimulate the heart. In general, the recordings are bipolar electrograms using a given pair of electrodes from a multipolar catheter. The resulting electrical signals are appropriately ampli-fied and filtered. Then, by use of a multi-channel recorder, they are displayed in real time on an oscilloscope while being recorded directly on paper and usually simultaneously on electromagnetic tape or CD-ROM. (The frequency range is typically between 50 and 1000 Hz.) The permanent recordings, produced either by direct means or by subsequent playback from the recording media, are recorded at speeds of 50 to 250 mm/sec to provide appropriate temporal resolution of the electrical events. Simultaneous recording of the electrical activity from cardiac structures throughout the heart produces high-frequency electrograms free of extraneous signals. These recordings allow a much more precise timing of the electrical activity as it traverses the heart than is possible from surface electrocardiogram (ECG) recordings. The resulting pathway, or pathways, of electrical activity provide a map of the flow of electrical current during normal and abnormal cardiac activation. With appropriate amplification and filtering, even recordings from the sinus node and accessory pathways are sometimes possible, in addition to the more routine atrial, His bundle, and ventricular electrograms.[5] Recordings from the area of the slow pathway in the AV node may show a potential called the slow pathway potential. This potential is used as a landmark for the placement of radio frequency catheter ablation lesions.

Intervals

Baseline recordings typically include the high right atrium, His bundle, right ventricular apex, and at least three surface leads. Figure 6–1 is a His bundle recording with only one other intracavitary lead, from the right atrium, and two surface leads. The displayed intracavitary signals are labeled according to their site of origin: the atrial signal (A), the His signal (H), and the ventricular signal (V). Recordings from the proximal and distal coronary sinus are obtained when studying patients with AV junctional tachycardias with or without known preexcitation. The specific location of additional leads (for example, high, middle, and low right atrium, right ventricular apex or outflow tract, and the coronary sinus) are also identified when appropriate (Fig. 6–2).

In addition to recording the His bundle potential (the term "spike" is synonymous with "potential"), the His bundle lead records the electrogram from the low right atrium and the high right ventricular septum. The AV node's conduction time is reflected by the interval from the onset of the low right atrial signal to the onset of the His potential (A-H interval). The AV node conducts more slowly than the infranodal conduction tissues and a normal A-H interval is 60 to 120 milliseconds. This interval is influenced by heart rate and autonomic tone as well as by drugs and disease processes that affect AV nodal conduction.

The interval from the first high-frequency component of the His potential to the earliest ventricular activation in any surface or intracardiac lead denotes the time required to traverse the His-Purkinje system and activate the ventricle (H-V interval). This interval (normally 35 to 55 milliseconds) is relatively independent of heart rate, medication, or autonomic tone. It tends to be more fixed than the A-H interval and, when prolonged, usually reflects a degenerative disease process such as fibrosis or erosion of the conduction tissue. When determination of the location and electrical characteristics of an accessory pathway is required, an additional multipolar coronary sinus catheter is used to record electrograms from the posterolateral left AV groove, and a modified Brockenbrough catheter is used to map around the tricuspid annulus. The interval from the His potential to the onset of the QRS in patients with ventricular preexcitation will be short because the ventricle is "preexcited" through an accessory pathway. The onset of the ventricular activation as seen in the coronary sinus is earliest at the site closest to the accessory pathway.

Programmed Electrical Stimulation

Programmed electrical stimulation of the heart requires a special stimulating device capable of sensing the patient's own electrical activity and of stimulating the cardiac chambers in a predictable fashion. The purpose of introducing timed electrical impulses is to measure the functional characteristics of pacemaker and conduction tissues and to induce clinically relevant arrhythmias. The characteristics of sinus node impulse formation and conduction, and the function of the AV conduction system, can be determined by PES. Arrhythmias that are identical to clinical arrhythmias can be induced by single, double, or several trains of properly timed extrastimuli. Patients with unexplained clinical syndromes such as syncope, angina, or heart failure that could be caused by arrhythmias may undergo PES because of the ability of this technique to induce arrhythmias and to reproduce their clinical picture.

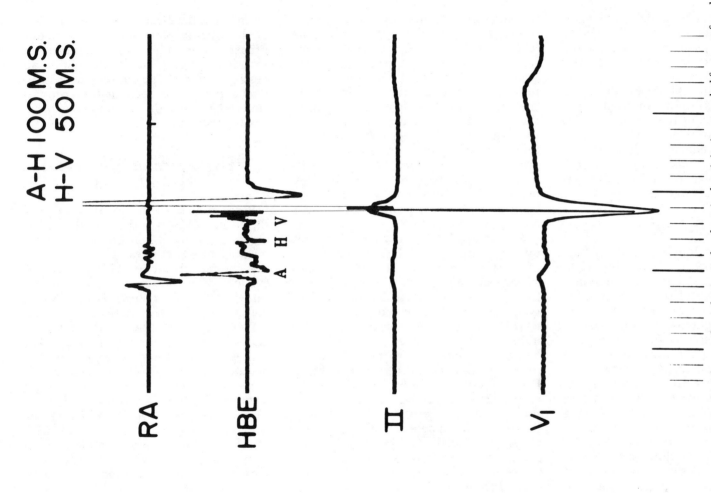

FIGURE 6–1. In this electrophysiologic study, electrical activity is recorded from surface leads V_1 and II, the high right atrium (RA), and the His region (His bundle electrogram [HBE]). The interval from the first high-frequency spike of atrial activity (HBE—A) to the onset of the first high-frequency spike of His region activity (HBE—H) is the A-H interval (normally 60 to 120 milliseconds). The H-V interval is the interval from the first high-frequency portion (H) of the His region recording to the onset of ventricular activity in any lead (normally 35 to 55 milliseconds). M. S. = milliseconds.

126

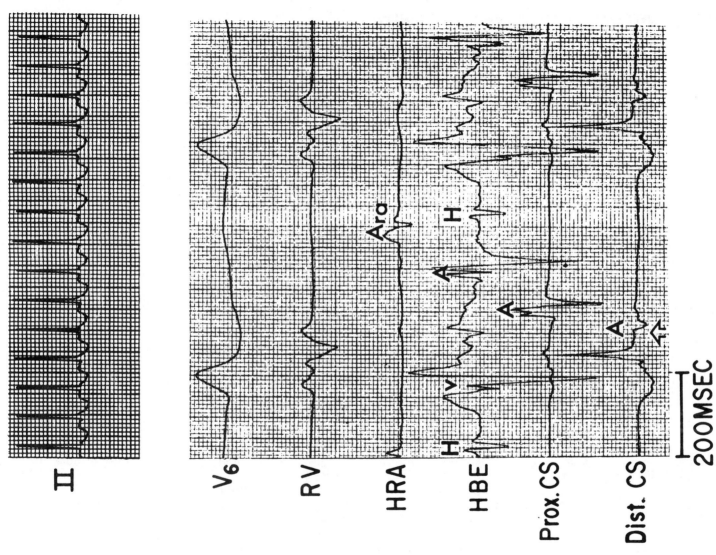

FIGURE 6–2. This electrophysiologic study was obtained during an atrioventricular reciprocating tachycardia (AVRT). A surface lead II during tachycardia is shown at the top. The atrial activation sequence (labeled A in the lower three tracings and A_{ra} in the high right atrial recording [HRA]) during AVRT shows the earliest site of activation to be in the distal coronary sinus (Dist. CS, arrow), confirming not only retrograde preexcitation but also its anatomic location in the left lateral free wall. Prox. CS = proximal coronary sinus; H = His potential; HBE = His bundle electrogram; RV = right ventricular lead; V_6 = surface lead.

Table 6–2. USE OF PROGRAMMED ELECTRICAL STIMULATION

TYPE OF ARRHYTHMIA	PROBLEM EVALUATED	STIMULATION PROTOCOL
Bradyarrhythmias	Sinus node function	Sinus node recovery time
	AV conduction	A-H and H-V intervals; atrial pacing; premature atrial stimulation
Tachyarrhythmias	Sinus node, atrial, or AVNR	Rapid atrial pacing; premature atrial stimulation, isoproterenol
	Preexcitation—pathway localization	Mapping of atrial activation sequence during ventricular pacing and AVRT
	AVRT	Premature atrial and ventricular stimulation
	Atrial fibrillation	Rapid atrial pacing
	Ventricular tachycardia and ventricular fibrillation	Premature ventricular stimulation (S_2, S_3, S_4);* burst rapid ventricular pacing; premature atrial stimulation†

AV = atrioventricular; AVNR = atrioventricular nodal reentry; AVRT = atrioventricular reciprocating tachycardia.

*S_2, S_3, or S_4 indicates the number of premature beats inserted during sinus or paced rhythm.

†Atrial stimulation may rarely induce ventricular tachycardia.

Programmed electrical stimulation protocols differ from laboratory to laboratory and vary with the clinical problem. A complete evaluation could include some or all of the studies outlined in Table 6–2. The patient being studied for bradyarrhythmias, for example, could undergo an evaluation of the function of the sinus node and AV conduction system. Patients with suspected vasodepressor syncope are also subjected to a tilt table study to attempt to elicit a withdrawal of sympathetic tone and enhanced parasympathetic tone. In patients with supraventricular arrhythmias, PES may be used to induce the clinical arrhythmias or to demonstrate evidence of dual AV nodal pathways or an accessory pathway. Premature atrial stimulation can induce a wide variety of arrhythmias, including sinus, atrioventricular nodal, and atrial reentry, in addition to the atrioventricular reciprocating tachycardias (AVRTs) seen in patients with an accessory AV connection. Rapid atrial pacing may also be used to induce these arrhythmias and atrial fibrillation. Atrial pacing with or without induced atrial fibrillation allows an analysis of the rate of the ventricular response, a particularly important measurement in the evaluation of patients with complete or partial AV bypass tracts. Ventricular stimulation protocols are used to induce ventricular tachycardia or fibrillation and may be used to induce AVRT in patients with accessory pathways.

The protocols for atrial stimulation and ventricular stimulation differ, but both are designed to induce clinical arrhythmias while inducing the fewest number of arrhythmias that are isolated "laboratory phenomena" and therefore have no clinical significance (termed *nonclinical arrhythmias*).

Programmed electrical stimulation has been used to try to determine the electrophysiologic mechanism of a variety of ventricular tachycardias. Reentrant ventricular tachycardia may be inducible with appropriately timed premature ventricular beats (up to four). Ventricular tachycardia due to abnormal automaticity, on the other hand, is not inducible with PES but may be initiated with isoproterenol. Ventricular tachycardia due to delayed afterdepolarizations can be triggered by rapid atrial or ventricular pacing, and occasionally by PES. A number of criteria have been developed to distinguish the three mechanisms, but often, definitive identification is not possible.[6] For the purposes of this text, any clinical tachyarrhythmia that can be initiated by properly timed atrial or ventricular stimuli is therefore presumed to be reentrant, and this definition serves as the basis for interpreting the clinical response to PES and for guiding therapy. Whereas arrhythmias due to enhanced or abnormal pacemaker activity, such as accelerated junctional or ventricular rhythms, are not inducible with PES, they may be induced and studied during EPS by the infusion of agents (e.g., isoproterenol) that increase automatic pacemaker activity.

In the laboratory, in addition to precise arrhythmia diagnosis, the hemodynamic consequences of any induced or spontaneously occurring arrhythmia can be carefully documented. The exact reproduction of all aspects of the actual clinical situation, of course, is not possible. For example, it is presumed that the increase in catecholamines during an arrhythmia occurring in the upright, ambulatory posture might result in a faster tachycardia than that observed in the laboratory. In fact, some investigators studying the ventricular response to atrial fibrillation in patients with an accessory AV connection administer isoproterenol to estimate more accurately what the ventricular rate might be in the patient's ambulatory clinical setting.[7] The electrophysiologic consequences of the arrhythmia are also noted to determine whether it is stable or whether it deteriorates into a faster, more dangerous rhythm.

A major component of any EPS commonly centers on the interpretation of the significance of induced arrhythmias. Nonclinical arrhythmias are particularly common during PES of the ventricle. Sustained monomorphic ventricular tachycardia is usually a clinical arrhythmia, particularly when it is identical to the patient's spontaneously occurring episodes. Programmed electrical stimulation may induce nonclinical arrhythmias, including polymorphic ventricular tachycardia, nonsustained ventricular tachycardia, ventricular tachycardia much faster than the clinically occurring arrhythmia, and ventricular fibrillation. These arrhythmias are particularly likely in patients with severe cardiac disease, and it is often difficult to determine their significance. Ventricular fibrillation may be a clinical arrhythmia in a patient resuscitated from a cardiac arrest, whereas it may be nonclinical if induced in a patient with slow, sustained ventricular tachycardia. Regardless of the clinical setting, these tachyarrhythmias must be interpreted cautiously and with the understanding that they may have no clinical significance.[8]

The protocols designed to study tachyarrhythmias usually begin with the least aggressive (e.g., one extrastimulus) and progress to the most aggressive (e.g., three or more extra stimuli). The progression is designed to minimize the induction of nonclinical arrhythmias and to maximize the likelihood of detecting a clinically significant arrhythmia. The more extrastimuli required to induce a tachyarrhythmia, the less likely it is to be a clinical arrhythmia.

Mapping

Any spontaneously occurring arrhythmias are carefully recorded and the patterns of activation and refractory periods of key structures are measured. Usually, however, PES is necessary to evaluate the functional properties of areas of interest, including refractory periods and the escape functions and rate limits of the sinus node, as well as other atrial and lower escape pacemakers (see Chapters 1 and 13); to map the pathway of depolarization of the heart; and to attempt to initiate arrhythmias that duplicate those occurring spontaneously.

The mapping of electrical activity as it passes through the heart is used to define the presence and location of accessory pathways and to determine the site of origin of atrial and ventricular tachycardias. The sequence of retrograde atrial activation during ventricular pacing or during an induced AVRT (see Fig. 6–2) identifies the location of an accessory pathway by defining the area of earliest retrograde atrial activation. This earliest site of atrial activation denotes the site of atrial insertion of the accessory pathway as it extends between the atrium and the ventricle.

Similarly, during atrial or ventricular tachycardias, recordings from multiple atrial or ventricular sites may allow identification of the earliest site of endocardial activation and, thereby, the approximate anatomic location of the arrhythmia. Recording from an atrial catheter is useful in identifying an area of slow conduction in atrial flutter to provide guidance for catheter ablation.

The localization of the AV node–His bundle, accessory pathways, and atrial foci, in particular, is quite accurate, and such maps are crucial in guiding attempts to alter or ablate their conduction.[9] Similarly, mapping during ventricular tachycardia can also localize its site of origin, but in general, this technology is less exact than the localization of supraventricular sites. However imperfect, the data from ventricular mapping studies are also used to guide attempts at ablation (most commonly by open surgical techniques), whose purpose is to prevent recurrences of ventricular arrhythmia.

CLINICAL USE OF ELECTROPHYSIOLOGIC STUDIES

Electrophysiologic studies can be used to evaluate both bradyarrhythmias and tachyarrhythmias.[10] The latter group constitute the major indication for EPS, as its use in evaluating bradyarrhythmias is extremely limited.

Bradyarrhythmias

Bradyarrhythmias may result from failure of either impulse formation or impulse conduction (see Chapter 1, pages 6 to 8, and 11 to 15). Sinus node dysfunction can result from failure of the sinus node to generate impulses (i.e., *sinus arrest*) or failure of impulses to conduct from the sinus node to the atrium (i.e., *sinus exit block*). The electrical activity of the sinus node itself is difficult to re-cord, although the ability to demonstrate sinus node activity has been reported and used to differentiate sinus exit block from sinus arrest. So far, this distinction has not proved to be clinically important.

When bradycardias do not occur spontaneously in patients undergoing EPS for sinus node dysfunction, assessment of sinus node function may require PES. With the use of a right atrial catheter, the atria are paced for 30-second intervals at several cycle lengths and then pacing is abruptly terminated. The time that it takes for the first sinus beat to escape after termination of pacing is the sinus node recovery time (SNRT). Because the SNRT is partially a function of the patient's underlying rate, the corrected sinus node recovery time (cSNRT) is reported. Normally, the pause following the termination of pacing should not exceed the prepacing sinus rate by more than 500 milliseconds.[11] For example, the SNRT of a patient with a basic sinus rate of 60 (PP interval 1000 milliseconds) would be expected to be less than 1500 milliseconds. Corrected sinus node recovery time may be prolonged, owing to intrinsic sinus node disease (e.g., fibrosis), or owing to medications that affect sinus node impulse formation, such as antiarrhythmic drugs, β-blockers or calcium blockers, and some antihypertensive agents. Unfortunately, these same factors may also affect conduction of the paced impulse into the sinus node, so that divining the effects of atrial pacing on sinus node function is sometimes more of an art than a science.

An abnormal cSNRT is not used as the sole indication for permanent pacing but as supportive evidence when other signs of sinus node dysfunction, particularly corresponding clinical symptoms, are present. Conversely, a normal cSNRT does not exclude clinically significant sinus node dysfunction. A close correlation with clinical status is crucial, because monitoring (particularly in the elderly) sometimes shows dramatic bradyarrhythmias that are asymptomatic and lack clinical significance. Electrophysiologic study, in particular, should not be used to evaluate sinus node function in such patients. Indeed, with very few exceptions,

the results of EPS should never be the sole determining factor in any decision regarding pacemaker insertion. Ambulatory ECG monitoring more accurately documents sinus node dysfunction by allowing a close correlation between the patient's spontaneously occurring symptoms, varying autonomic tone, and the rhythm status. For example, many episodes of sinus arrest are due to spontaneously occurring sudden increases in parasympathetic tone and cannot be reliably reproduced in the EPS laboratory.

AV Conduction

Electrophysiologic study is rarely clinically necessary in evaluating patients with AV conduction disturbances. Asymptomatic or even symptomatic patients with second- or third-degree AV block, or with intact AV conduction and fascicular block, rarely require EPS for diagnosis or guidance of therapy of bradyarrhythmias. The site of AV block and its implications for therapy can usually be determined from the scalar ECG (see Chapter 1, pages 11 to 15, and Chapter 14, pages 327 to 336). An EPS-guided evaluation of AV conduction, however, may be indicated for patients with unexplained syncope or for those in whom necessary drug therapy may provoke or worsen AV block.

Atrial pacing at incremental rates can be used to determine the refractory peri-

ods of the AV node and, in some instances, of the His-Purkinje system. The normal AV node under basal resting conditions conducts 1:1 to the ventricles at pacing rates up to about 130 beats per minute. Atrioventricular nodal block at slower rates may indicate dysfunction (Fig. 6–3), although conditioned athletes, and even some normal subjects with high resting vagal tone, may develop second-degree AV nodal block at lower rates. The refractory period of the AV node is determined by introducing progressively more premature atrial stimuli during pacing (or "driving") of the atria at a constant basic rate. Atrioventricular nodal conduction is affected by intrinsic disease, autonomic tone, and certain drugs, such as calcium blockers, β-blockers, and digitalis. Atrial premature stimuli are used to show the presence of two pathways in the AV node. Normal conduction down the AV node gradually increases the earlier the atrial premature beat arrives at the AV node. In patients with AV node reentry there are "dual" pathways: a slow pathway located near the entrance of the coronary sinus and a fast pathway near the His bundle. The fast pathway has a rapid conduction but a long refractory period, whereas the slow pathway has slow conduction but a short refractory period. Premature stimulation of the atria produces a "jump" of 750 msec from a fast pathway to a slow pathway when the conduction blocks in

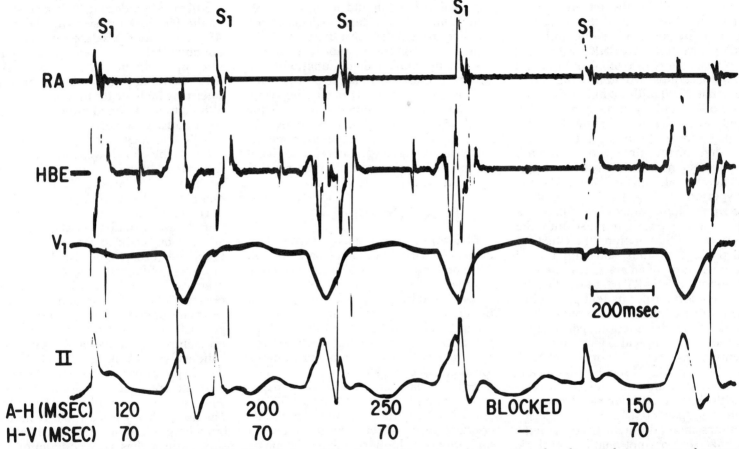

| A-H (MSEC) | 120 | 200 | 250 | BLOCKED | 150 |
| H-V (MSEC) | 70 | 70 | 70 | — | 70 |

FIGURE 6–3. This 69-year-old man with left bundle branch block and a history strongly suggestive of cardiovascular syncope underwent electrophysiologic study. The resting A-H interval was normal at 120 milliseconds, but the H-V interval was prolonged at 70 milliseconds (normally 35 to 55 milliseconds). During right atrial pacing at a basic cycle length (S_1-S_1) of 400 milliseconds (rate = 150 beats/min), progressive A-H interval prolongation led to block of the fourth S1 in the atrioventricular (AV) node. This response to atrial pacing is typical, in that block occurs in the AV node before it has a chance to block in the infranodal region. HBE = His bundle electrogram; RA = right atrial recording; S = stimulus; II and V_1 = surface electrocardiogram (ECG) leads.

the fast pathway, the A-H interval jumps by more than 50 msec and the premature atrial beat decreases by 10 msec.

His-Purkinje conduction is best evaluated by measurement of the H-V interval (normally 35 to 55 milliseconds), wherein prolongation reflects slowed conduction in the His bundle or in all three fascicles of the distal conduction system. In the presence of block in two of the "three" fascicles (i.e., some combination of the right bundle branch, the left anterior fascicle, and the posterior fascicle), a prolonged H-V interval indicates trifascicular block with slowed conduction in the remaining fascicle.[12]

Atrial pacing studies, as techniques of evaluating the refractory period of the His-Purkinje system (infranodal tissues), are generally unrewarding as a means for documenting infranodal block, for several reasons. The H-V interval is quite independent of the atrial or His pacing rate, and clinically significant infranodal block is rarely produced by such pacing. Also, determining the His-Purkinje refractory period is rarely possible, as the AV node's refractory period is the longer of the two and premature atrial impulses therefore block first in the AV node, never reaching the His-Purkinje system (see Fig. 6–3). Even when the study shows induced infranodal block, the information gained is rarely the sole determinant of the need for a permanent pacemaker. Just as with sinus node dysfunction, the indication for

pacing is highly dependent on corroborative clinical information (e.g., history, resting ECG, and results of ambulatory ECG monitoring).

Tachyarrhythmias

The most important use of EPS is in the evaluation of supraventricular and ventricular tachyarrhythmias, wherein it is used to determine the diagnosis, prognosis, and therapy, particularly when the requisite data are not available from routine clinical methods. Patients with known or potentially life-threatening arrhythmias constitute the largest number of candidates. Such patients should not be treated empirically because the consequences of treatment failure are serious. Patients with tachyarrhythmias unresponsive to conventional methods of treatment are another group who are candidates for EPS. Patients with unexplained syncope that is possibly due to a tachycardia are a third group (see Chapter 2, pages 34 and 51). Finally, an EPS-guided evaluation can immediately test the efficacy of additional drugs in treating the patient, as well as testing the patient's candidacy for implantable devices (antitachycardia pacemakers or cardioverters defibrillators), or catheter or surgical ablation. With a more accurate diagnosis and careful observation of the hemodynamic and electrical consequences of the tachycardia, a more accurate prognosis ensues.

SUPRAVENTRICULAR TACHYARRHYTHMIAS

Supraventricular arrhythmias, as outlined in Chapter 7, are divided into those originating solely in the atria and those involving the AV junction. When an accurate diagnosis and plan of therapy are possible from routinely available clinical information, such as surface rhythm strips, ambulatory ECG monitoring, and exercise provocation, EPS is not required to establish the diagnosis. Electrophysiologic study may be useful, however, when the diagnosis is unclear or when a decision regarding therapy requires observing the clinical consequences of the arrhythmia, or when both considerations are at issue. Therapy guided by EPS does frequently lead to a more precise and reliable treatment regimen, which may be mandatory with life-threatening arrhythmias.

Atrial arrhythmias due to reentrant mechanisms, including atrial flutter-fibrillation and the rarely occurring sinus node and tachycardias can be induced in the laboratory. Multifocal atrial tachycardia and automatic atrial tachycardias are not reentrant and therefore are not inducible with EPS. Induction of atrial flutter-fibrillation is carried out to assess the ability of the AV conduction system to slow the ventricular response adequately during the stress of a rapid atrial rate. Patients with ventricular preexcitation and a po-

A   Lead II   Control

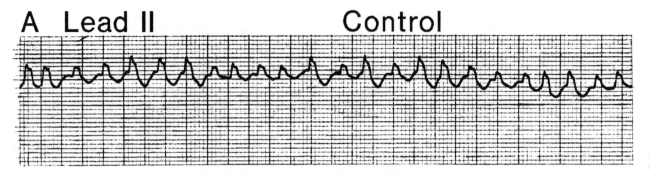

B   Lead II   After 1.0 gm Procainamide IV

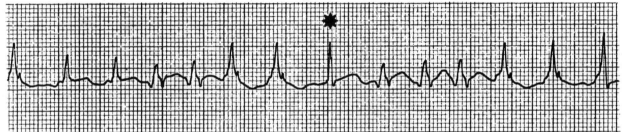

FIGURE 6–4. A 45-year-old man with syncope and ventricular preexcitation underwent electrophysiologic study. (*A*) During induced atrial fibrillation, the ventricular response was 300 to 320 beats per minute with preexcitation of each beat (note the wide QRS complexes). (*B*) After intravenous administration of 1 g of procainamide, the ventricular response slowed, with some loss of preexcitation (note particularly the narrow QRS complex marked by the asterisk). II = surface ECG lead.

tentially rapidly conducting accessory pathway can be studied to determine their fastest possible ventricular rate and to test different therapies acutely under controlled circumstances in the laboratory (Fig. 6–4). A rapidly conducting accessory pathway may allow ventricular rates to exceed 300 beats per minute and may therefore cause syncope or sudden death (see Chapter 10, pages 224 to 225 and 230, and Chapter 11, pages 246 to 249 and 255 to 256). Even without a demonstrable accessory pathway, some patients experience rapid conduction over normal pathways with extremely rapid and hemodynamically significant ventricular responses to atrial fibrillation. Such patients also can be studied in the laboratory and their response to drugs determined.[13]

When "atrial tachycardia with block" is due to focal atrial reentry (or rarely, atrioventricular nodal reentry [AVNR]), it may be inducible, but these varieties of tachycardia are uncommon and even less frequently require aggressive evaluation. Similarly, sinus nodal reentry may be induced by PES but is generally nonsustained, is uncommon, and is even more rarely a significant clinical problem. Atrial tachycardias due to accelerated pacemakers (e.g., digitalis-induced ectopic atrial tachycardia) are not inducible by PES.

Electrophysiologic study provides an accurate understanding of AV junctional reentry tachycardias, including those due to AVNR and those due to reentry using an accessory pathway (AVRT). Programmed electrical stimulation induces these tachycardias in susceptible individuals, and they are usually easily distinguished from each other. For example, patients with AVNR tachycardias usually have evidence of dual AV nodal pathways (see Chapters 1 and 11), which can be exposed by introducing premature atrial beats. The fast pathway conducts premature atrial impulses until it blocks, forcing conduction over the more slowly conducting pathway to become manifest, producing an abrupt transition in the AV nodal conduction time. This transition can be easily detected by measuring the A-H intervals during programmed atrial pacing. With increasingly more premature atrial beats, the A-H interval smoothly and progressively lengthens until there is an abrupt prolongation (more than 50 milliseconds), indicating the switch from the fast to the slow pathway and showing that dual AV nodal pathways are present (Fig. 6–5). The initiation of an AVNR tachycardia often coincides with this jump from the fast pathway to the slow pathway.

The AVRTs using an accessory pathway are also easily inducible during PES. The properties of the accessory pathway are, in most cases, analogous to the fast pathway in the AV node, with a fast conduction velocity but a long refractory period. Premature atrial or ventricular stimulation typically blocks in the accessory pathway, while conduction through the AV node–His-Purkinje system occurs normally. When this normal antegrade impulse conducts through the ventricle, engages the accessory pathway, and finds it recovered, retrograde conduction into the atria occurs, which may trigger a reentrant arrhythmia (see Fig. 6–4). As has already been mentioned, during induced AVRT, the location of the accessory pathway, as reflected by the earliest site of retrograde atrial activation, can be identified and can provide key information if surgery or catheter ablation of the pathway is being considered.

VENTRICULAR TACHYCARDIA AND VENTRICULAR FIBRILLATION

The most common clinical indication for EPS is in guiding the management of ventricular arrhythmias. Wellens and co-workers first demonstrated that ventricular tachycardia could be induced with PES in patients with clinical ventricular tachycardia.[14] These investigators, as well as Josephson and associates,[15] used EPS to study patients with cardiac arrest and sustained and nonsustained ventricular tachycardia and to show that ventricular tachycardia is most likely due to a reentry mechanism. The difficulty in assigning a mechanism to clinical arrhythmias is outlined in detail by Akhtar.[16]

Technical Considerations. A consensus protocol for ventricular stimulation in patients with known or suspected ventricular tachycardia has not been established. In general, stimulation at two sites in the right ventricle, at an amplitude twice the diastolic threshold for ventricular capture, is carried out at two or three basic driving rates with up to at least three extrastimuli (S2, S3, and S4). More aggressive protocols, with more than three extrastimuli and higher voltages, produce a greater number of nonclinical arrhythmias but also induce more clinically significant responses. If right ventricular stimulation does not yield a positive response, isoproterenol may be infused and the protocol repeated. Patients who have been resuscitated from sudden death due to ventricular fibrillation and in whom an aggressive right-sided EPS is negative may be candidates for PES of the left ventricle; an additional 5% to 10% of such patients may have a clinical arrhythmia induced in this way.

Programmed ventricular stimulation consists of the introduction of precisely timed ventricular stimuli during spontaneous sinus rhythm or during a paced

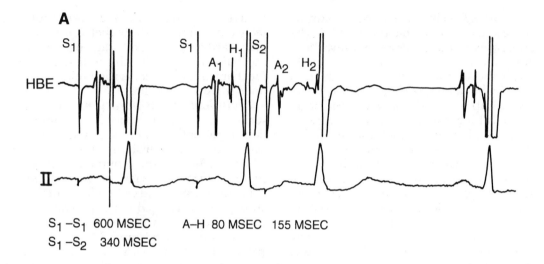

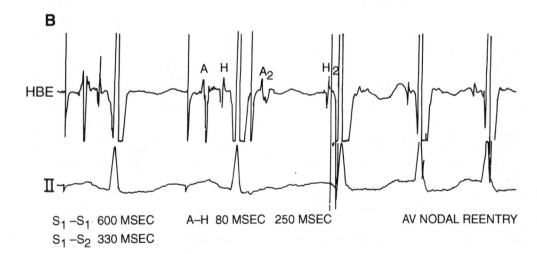

FIGURE 6–5. Leads II and HBE during an electro-physiologic study are shown in a patient with atrio-ventricular nodal reentry (AVNR). The control A-H interval (A_1-H_1) is normal at 80 milliseconds. (*A*) During atrial pacing at a cycle length of 600 milli-seconds, an atrial extrastimulus (S_2; S_1-S_2 interval = 340 msec) conducts with a prolonged A-H inter-val (A_2-H_2 = 155 msec). (*B*) When S_2 is introduced just 10 milliseconds earlier, the A-H interval sud-denly increases by an additional 95 milliseconds (A_2-H_2 = 250 msec), unmasking a second nodal pathway. This sudden prolongation coincides with the onset of an AVNR.

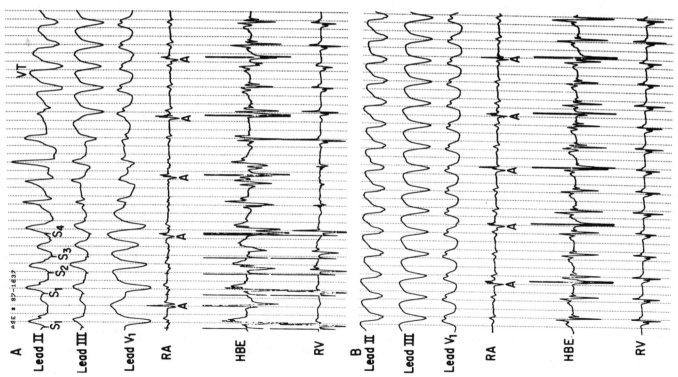

FIGURE 6–6. This 45-year-old man with classic cardiac syncope but no significant arrhythmia on ambulatory ECG monitoring underwent electrophysiologic study. As shown in (*A*), the right ventricular apex (RV) was driven at a basic cycle length (S_1-S_1) of 400 milliseconds during monitoring of surface leads II, III, and V_1. Three extrastimuli (S_2, S_3, S_4) initiated a sustained episode of rapid, wide-QRS tachycardia at 220 beats per minute, which was initially polymorphic but rapidly became monomorphic (*B*). The ventricular origin of this tachycardia was proved by AV dissociation (note the atrial activity [A], which is independent of ventricular activity in the right atrial lead [RA]) and by the absence of a His potential preceding the wide QRS complexes in the His bundle electrogram lead (HBE).

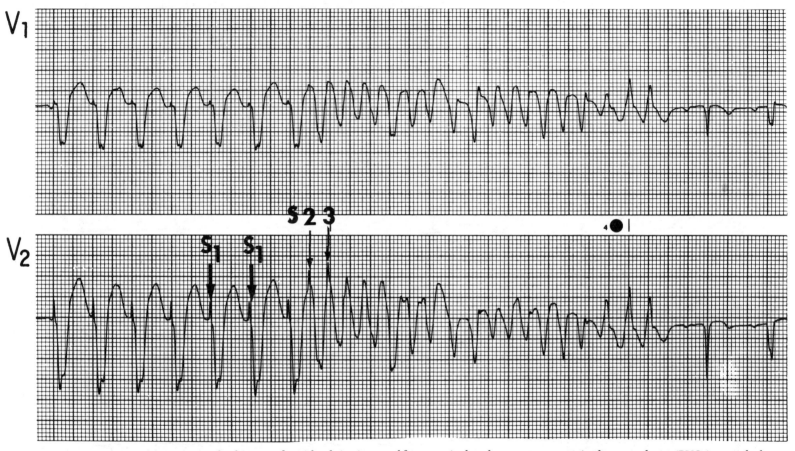

FIGURE 6–7. A 52-year-old woman with a history of rapid palpitations and frequent isolated premature ventricular complexes (PVCs) on ambulatory ECG monitoring underwent electrophysiologic study. Simultaneous surface leads V_1 and V_2 are shown during programmed electrical stimulation at a driven S_1-S_1 interval of 400 milliseconds. Two extrastimuli (S_2 and S_3) induce a 2.5-second run of polymorphic ventricular tachycardia that terminates spontaneously. This ventricular arrhythmia is considered to have no clinical significance (i.e., it is a "nonclinical arrhythmia"), neither explaining the patient's symptoms nor indicating a need for treatment.

atrial or ventricular rhythm.[17] The right ventricular apex is stimulated first, and if no sustained arrhythmia is induced, the right ventricular outflow tract is stimulated. The ventricles are paced at a constant cycle length (e.g., S_1-S_1 interval of 600 milliseconds) for 8 or 10 beats, and one to three or more premature ventricular stimuli are introduced after the last driven beat (S_1). The first extrastimulus (S_2) is inserted progressively closer to the basic driving stimulus (S_1-S_2) until it fails to capture the ventricle (i.e., the effective refractory period [ERP] is reached). The basic ventricular paced rate S_1-S_1 is then shortened to 400 milliseconds, and the process is repeated. The S_1-S_2 interval is adjusted to 50 milliseconds above the previously determined ERP and an S_3, and later an S_4, are inserted at progressively shorter intervals until all three extrastimuli are blocked.

Estimation of Clinical Significance.
The criterion for a positive result is the development of sustained monomorphic ventricular tachycardia (of 30 seconds or more) identical to the patient's clinical arrhythmia (Fig. 6–6). This rhythm can be induced in 60% to 90% of patients with clinically occurring sustained ventricular tachycardia, but the success rate varies with the underlying disease process. Patients with coronary heart disease and clinical ventricular tachycardia are inducible 90% of the time, whereas patients

with a nonischemic, congestive cardiomyopathy are inducible only 60% of the time. An even smaller rate of induction is seen with normal or nearly normal hearts (e.g., mitral valve prolapse).

Nonsustained ventricular tachycardia (with runs less than 30 seconds), polymorphic ventricular tachycardia, and ventricular fibrillation are nonspecific responses (Fig. 6–7), and as already mentioned, the more aggressive the stimulation protocol is, the more likely is the development of a nonclinical arrhythmia.

Chapter 12 addresses the interpretation of these studies in deciding therapy for patients with ventricular tachycardia.

REFERENCES

1. Durrer D, Schoo L, Schuilenburg RM, and Wellens HJJ: The role of premature beats in the initiation and the termination of supraventricular tachycardia in the Wolff-Parkinson-White syndrome. Circulation 36:644–662, 1967.
2. Coumel P, Cabrol C, Fabiato A, Gourgon R, and Slama R: Tachycardie permanente par rhythm réciproque. I. Preuves du diagnostic par stimulation auriculaire et ventriculaire. II. Traitement par l'implantation intracorporelle d'un stimulateur cardiaque avec entraînement simultané de l'oreillette et du ventricule. Arch Mal Coeur 60:1830–1864, 1967.
3. Scherlag, BJ, Lau SH, Helfant RH, Berkowitz WD, Stien E, and Damato AN: Catheter technique for recording His bundle activity in man. Circulation 39:13–18, 1969.
4. Wellens HJJ and Brugada P: Treatment of cardiac arrhythmias: When, how and where? J Am Coll Cardiol 14:1417–1428, 1989.
5. Jackman WM, Friday KJ, Yeung-Lai-Wah JA, et al: New catheter technique for recording left free wall accessory atrioventricular pathway activation: Identification of pathway fiber orientation. Circulation 78:598–611, 1988.
6. Josephson ME, Horowitz LN, Farshidi A, and Kastor JA: Recurrent sustained ventricular tachycardia. I. Mechanisms. Circulation 42:216–226, 1972.
7. German LD, Gallagher JJ, Broughton A, Guarnieri T, and Trantham JL: Effects of exercise and isoproterenol during atrial fibrillation in patients with Wolff-Parkinson-White syndrome. Am J Cardiol 51:1203–1206, 1983.
8. Cooper MJ, Hunt LF, Richards DA, Denniss AR, Uther JB, and Ross DL: Effect of repetition of extrastimuli on sensitivity and reproducibility of mode of induction of ventricular tachycardia by programmed stimula-

tion. J Am Coll Cardiol 11:1260–1267, 1988.

9. Schlüter M, Geiger M, Siebels J, Duckeck W, and Kuck K-H: Catheter ablation using radiofrequency current to cure symptomatic patients with tachyarrhythmias related to an accessory atrioventricular pathway. Circulation 84:1644–1661, 1991.

10. Zipes DP, Akhtar M, Denes P, et al (Report of Joint ACC/AHA Task Force on Assessment of Cardiovascular Procedures Subcommittee to Assess Clinical Intracardiac Electrophysiologic Studies): Guidelines for clinical intracardiac electrophysiologic studies. J Am Coll Cardiol 14:1827–1842, 1989.

11. Benditt DG, Gornick CC, Dunbar D, Almquist A, and Pool-Schneider S: Indications for electrophysiologic testing in the diagnosis and assessment of sinus node dysfunction. Circulation 75:1193–1201, 1987.

12. Kaul U, Dev V, Narula J, Malhotra AK, Talwar KK, and Bhatia ML: Evaluation of patients with bundle branch block and "unexplained" syncope: A study based on comprehensive electrophysiologic testing and ajmaline stress. PACE 11:289–297, 1988.

13. Klein GJ, Bashore TM, Sellars TD, Pritchett ELC, Smith WM, and Gallagher JJ: Ventricular fibrillation in the Wolff-Parkinson-White syndrome. N Engl J Med 301:1080–1085, 1979.

14. Wellens HJJ, Schuilenburg RM, and Durrer D: Electrical stimulation of the heart in patients with ventricular tachycardia. Circulation 42:216–226, 1972.

15. Josephson ME, Horowitz LN, Farshidi A, and Kastor JA: Recurrent sustained ventricular tachycardia. I. Mechanisms. Circulation 57:431–440, 1978.

16. Akhtar M: Clinical spectrum of ventricular tachycardia. Circulation 82:1561–1573, 1990.

17. Wyndham CRC: Role of invasive electrophysiologic testing in the management of life-threatening ventricular arrhythmias. Am J Cardiol 62(Suppl 14):13I–17I, 1988.

THE IMPORTANT ARRHYTHMIA PROBLEMS: TACHYCARDIAS

Premature Beats

BARRY W. RAMO, MD

The most common arrhythmia problem confronting clinicians is the management of patients having premature beats. Premature beats are ubiquitous and a source of concern for patients and physicians alike because they can either trigger or be the first beat of significant, sometimes life-threatening tachyarrhythmias. This fact has prompted the indiscriminate treatment of patients with premature ventricular complexes (PVCs); many receive potentially dangerous, inappropriate drugs, and others receive medications they do not need. The proper management of premature beats depends on establishing the correct diagnosis and understanding the natural history of the arrhythmia with and without treatment.

This chapter discusses the mechanism, classification, diagnosis, and treatment of premature beats to provide a rational basis for therapeutic decisions. Many of these principles, however, are also applicable to the diagnosis and management of the tachyarrhythmias detailed in Chapters 9 through 12.

CLASSIFICATION

Premature beats (complexes) are classified according to their site of origin (Fig. 7–1): atrial, junctional, or ventricular. This classification is the same one used to classify tachyarrhythmias. Premature atrial complexes (PACs) and premature junctional complexes (PJCs) originate above the ventricle and thus can be classified together as *supraventricular*. The pathway of ventricular excitation from PACs and PJCs is usually the same as for normal sinus beats, and the QRS configuration generated by supraventricular beats, therefore, is also the same. Premature supraventricular beats, however, can conduct with aberration (that is, with functional block in a portion of the intraventricular conduction system), producing an abnormal QRS configuration and complicating the differential diagnosis of wide premature beats. This complication is a particular problem with aberrated atrioventricular (AV) junctional premature beats; without a preceding P wave, they frequently cannot be reliably differentiated from PVCs on the surface electrocardiogram (ECG).

MECHANISMS

The mechanisms responsible for premature heart beats and tachyarrhythmias are discussed in detail in Chapter 1. Briefly, premature beats may be due to enhanced automaticity in tissues normally capable of generating impulses, to abnormal automaticity in tissues that do not normally generate impulses, to triggered automaticity, and to reentry. Defining the precise electrophysiologic mechanism of single premature beats is usually not possible and is not as important in diagnosis or therapy as it is when considering sustained tachyarrhythmias. A premature beat, however, can be the first beat of an automatic or reentrant tachycardia and may demand attention in certain clinical situations. Thus, a PAC can induce atrial fibrillation or nodal reentry, and a PVC can trigger ventricular tachycardia, ventricular fibrillation, or a supraventricular tachycardia. Furthermore, these various arrhythmias can result regardless of the mechanism of the inciting premature beat itself.

Concealed Conduction

In addition to causing tachyarrhythmias, premature beats may affect the function of other pacemakers and subsequent conduction. The ability of a premature beat to depolarize the sinus node determines when the next sinus beat is formed. When the sinus node is depolarized prematurely, it is reset, and spontaneous diastolic depolarization starts over from the time of premature depolarization. If there is only resetting, the next cycle is the same as the prior PP interval, but if overdrive suppression occurs, the next sinus beat is delayed. A PVC that conducts retrograde into the AV node can cause the next P wave either to block or to conduct with a longer PR interval because partial depolarization of the AV node from a retrograde direction increases its refrac-

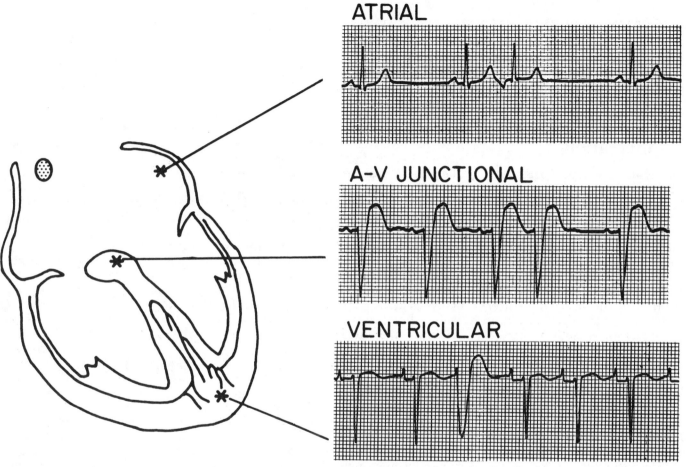

ATRIAL

A-V JUNCTIONAL

VENTRICULAR

FIGURE 7–1. There are three potential sites of origin of premature beats: atrial, atrioventricular (AV) junctional, and ventricular. Premature atrial complexes (PACs) (top tracing) are initiated by a premature P wave and may block in the AV node or conduct to the ventricle with a QRS configuration that is the same or different from the patient's normal QRS configuration. Premature junctional complexes (PJCs) (middle tracing) originate from the distal AV node and His bundle and are diagnosed only when there is no preceding P wave *and* the QRS complex is unchanged from the patient's normal QRS complex. Premature ventricular complexes (PVCs) (bottom tracing) are defined by premature wide QRS complexes that are both different from the patient's normal QRS complexes *and* not preceded by premature P waves.

toriness to the next on-time P wave. Such effects on impulse formation and conduction, which cannot be seen directly on the ECG but are inferred, are referred to as *concealed conduction* (Fig. 7–2).

Aberration

Supraventricular premature beats may produce aberration via a variety of mechanisms. As long as the bundle branch system is activated slowly enough to allow full recovery of all the parts prior to the next impulse, normal ventricular activation ensues. When a portion of the bundle branch system has a longer refractory period than other portions, however, a PAC (or an increase in the heart rate) may allow impulses to engage that portion of the distal conduction system during its longer refractory period, thus blocking the impulse and producing an abnormal (aberrant) pattern of ventricular activation. When the increase in the refractoriness of a part of the bundle branch system is relatively fixed, aberration results each time that a PAC is sufficiently premature to encounter this increased refractoriness (Fig. 7–3). The refractory period of the bundle branch system is also dynamically dependent on the prior RR interval. When this RR interval lengthens, the refractory periods of the bundle branch systems of subsequent beats also lengthen. A PAC following a long prior RR interval, therefore, is even more likely to encounter refrac-

toriness in a portion of the bundle branch system and conduct with aberration (see Fig. 7–3A). Thus, a pattern of long cycles followed by short cycles, with wide beats terminating the short cycles, is likely to be aberration. Such long and short cycles may be observed together with sinus rhythm and PACs, but are particularly likely to be observed with atrial fibrillation (the Ashman phenomenon [Fig. 7–4A]). Bundle branch block resulting from spontaneous phase-4 depolarization of the distal conducting system occurs at very slow heart rates and is not relevant to mechanisms of aberration of premature beats (see Chapter 4, page 82).

Premature junctional complexes normally result in an unchanged QRS configuration but can produce aberration by means of the same mechanism as for PACs. They can also produce asynchronous ventricular activation because of preferential conduction down one portion of the bundle branch system. Preferential activation may result from the premature His focus being located near the branch point of a fascicle, or from preferential spread of the impulse to the fascicle from a location higher in the His bundle (longitudinal dissociation). Atrial activity associated with AV junctional beats is typically nonexistent (that is, retrograde ventriculoatrial block occurs) or is hidden by being buried within the QRS complex or the ST-T waves. Premature ventricular complexes can produce the same type of

atrial activity, and without intracardiac leads, the diagnosis of premature junctional beats with aberration (i.e., a QRS complex different from the patient's normal QRS complex and more than 0.12 second) usually cannot be made. Therefore, any wide premature QRS complex with no preceding P wave and with morphologic features that differ from those of the QRS configuration of normal conduction should be considered ventricular in most clinical settings. Not uncommonly, PJCs with aberration are diagnosed incorrectly to avoid treating PVCs.

Figure 7–3 illustrates a clinical example of aberrant conduction with PACs that conduct normally, others that conduct with aberration, and still others that are not conducted or blocked. With PACs, AV block may be partial with a prolonged PR interval, or it may be complete. Figure 7–4B illustrates the typical inverse relationship between the RP interval and the subsequent PR interval. The closer the preceding P wave is to the previous QRS complex (that is, the shorter the RP interval), the longer the next PR interval is. The likelihood of aberrant conduction increases as the RP interval (and therefore the RR interval) shortens, since the earlier the ventricles are activated, the more likely the impulse will find a portion of the bundle branch system still refractory. With blocked PACs, the site of block is usually in the AV node and results in an unexpected pause in the rhythm. With

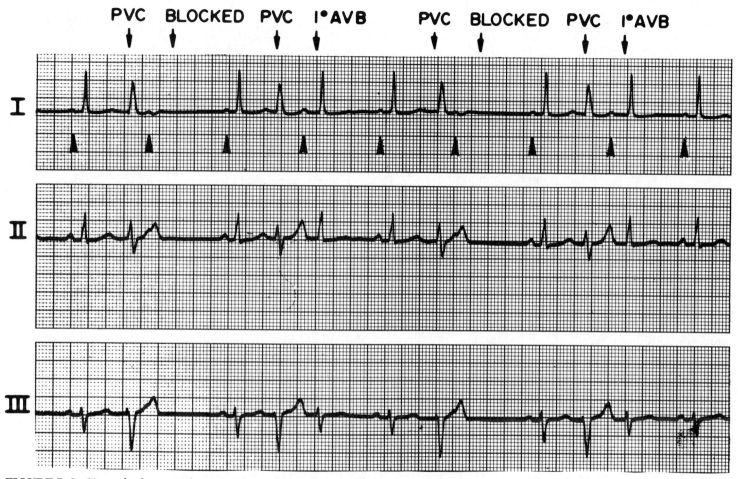

FIGURE 7–2. Sinus rhythm at 68 beats per minute is present in association with premature ventricular complexes (PVCs). The first and third PVCs cause transient AV dissociation because their retrograde concealed conduction entirely blocks subsequent antegrade AV conduction of the on-time P wave. The second and fourth PVCs, however, occur slightly earlier and are therefore interpolated; their "concealed" retrograde ventriculoatrial (VA) conduction results only in a prolonged (first-degree) antegrade AV conduction time of the next on-time sinus beat.

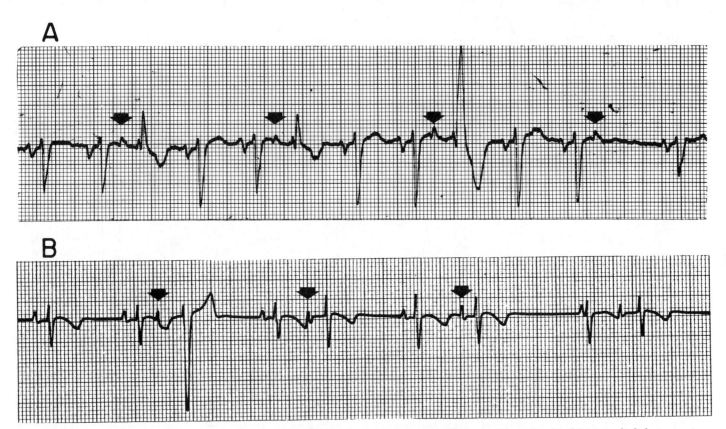

FIGURE 7–3. (*A*) These PACs (arrows) cause varying PR intervals and degrees of aberration. The third PAC is slightly more premature, with a slightly longer PR interval. The more complete right bundle branch aberration occurs despite a longer coupling interval to the prior conducted beat, because the RR interval preceding the prior conducted beat is slightly longer than the corresponding intervals preceding the first two PACs. The fourth PAC is so premature that it is completely blocked in the AV node. (*B*) These PACs (arrows) vary more obviously in degree of prematurity, resulting in greater variations in the PR intervals and in the morphologic characteristics of the conducted QRS complexes. The first PAC is the earliest, with the longest PR interval (i.e., short RP interval = long PR interval) and the greatest aberration of the QRS complex (note the increased width of the QRS complex and the marked difference in terminal forces). The second PAC is later, with a less prolonged PR interval (i.e., longer RP interval = shorter PR interval). The lateness of this PAC more than compensates for any shortening of the PR interval and results in a longer QRS coupling interval. These events allow time for complete recovery of the conduction system, so that no aberration occurs. The third PAC is even later, with no change in either the PR interval (i.e., longest RP interval = shortest PR interval) or the morphologic features of the conducted QRS complex.

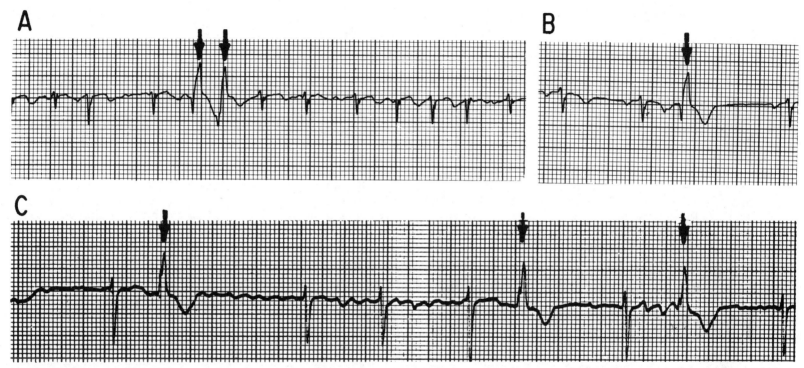

FIGURE 7–4. Atrial fibrillation with premature wide QRS complexes can be due to aberrant conduction or to PVCs. (*A*) The underlying rhythm is atrial fibrillation with rapid AV conduction. The two wide QRS complexes (arrows) follow a long cycle and do not have a subsequent compensatory pause, two features suggesting aberration. (*B*) The diagnosis is established by finding, during sinus rhythm, an identical wide QRS complex caused by a PAC (arrow). (*C*) In this example of atrial fibrillation, the premature wide QRS complexes (arrows) demonstrate two features typical of PVCs. The first is fixed coupling to the prior normal QRS complexes, presumably because intraventricular reentry imparts an element of "regularity" to a rhythm that is otherwise totally irregular. The second is the occurrence of relative compensatory pauses following each wide QRS complex due to retrograde concealed AV nodal conduction, which blocks subsequent antegrade atrial impulses.

such atrial pauses, the ST segment and T wave should be carefully scrutinized for a hidden blocked premature P wave, as the diagnosis of sinus arrest is often made incorrectly; more than one lead should always be checked for hidden P waves before such a diagnosis is made (see Fig. 5–3).

Premature ventricular complexes originate below the His bundle and are different from the normally conducted QRS complex.[1] The QRS duration of PVCs is always prolonged (0.12 second or more, and frequently more than 0.14 to 0.16 second) because ventricular activation is spread slowly by means of muscle-to-muscle conduction. In some leads, the premature QRS complex may look like the normal QRS complex, so one should always look at more than one lead to be certain that there is not a difference (Fig. 7–5). All premature QRS complexes that are different from the normal QRS complex and not preceded by a premature P wave should be considered PVCs.

CLINICAL METHODS OF DIAGNOSIS

Premature Atrial and Ventricular Complexes

A systematic approach to diagnosing premature beats can be accomplished by answering the following questions (Fig. 7–6):

1. Is the QRS configuration the same as or different from the normally conducted QRS complex?
2. Is there a premature P wave preceding the premature QRS complex?

An answer of yes to the first question indicates a supraventricular origin. An answer of no leaves unresolved the question of ventricular origin versus supraventricular with aberration. An answer of yes to the second question also identifies a supraventricular origin. Both questions are independent of QRS width, because a PVC may be narrow in one lead and wide in another (see Fig. 7–6).

Aberration vs. Ectopy During Atrial Flutter-Fibrillation

The diagnosis of premature wide-QRS beats (ventricular ectopy versus aberration) during atrial flutter or fibrillation is a difficult challenge. Much of the solution to this diagnostic problem lies in using logic based on an understanding of the mechanisms of aberrant conduction and PVCs. The ECG often must be regarded as one of a number of clinical tests and not the whole answer. This differential diagnosis is discussed in more detail in Chapters 10 and 12, and three helpful questions follow. The two questions in the previous section and those in Figure 7–6 should also be answered before a diagnosis is established.

1. What is the rate of the underlying ventricular response? Aberrant conduction generally occurs when AV nodal conduction is rapid and the average ventricular response is greater than 100 to 120 beats per minute. Ventricular premature beats tend to occur when the degree of AV block is greater and the ventricular rate is slower.
2. What are the morphology, width, and coupling intervals of the wide QRS complexes? PVCs tend to occur with fixed coupling intervals and may even produce a bigeminal or trigeminal pattern. The wide beats also tend to be followed by relative pauses that are due to retrograde concealed conduction into the AV node, causing increased refractoriness to subsequent antegrade impulses (see Fig. 7–4C). Aberrantly conducted beats also tend to display typical conduction system blocks (i.e., right bundle branch block [RBBB], left bundle branch block, or left anterior or posterior fascicular block). Aberrated beats, particularly with an RBBB pattern (rSR′), are also rarely more than 0.14 second unless there is ventricular preexcitation or therapy

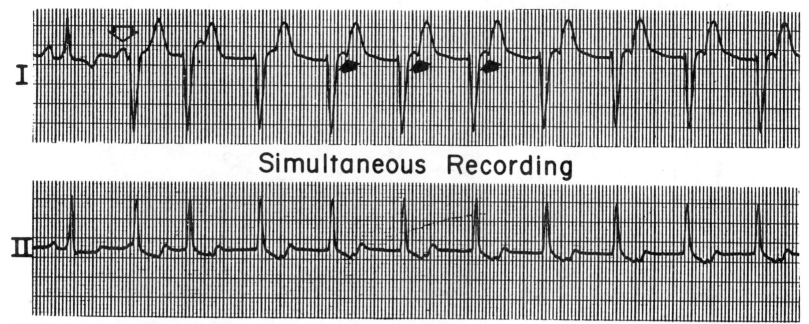

FIGURE 7–5. Sinus rhythm (first beat) is interrrupted by a slightly faster rhythm. In lead II, the configuration of the accelerated rhythm is similar to that of the normally conducted beat. In lead I, however, a marked difference in QRS configuration is obvious. A transient period of AV dissociation (note P merging with the QRS complex of second beat [open arrow]) at the beginning of the run identifies an accelerated ventricular rhythm, which is also more clearly defined by lead I. By the fourth beat of the tachycardia, there is retrograde atrial capture with P waves following each QRS complex (solid arrows).

with a class I drug. Unfortunately, ventricular beats can mimic all of these patterns and can also be less than 0.14 second.

3. What does an analysis of premature wide QRS complexes during periods of sinus rhythm demonstrate? Periods of sinus rhythm occurring before or after the resolution of atrial fibrillation often reveal easily diagnosed premature beats. If the wide-QRS beats during atrial fibrillation are conducted with a QRS complex identical to those of premature atrial beats during sinus rhythm, they are likely to be aberrant (see Fig. 7–4*A* and *B*). Conversely, wide-QRS premature beats during atrial fibrillation having morphologic characteristics similar to those of PVCs during sinus rhythm are likely to be PVCs. Often one has only to look in the

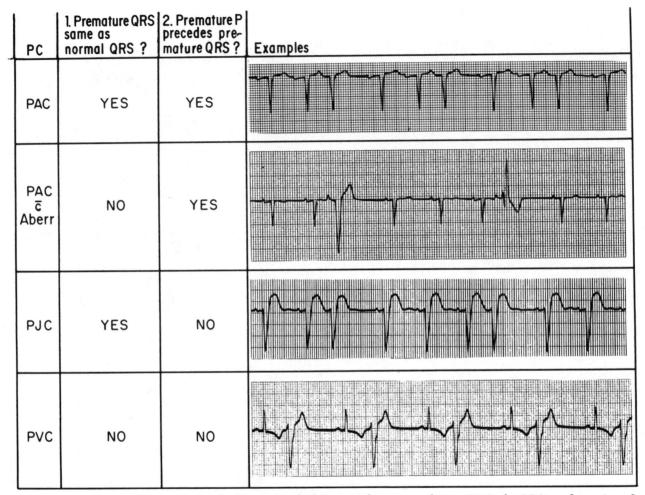

PC	1. Premature QRS same as normal QRS ?	2. Premature P precedes premature QRS ?	Examples
PAC	YES	YES	
PAC c̄ Aberr	NO	YES	
PJC	YES	NO	
PVC	NO	NO	

FIGURE 7–6. Two questions are key in diagnosing the location of premature beats: (1) "Is the QRS configuration of the premature beat the same as the normally conducted QRS configuration?" and (2) "Does a premature P wave precede the premature QRS complex?" In the top tracing, for example, the answer to both questions is yes, and the premature beats, therefore, are atrial. One should be careful in diagnosing premature junctional complexes (PJCs) (third tracing), since premature atrial complexes (PACs) could be missed by confining the search to this one rhythm strip. PVC = premature ventricular complex.

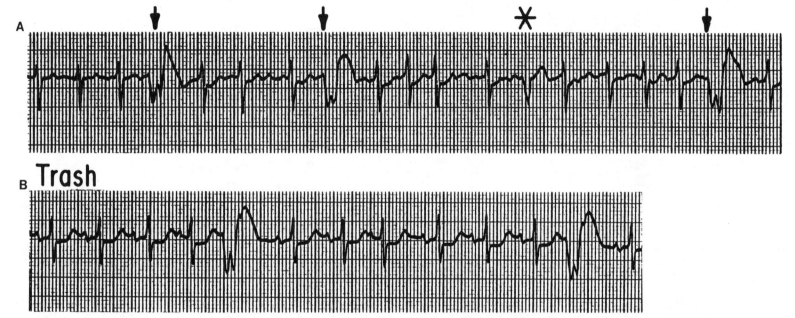

FIGURE 7–7. (*A*) In this run of atrial fibrillation from a patient on quinidine therapy, the wide QRS complexes (arrows) show several features suggestive of PVCs, including their width (0.16 second—a suggestive, but not diagnostic, finding when it occurs with class I drug therapy), a probable fusion beat (asterisk), and fixed coupling, but they are not consistently followed by relative pauses. The ventricular response is rapid, however, compatible with high sympathetic tone. Thus, the absence of relative pauses may indicate either that the wide QRS complexes are due to aberration or that they are ventricular with retrograde concealed conduction blunted by high sympathetic tone. (*B*) Through a diligent search (involving, in this case, going through the trash), the matter was resolved by finding an example of sinus rhythm with premature wide beats identical to those occurring during atrial fibrillation. With no preceding P waves apparent, the answer to both questions posed in Figure 7–6 became no, confirming the ventricular origin of these premature wide beats.

trash where the previous strips have been deposited (Fig. 7–7).

INTERACTION WITH THE AUTONOMIC NERVOUS SYSTEM

At times, premature beats are related to the level of sympathetic tone and appear only during the stress of exercise or daily activities. In other patients, slower heart rates during rest or sleep allow the emergence of premature beats. The use of an autonomic maneuver such as carotid massage is helpful in patients with atrial fibrillation; the aberrantly conducted beats disappear or diminish as the rate is slowed. On the other hand, the frequency of PVCs may increase in patients whose ventricular rate has been slowed.

INVASIVE ELECTROPHYSIOLOGIC TESTING

Electrophysiologic testing is rarely indicated in patients with isolated PVCs, although a His bundle recording of the premature beats can provide a precise diagnosis of the origin of these beats. Chapter 6 (pages 135 to 139) discusses the role of electrophysiologic testing in the induction of tachyarrhythmias in high-risk patients with ventricular ectopy.

CLINICAL FEATURES

Premature Supraventricular Beats

PREDISPOSING CLINICAL SETTINGS

For all practical purposes, PACs and PJCs can be considered together. Their presence does not necessarily imply organic heart disease, and alone they are rarely of clinical significance, although they can be a terrible nuisance for the patient. On occasion, they may trigger hemodynamically significant supraventricular tachycardias. Premature atrial complexes may be seen in diseases that cause atrial dilation, such as heart failure, mitral valve disease, and chronic obstructive pulmonary disease with cor pulmonale. In the setting of acute myocardial infarction, PACs may reflect incipient congestive heart failure and herald atrial fibrillation (Fig. 7–8). They are often encountered with anesthesia and surgery and are particularly common after coronary bypass surgery and valve surgery. Metabolic factors and drugs may trigger premature supraventricular beats. Sympathomimetic agents used for rhinitis, si-

nusitis, or asthma, as well as alcohol, may be responsible. Caffeine, though frequently incriminated, is more rarely a culprit in causing premature beats. Premature atrial complexes can trigger recurrent atrial flutter-fibrillation in these and other settings. In all clinical situations, suppressing them may prevent the tachyarrhythmia.

NATURAL HISTORY

In general, the natural history of premature supraventricular beats reflects that of the underlying heart disease, if any.

TREATMENT

The initial treatment reassures patients about the benign nature of their arrhythmia. If intolerable symptoms persist despite such reassurance, a trial of discontinuing stimulants such as caffeine, alcohol, and nicotine may be undertaken, although commonly the premature beats continue unabated despite significant modifications in lifestyle. When the premature beats are associated with recurrent paroxysmal supraventricular tachycardias, such as atrial flutter-fibrillation or AV junctional reentry, drug therapy may be indicated. When the premature beats are isolated and symptoms are intolerable, pharmacologic therapy may be indicated. The most benign antiarrhythmic drug is a β-blocker, and its administration is begun with a low dose (e.g., proprano-

A

V_1-V_2-V_3 V_4-V_5-V_6

B

I-II-III

C

I-II-III

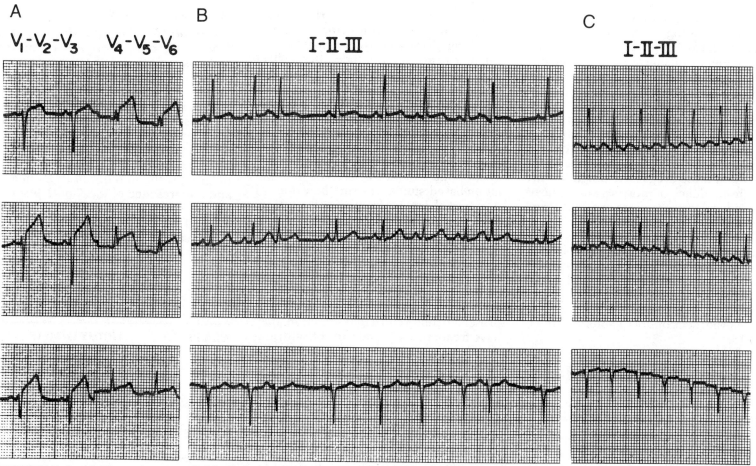

FIGURE 7–8. (*A*) These six precordial leads from a patient with acute anterior myocardial infarction show sinus rhythm. (*B*) At a later time, these simultaneous limb leads show sinus rhythm with two PACs. (Note the deformity of the T wave preceding each premature beat in lead I.) (*C*) Still later, these simultaneous limb leads show atrial flutter-fibrillation. This common sequence occurs in patients with large infarctions that cause significant left ventricular dysfunction and atrial distention.

lol, 10 mg bid to qid), with subsequent titration according to the patient's symptoms. β-blockers may have no effect on the frequency of supraventricular ectopy itself but can blunt the sympathetic response to the perception of the premature beats and improve symptomatic status. Treatment of isolated supraventricular ectopy with the more potent antiarrhythmic drugs such as the class Ia and class Ic agents should be tempered by the possibility that these drugs have a significantly higher incidence of more serious noncardiac side effects, are more expensive, and most important, are potentially proarrhythmic (and even lethal).[2] Unless the supraventricular ectopy cannot be tolerated by the patient or is related to paroxysmal tachycardias, drug therapy should not be undertaken. The use of drugs for supraventricular tachycardias is discussed in the relevant sections of Chapters 9, 10, 11, and 15.

Premature Ventricular Complexes

PREDISPOSING CLINICAL SETTINGS

Premature ventricular complexes are found in most individuals monitored for a sufficiently long period, and the clinical setting in which they occur is the important factor in determining whether therapy is necessary. Although frequent in the general population, PVCs are even more frequent in patients with underlying heart disease. In patients with chronic obstructive lung disease, cardiomyopathy, and valvular heart disease, they often reflect underlying ventricular dysfunction, hypoxia, increased sympathetic tone, metabolic-drug interaction, or any combination of these factors. Hypoxia, acidosis, and sepsis are commonly associated with PVCs, even without intrinsic heart disease. In coronary artery disease, the frequency and complexity of PVCs in population-based studies mirror the extent of myocardial damage from prior infarction. However, the factors explaining why two patients with similar degrees of ventricular dysfunction, the same infarction site, and other similar clinical descriptors may have a markedly disparate frequency and complexity of ventricular ectopy remain obscure. In addition, patients with well-preserved left ventricular function may have frequent PVCs and runs of ventricular tachycardia. Premature ventricular complexes are a marker for the risk of sudden death, but whether they are independent risk factors (or simply reflect the extent of ventricular dysfunction) is more controversial. At best, they are poor predictors of sudden death. Even with more complex ventricular ectopy, specific antiarrhythmic drug treatment does not favorably affect the natural history; indeed, the opposite has been shown, with a higher mortality in the subgroups treated with encainide and flecainide.[2]

NATURAL HISTORY

Prognostic Stratification by Electrocardiogram.
There are a number of prognostic ECG classification systems for grouping PVCs according to the risk for the development of sudden death. The Lown classification (Table 7–1) is one of the most widely referenced systems.[3] It is based on the number of PVCs per minute, the constancy of their morphologic features, and in the more ominous prognostic groups, the number of PVCs in a row and the presence of the R-on-T phenomenon (the R wave of the QRS complex falls on the T wave of the preceding beat). This classification evolved from a study of

Table 7–1. CLASSIFICATION OF VENTRICULAR ARRHYTHMIAS

CLASS	ARRHYTHMIAS
0	No to rare ventricular beats
1	Occasional isolated beats ($<$ 30/hr)
2	Frequent beats ($>$ 30/hr)
3	Multiform beats
4A	Couplets (2 in succession)
4B	Salvos (3 or more in succession)
5	Early beats (R on T)

Source: Reproduced with permission. From Lown B and Wolf M. Approaches to sudden death from coronary heart disease. Circulation 44:130–142, 1971. Copyright 1971, American Heart Association.

Table 7–2. CLASSIFICATION OF VENTRICULAR ARRHYTHMIAS

	Classification		
	BENIGN	**POTENTIALLY MALIGNANT**	**MALIGNANT**
Arrhythmias present	PVCs, pairs, nonsustained VT	PVCs, pairs, nonsustained VT	Sustained and nonsustained VT, torsades de pointes, VF
Nature of heart disease	None	Coronary, hypertensive, valvular, and idiopathic	Coronary, hypertensive, valvular, and idiopathic
Left ventricular function	Normal to mildly impaired	Normal to severely impaired	Moderately to severely impaired (normal function uncommon)
Hemodynamic/ electrical significance	None	None	Syncope/sudden death
Treatment objectives	Reduce symptoms	Reduce risk for sudden death	Reduce risk for sudden death

PVCs = premature ventricular complexes; VF = ventricular fibrillation; VT = ventricular tachycardia.

Source: Adapted with permission from the American College of Cardiology (Morganroth J, et al: Journal of the American College of Cardiology, 8:607–615, 1986).

acute myocardial infarction patients and suffers from the lack of a prospective clinical correlation in determining risks. For example, two patients with runs of nonsustained ventricular tachycardia, one with an ischemic cardiomyopathy and an ejection fraction of 20% and the other with mitral valve prolapse and a normal left ventricle, would have the same arrhythmia classification. This classification therefore appears to be of limited clinical usefulness.

Prognostic Stratification by ECG and Clinical Data. The classification of ventricular arrhythmias proposed by Morganroth and colleagues (Table 7–2) is a more clinically useful prognostic system,

because it is based on patient symptoms, the presence of underlying heart disease, and the risk for sudden death or ventricular tachycardia.[4] Benign ventricular arrhythmias are frequent PVCs or repetitive PVCs (pairs or runs of nonsustained ventricular tachycardia) occurring without evidence of organic heart disease. These patients have no hemodynamically important symptoms but may have the nuisance symptom of palpitations. Because they have virtually no risk for sudden death, they have an excellent prognosis without therapy. Patients in the malignant subgroup have a history of hemodynamically significant ventricular arrhythmias causing syncope or sudden death and re-

quire therapy. In the potentially malignant subgroup are a much more heterogenous array of patients with organic heart disease who have similar arrhythmias, including frequent PVCs and nonsustained ventricular tachycardia. Some may have minimal left ventricular dysfunction (with a low risk for sudden death), and others, severe left ventricular dysfunction (with a much higher risk). Chapters 6 and 12 discuss the role of ambulatory ECG monitoring and electrophysiologic study in further risk stratification of such patients.[5]

Table 7–3 outlines an approach to considering the significance of premature ventricular beats as well as nonsustained

Table 7–3. SIGNIFICANCE OF CARDIAC ARRHYTHMIAS

1. Is the arrhythmia a nuisance?
   a. The patient is unable to tolerate the palpitations.
   b. There is a strong fear that the arrhythmia will lead to or is the result of heart disease.
   c. The physician is concerned that the arrhythmia will lead to heart disease or sudden death.

2. Is the arrhythmia hemodynamically or electrically significant?
   a. It has the potential to increase myocardial oxygen demands and worsen or cause ischemia.
   b. It has the potential for producing hypotension.
   c. It has the potential for producing sudden death.

and sustained ventricular tachycardias. The classification of patients into one of these categories requires a knowledge of the arrhythmias' natural history in given clinical settings, information that can be obtained using the Morganroth classification. These data allow the development of a rational approach to the use of diagnostic methods such as ambulatory ECG monitoring, exercise testing, and electrophysiologic testing in the management of patients with PVCs. The subject is discussed in greater detail, with reference to ventricular tachycardia, in Chapter 12. The natural history and treatment of PVCs in certain common clinical settings is discussed in the following sections.

NO HEART DISEASE. Ventricular tachycardia and ventricular fibrillation can occur in patients with normal hearts, but their occurrence is extremely rare. Studies of the natural history of isolated PVCs in patients with normal hearts indicate that the incidence of sudden death and ventricular tachycardia is the same as in patients with no PVCs. Unless proof to the contrary is found, ventricular ectopy in this population should not be considered to have prognostic significance.

MITRAL VALVE PROLAPSE. The theory that ventricular arrhythmias are related to sudden death in the setting of mitral valve prolapse (MVP) has caused more harm than good. The publicity concerning the connection between MVP, PVCs, and sudden death (no matter how infrequent) has created enormous anxiety and irreparable harm to significant numbers of patients. When one considers that MVP affects 6% to 15% of the population, the incidence of sudden death is minuscule, with fewer than 100 documented cases. Patients with MVP and PVCs should be reassured that they have an excellent prognosis. Any patient with syncope or symptoms suggestive of a sustained tachycardia, on the other hand, should be carefully evaluated, and the exact nature of any arrhythmia must be determined, independent of the presence or absence of MVP.

Jeresaty[6] has developed a general clinical picture of patients with MVP who are at risk for sudden death. In general, one or more of the following findings were present:

1. *History:* presyncope or syncope
2. *Auscultation:* an apical late systolic or holosystolic murmur
3. *ECG:* ST-T wave abnormalities in the inferior or precordial leads, or in both, with frequent PVCs

4. *Catheterization:* pronounced cineangiographic prolapse with mild to moderate mitral valve regurgitation on left ventriculography

Patients with familial prolapse may constitute another subgroup at higher risk for sudden death, and some reported cases of sudden death have occurred during class Ia drug therapy; the possibility of a proarrhythmic effect should be considered likely. Without these findings, one can be comfortable in reassuring the asymptomatic patient and the referring physician that there is no chance that this condition will cause sudden death.

ISCHEMIC HEART DISEASE
Acute Myocardial Ischemia or Infarction. With the advent of coronary care units (CCUs) in the mid-1960s, continuous ECG monitoring during acute myocardial infarction became possible. The concept of "warning" ventricular arrhythmias was developed to predict the appearance of significant ventricular arrhythmias such as ventricular tachycardia or fibrillation. The term "warning arrhythmias" was used to refer to PVCs of a certain form and frequency, such as the R-on-T phenomenon, multiform PVCs, ventricular couplets, and greater than six PVCs per minute. These were considered harbingers of ventricular fibrillation. Subsequent studies, however, showed that at least 50% of patients developing ventricular fibrillation did so without warning arrhythmias,

and many patients with such warning arrhythmias did not subsequently develop ventricular fibrillation. Waiting for warning arrhythmias to administer therapy provides a false sense of security and sometimes results in inappropriate withholding of therapy.

Unfortunately, the concept of warning arrhythmias was also used to characterize the significance of arrhythmias occurring outside the setting of acute myocardial infarction. There is no valid basis for this extrapolation, and its use led to many patients with benign arrhythmias being treated with potentially lethal antiarrhythmic drugs. We are presently trying to "unlearn" this dogma of the 1960s to avoid such unnecessary treatment.

Postmyocardial Infarction. Studies in patients recovered from acute myocardial infarction have shown that the major determinant of long-term survival is the status of left ventricular function. Initial studies indicated that the ventricular ectopy was simply a marker of the degree of underlying left ventricular dysfunction and did not connote additional prognostic significance, but other studies have indicated that ventricular ectopy identifies an additional risk for sudden death even when the degree of left ventricular dysfunction is considered. The highest-risk groups appear to be those with ejection fractions less than 40% and PVCs more frequent than 30 per hour.

MISCELLANEOUS CLINICAL CONDITIONS. Patients with congestive cardiomyopathy, particularly those with more severe left ventricular dysfunction, have a high incidence of sudden death. It is not clear, however, that ventricular ectopy is an independent risk factor for sudden death. With hypertrophic cardiomyopathy, frequent ventricular ectopy may help identify patients at increased risk for sudden death, although the data are more convincing in those with ventricular tachycardia. A cause-effect relationship between ventricular arrhythmias and sudden death, however, remains unproved. In the setting of digitalis therapy, PVCs should be considered a manifestation of digitalis toxicity until proved otherwise. Similarly, frequent ventricular ectopy in the setting of therapy with a class Ia and Ic agent may reflect a proarrhythmic effect (see Chapter 15, pages 353 to 354). In both situations, iatrogenic life-threatening arrhythmias could develop, and the need for the particular therapy or its potential role in causing the ventricular arrhythmias, or both factors, should be carefully evaluated.

METHODS OF TREATMENT

General Principles. In patients with organic heart disease, whenever possible, correction of the underlying problem should be the initial therapy of ventricular ectopy. For example, treatment of congestive heart failure may diminish sympathetic tone and markedly improve ventricular ectopy. Similarly, improving oxygenation in patients with congestive heart failure or chronic obstructive lung disease, correcting hypokalemia and hypomagnesemia, and recognizing toxicity from digitalis and antiarrhythmic agents are important goals.

Specific Clinical Conditions

NO HEART DISEASE. Unless the ventricular ectopy can be shown to be a factor in precipitating significant ventricular arrhythmias or causing incapacitating palpitations, these patients should not be treated with antiarrhythmic drugs. Cosmetic treatment of patients with antiarrhythmic drugs on the basis of an ambulatory ECG recordings is dangerous and may worsen ventricular arrhythmias and even cause sudden death. These patients initially should be reassured that their palpitations do not carry prognostic significance. Just as with supraventricular ectopy, a trial of avoiding stimulants such as alcohol, nicotine, and caffeine may be warranted. Exercise conditioning, biofeedback, and avoidance of stress might be attempted, depending on the individual circumstances. When incapacitating palpitations persist and antiarrhythmic drug therapy is undertaken, it should be initiated with the most benign agent available; β-blockers are the first choice. Class Ib agents are reasonable alternative antiarrhythmic agents. The clinician should follow the same guidelines as outlined for the use of these drugs with supraventricular ectopy, bearing in mind that all antiarrhythmic drugs have the potential for proarrhythmia (see Chapter 15). Use of class Ia and class Ic agents carries an additional risk for side effects and ventricular proarrhythmia. Class Ic drugs are quite effective in suppressing PVCs but have the highest (or perhaps the most carefully studied) risk of proarrhythmia. Chapter 15 discusses the use of these and other agents in treating ventricular arrhythmias.

MITRAL VALVE PROLAPSE. The same measures used for the treatment of PVCs in patients with normal ventricular function also apply to most patients with MVP. With significant mitral regurgitation and left ventricular dysfunction, the risk of sudden death may be higher, although there are no data that antiarrhythmic therapy alters the natural history of this rare complication. When the PVCs can be shown to be related to a significant ventricular tachyarrhythmia, therapy should be guided by careful electrophysiologic evaluation (see Chapters 6 and 12).

ISCHEMIC HEART DISEASE

Acute Myocardial Ischemia or Infarction. The indications for prophylactic lidocaine in all patients with suspected acute myocardial infarction who do not demonstrate bradyarrhythmias have not been settled, although the drug has been used with considerable frequency. The administration of a loading dose followed by a continuous infusion of 2 to 4 mg per minute will usually suppress the development of ventricular fibrillation, although the higher maintenance dose is frequently accompanied by side effects (usually neurologic) that resolve when the infusion rate is decreased (see Chapter 15, pages 363 to 364).

Although prophylactic lidocaine during acute myocardial infarction prevents primary ventricular fibrillation, there are no data that the overall CCU mortality rate is improved. Indeed, a meta-analysis of 14 randomized controlled trials of prophylactic lidocaine during the prehospitalization (six trials) or early hospital phase (eight trials) of acute myocardial infarction was unable to show any survival benefit for the drug in either group.[7] Although lidocaine prophylaxis did no harm in the prehospitalization-phase group, there was a significant adverse effect on treatment-phase mortality in the hospital-phase group. Although bradyarrhythmic complications of lidocaine therapy are well documented, even in patients without myocardial infarction, any cause-effect relation between lidocaine, bradyarrhythmias, and increased mortality remains unproven. Interestingly, this same meta-analysis was unable to show any adverse effects of lidocaine prophylaxis on total mortality for the hospital-phase group.[7] Logically, if the patient is in a setting where careful and continuous observation of the monitored rhythm is not possible, prophylactic lidocaine should be used for the first 24 hours to reduce the chance of ventricular fibrillation. Where careful monitoring is available, it might be reasonable to treat such patients with lidocaine only after ventricular arrhythmias develop, recognizing the possible incidence of ventricular fibrillation and the need for resuscitation. I prefer to use prophylactic lidocaine in the high-risk patient because some data suggest that the long-term prognosis is better in patients with acute infarction who do not develop ventricular fibrillation. Lidocaine does not have to suppress all ventricular ectopic activity to be effective in preventing ventricular fibrillation. Although not tested, many centers administer a reduced drip (e.g., 2 mg per minute) in an attempt to protect against the development of primary ventricular fibrillation while minimizing the incidence of neurologic side effects.

Postmyocardial Infarction. As mentioned earlier, data conflict about whether PVCs in this clinical setting carry prognostic significance independent of the extent of left ventricular dysfunction. The only drugs that have been shown to have a favorable impact on the natural history of postmyocardial infarction patients

are β-blockers. The mechanism of this protection is unclear, because patients under study were not selected for randomization on the basis of ventricular ectopy.

Postmyocardial infarction patients with single PVCs, in contrast to more complex ventricular ectopy, should not be treated with antiarrhythmic drugs for "prophylaxis" against sudden death, although all such patients, by virtue of their postmyocardial infarction status, may be candidates for treatment with β-blockers. As mentioned previously, antiarrhythmic drug therapy not only failed to reduce the risk of sudden death in postinfarction patients with PVCs and nonsustained ventricular tachycardia, it actually increased the mortality rate.[2] When intolerably symptomatic PVCs occur, nonpharmacologic approaches (correction of electrolyte imbalance, treatment of congestive heart failure, elimination of unnecessary drug therapy), in addition to the other measures mentioned earlier (see Chapter 7, pages 159 to 160), should be used first.

The use of the more potent antiarrhythmic agents should be reserved for those with more complex ventricular ectopy and should be guided by careful selection criteria designed to identify patients at high risk for sudden death, such as the extent of left ventricular dysfunction and coronary disease. In certain high-risk patients, recording high-amplitude ECGs to

search for late potentials in the terminal portions of the QRS complex (ECG signal averaging) or looking for decreased heart-rate variability on ambulatory monitoring may help further to define risk. Alternatively, electrophysiologic testing may provide the best guidelines for antiarrhythmic therapy. The latter approach is best discussed in more detail in Chapters 6 and 12 and is currently being evaluated in postinfarction patients with nonsustained ventricular tachycardia and reduced left ventricular function (the Multicenter Unsustained Tachycardia Trial).

MISCELLANEOUS CLINICAL CONDITIONS. No data have yet shown any benefit for antiarrhythmic drug therapy in patients with congestive cardiomyopathy who have asymptomatic PVCs. As in certain subsets of patients with ventricular arrhythmias and chronic ischemic heart disease, an automatic implantable cardioverter-defibrillator, in combination with antiarrhythmic drug therapy, may have a palliative role. There are also no prospective, controlled trials showing that antiarrhythmic drugs prevent sudden death in patients with hypertrophic cardiomyopathy and PVCs.

Life-threatening ventricular arrhythmias due to digoxin toxicity may necessitate therapy with digoxin antibodies, although lidocaine, procainamide, and dilantin may also be effective, are more readily available, and are much less expensive. The key to preventing this problem lies in recognizing that PVCs may be an early manifestation of digitalis toxicity and discontinuing the drug at that point. The key to treating proarrhythmia problems from other antiarrhythmic drugs lies in recognizing their potential to cause or worsen the very arrhythmia that one is trying to suppress or prevent in the first place, and discontinuing the drug.[1,8]

REFERENCES

1. Moulton KP, Medcalf T, and Lazzara R: Premature ventricular complex morphology: A marker for left ventricular structure and function. Circulation 81:1245–1251, 1990.

2. The Cardiac Arrhythmia Suppression Trial (CAST) Investigators: Preliminary report: Effect of encainide and flecainide on mortality in a randomized trial of arrhythmia suppression after myocardial infarction. N Engl J Med 321:406–412, 1989.

3. Lown B and Wolf M: Approaches to sudden death from coronary heart disease. Circulation 44:130–142, 1971.

4. Morganroth J, Anderson JL, and Gentzkow GD: Classification by type of ventricular arrhythmia predicts frequency of adverse cardiac events from flecainide. J Am Coll Cardiol 8:607–615, 1986.

5. Kharsa MH, Gold RL, Moore H, Yazaki Y, Haffajee CI, and Alpert JS: Long-term outcome following programmed electrical stimulation in patients with high-grade ventricular ectopy. PACE 11:603–609, 1988.

6. Jeresaty RM: Mitral Valve Prolapse. Raven Press, New York, 1979, pp 218–219.

7. Hine LK, Laird N, Hewitt P, and Chalmers TC: Meta-analytic evidence against prophylactic use of lidocaine in acute myocardial infarction. Arch Intern Med 149:2694–2698, 1989.

8. Velebit V, Podrid P, Lown B, Cohen BH, and Grayboys TB: Aggravation and provocation of ventricular arrhythmias by antiarrhythmic drugs. Circulation 65:886–894, 1982.

CHAPTER 8

A General Approach to the Diagnosis of Tachyarrhythmias

BARRY W. RAMO, MD

OUTLINE

The correct diagnosis of tachyarrhythmias requires an understanding of the electrophysiologic basis of arrhythmias, a thorough appreciation of the patient's overall clinical problem, and a systematic approach to the electrocardiogram (ECG). Electrocardiographic diagnosis requires, first, the localization of the arrhythmia to a specific area of the heart, and then an attempt to identify its mechanism. Often (as discussed in Chapter 4), because a precise ECG diagnosis cannot be made initially, the clinician must intervene with a vagal maneuver or a drug that selectively affects a specific locus; then, the clinician must reevaluate the clinical situation and the ECG. This chapter presents an overview of the tachyarrhythmias, which are discussed in detail in Chapters 9 through 12.

CLASSIFICATION

Site and Mechanism

Tachyarrhythmias are classified according to one of three locations (atrial, atrioventricular [AV] junctional, and ventricular) and one of two mechanisms (enhanced automaticity versus reentry) (Figure 8–1). A third mechanism, triggered automaticity, has been demonstrated in isolated tissues and may play a role in the genesis of clinical arrhythmias, but its clinical importance remains to be established. The site and mechanism of an arrhythmia are interdependent, because knowing the location of an arrhythmia allows one to speculate more precisely about its mechanism, and conversely, knowing the most likely electrophysiologic mechanism helps to localize it.

Narrow- vs. Wide-QRS Tachycardia

The division of tachyarrhythmias into two broad groups of narrow-QRS versus wide-QRS tachycardia is a helpful initial step in localizing their origin (Table 8–1).

A narrow-QRS tachycardia (less than 0.12 second) is always supraventricular, originating in either the atria (including the sinus node) or the AV junction. The latter site includes tachycardias that incorporate an accessory pathway or the AV node, or both, in their reentry loops (i.e., paroxysmal AV junctional tachycardia, or premature junctional tachycardia [PJT]). The QRS configuration is the same as that of the normally conducted QRS complex unless aberration occurs, but the QRS width is less than 0.12 second.

A wide-QRS tachycardia results when the ventricles are depolarized sufficiently differently from normal to result in a QRS duration of 0.12 second or more. A given rhythm strip may show a QRS duration of less than 0.12 second in some leads and 0.12 second or more in others, because the first or last portion, or both portions, of the QRS complex are isoelectric in certain leads. Because wide-QRS tachycardias can originate in any of the three locations, it is critical to consider how the QRS configuration of a wide-QRS tachycardia compares morphologically with the patient's normal QRS complexes. Such a comparison may allow the rapid differentiation of aberration from ventricular tachycardia (VT) (Fig. 8–2).[1]

Use of Interventions

In some cases, precise diagnosis necessitates an intervention designed to slow AV nodal conduction, terminate the arrhythmia, or change the atrial rate. A vagal maneuver, for example, may slow the sinus pacemaker, increase AV block, terminate AV junctional reentry tachycardias, or speed intra-atrial conduction (Table 8–2; see Chapter 4). When vagal maneuvers fail with a narrow-QRS tachycardia, drugs such as adenosine, β-blockers, or calcium-channel blockers may be used to the same end. Experience with adenosine has shown that it can also be used to help in the diagnosis of wide-QRS tachycardias because of its minimal and short lived hemodynamic effects (see Chapter 15, pages 389 to 390).

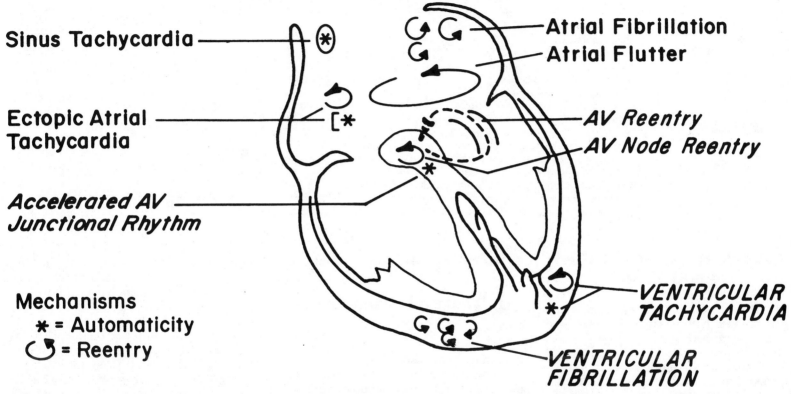

FIGURE 8–1. The sites and mechanisms of common tachycardias. The site may be either ventricular (defined as originating below the His bundle) or supraventricular (all others). The latter group can be divided into atrial and atrioventricular (AV) junctional subgroups. Tachycardias that incorporate an AV bypass tract (AV reentry) are considered AV junctional because the AV node is virtually always included in the reentry loop. The term "ectopic" includes both automatic and focal reentry varieties of atrial tachycardias. Atrial fibrillation is illustrated as consisting of multiple sites of reentry, whereas atrial flutter is depicted as a more organized and larger reentry circuit. Ventricular tachycardia may be due to automaticity or reentry; ventricular fibrillation is depicted as involving multiple sites of reentry.

**Table 8–1. DIFFERENTIAL DIAGNOSIS OF
TACHYARRHYTHMIAS BASED ON QRS WIDTH**

Narrow QRS Complex (<0.12 second):
　　Sinus tachycardia
　　Automatic atrial tachycardia
　　Multifocal atrial tachycardia
　　Atrial reentry tachycardia
　　Atrial flutter-fibrillation
　　Paroxysmal AV junctional tachycardia (atrioventricular nodal reentry and AVRT)
　　Accelerated AV junctional rhythm (nonparoxysmal junctional tachycardia)
Wide QRS Complex (≥0.12 second):
　　Any atrial or AV junctional tachycardia with aberration
　　Atrial fibrillation with ventricular preexcitation
　　AVRT with antidromic conduction
　　Ventricular tachycardia including torsades de pointes

AV = atrioventricular; AVRT = atrioventricular reciprocating tachycardia.

ELECTROCARDIOGRAPHIC ANALYSIS

Chapter 1 outlines a systematic approach to arrhythmias that can be applied to the diagnosis of tachyarrhythmias. This approach provides a logical sequence of steps to be used in refining the differential diagnosis. It consists of answering the following questions:

1. Is there a normal sinus beat?
2. What are the atria doing?
3. What are the ventricles doing?
4. What is the AV relationship?
5. What are the characteristics of the tachycardia's onset, termination, interruption, and response to interventions?

Is There a Normal Sinus Beat?

Identification of one (ideally two) normal sinus beats establishes the patient's heart rate, wave-form characteristics, and intervals. Brief runs of sinus rhythm may also be found by examining rhythm strips taken before the arrhythmia became sustained or after it terminated.

What Are the Atria Doing?

The answer to this question identifies atrial rate and regularity. Morphologic comparison of the P waves with the sinus P waves determines whether the atria are being activated normally or abnormally, or if atrial flutter-fibrillation is present. This task is difficult, however, when the P waves are superimposed on the prior QRS complex, ST segment, or T wave. If all else fails in determining what the atria are doing, the clinician might try using the right side of the brain. Turning the ECG strip 90° to its normal orientation allows an analysis of the strip from an entirely new perspective, and the subtle changes of dissociated P waves variably deforming the ST-T segments may become more manifest (Fig. 8–3). One should note whether such atrial activity "marches

FIGURE 8–2. The mechanisms for supraventricular tachycardia resulting in a wide-QRS tachycardia. (*A*) A wide-QRS tachycardia at a rate of 130 beats per minute stops abruptly. The QRS configurations during tachycardia and following restoration of sinus rhythm are identical, indicating a supraventricular origin with preexisting bundle branch block. (*B*) A sinus beat is followed by a premature atrial complex (PAC) (arrow), which initiates an irregular tachycardia that is first wide and later narrow. The initiation by a PAC and the morphologic conversion from wide to narrow QRS complexes are typical of a supraventricular origin and identify the wide beats as tachycardia-dependent aberration. (*C*) An irregularly irregular wide-QRS tachycardia at a rate of 300 beats per minute is terminated by cardioversion (100 watt-seconds [W.S.]). After 30 seconds, regular sinus rhythm is evident (P waves [P] are diminutive but present), with features typical of preexcitation (short PR interval and slurred upstroke of the QRS complex [delta wave indicated by arrow]). Atrial fibrillation with preexcitation is thus identified as the mechanism for the wide-QRS tachycardia.

A FIXED ABERRATION

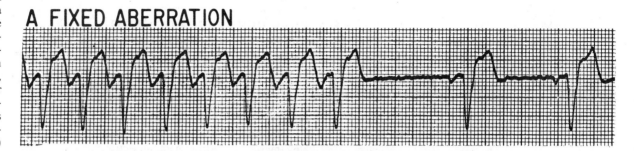

B TACHYCARDIA-DEPENDENT ABERRATION

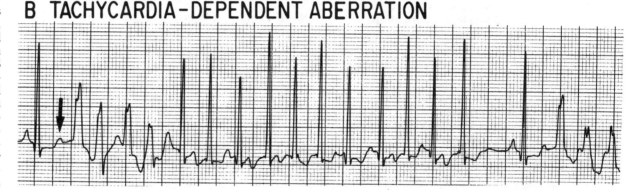

C PREEXCITATION

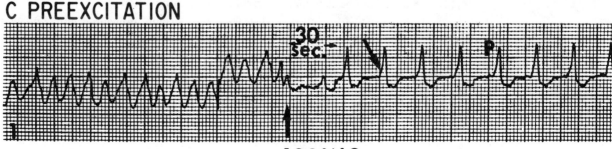

30 sec

100 W.S.

Table 8–2. POSSIBLE EFFECT OF VAGAL STIMULATION ON TACHYARRHYTHMIAS

LOCATION	ATRIAL RATE	VENTRICULAR RATE	TERMINATES
Atrium			
Sinus tachycardia	Slows	Follows atrial rate	No
Automatic atrial tachycardia	No effect*	Slows AV conduction	No
Multifocal atrial tachycardia	No effect	Slows AV conduction†	No
Atrial reentry tachycardia	No effect	Slows AV conduction	No‡
Atrial flutter-fibrillation	No effect or speeds	Slows AV conduction	No
AV Junction			
Accelerated junctional rhythm	Slows§	No change	No
Atrioventricular nodal reentry and atrioventricular reciprocating tachycardia	No change¶	No change¶	Yes
Ventricle			
Sustained ventricular tachycardias	Slows§	No change	No
Torsades de pointes	Slows	Exacerbates	No

AV = atrioventricular.

*This area would not be expected to respond to vagal stimulation.

†Typical clinical situation of high-adrenergic tone usually prevents significant ventricular slowing.

‡Sinoatrial nodal reentry may terminate, but focal atrial reentry in other locations does not terminate in response to increased vagal tone.

§With AV dissociation, atrial rate remains responsive to autonomic balance; with ventriculo-atrial association, the retrograde block may be increased.

¶Rates may slow transiently before terminating.

Intra-atrial Lead

V_1 Turned 90°

Simultaneous

V_1

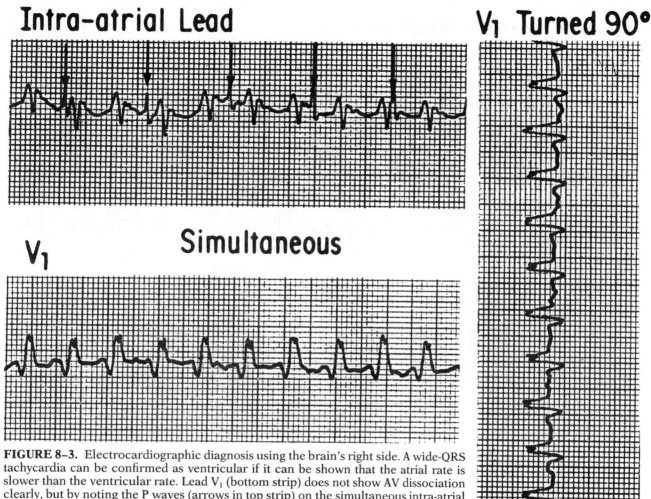

FIGURE 8–3. Electrocardiographic diagnosis using the brain's right side. A wide-QRS tachycardia can be confirmed as ventricular if it can be shown that the atrial rate is slower than the ventricular rate. Lead V_1 (bottom strip) does not show AV dissociation clearly, but by noting the P waves (arrows in top strip) on the simultaneous intra-atrial electrogram, one can discern the changes in the surface electrocardiogram (ECG) because of the superimposed P waves. Turning the tracing 90° (vertical strip on right) allows concentration on the subtle variations in wave form. This strategy may enhance detection of atrial activity that has a changing relationship with the ventricular activity, thus defining AV dissociation and confirming ventricular tachycardia.

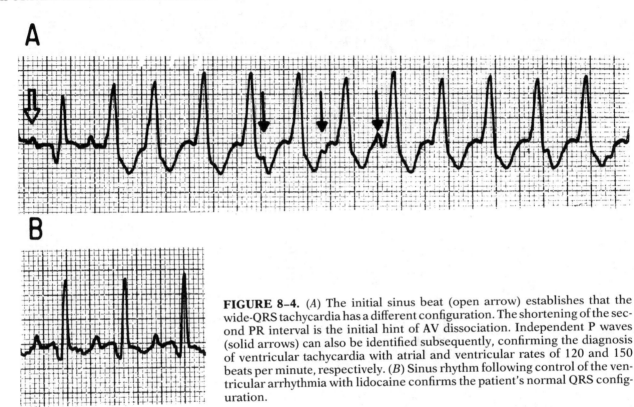

FIGURE 8–4. (*A*) The initial sinus beat (open arrow) establishes that the wide-QRS tachycardia has a different configuration. The shortening of the second PR interval is the initial hint of AV dissociation. Independent P waves (solid arrows) can also be identified subsequently, confirming the diagnosis of ventricular tachycardia with atrial and ventricular rates of 120 and 150 beats per minute, respectively. (*B*) Sinus rhythm following control of the ventricular arrhythmia with lidocaine confirms the patient's normal QRS configuration.

through," as variable retrograde ventriculoatrial (VA) conduction from a ventricular focus may simulate AV dissociation (although both characteristics have the same significance).[2] If the atrial rate is faster than the ventricular rate and AV association is evident, the atria must be driving the ventricles. On the other hand, if the patient has a wide-QRS tachycardia and the atrial rate is slower than the ventricular rate, VT is established (Fig. 8–4).

What Are the Ventricles Doing?

By determining the width of the QRS complex and by comparing its morphologic characteristics with those of the patient's normal QRS complex, one can rapidly evaluate the possibility of aberration. If the QRS complex is wide, 12-lead ECGs during the tachyarrhythmia and sinus rhythm should be compared. If the QRS complex is narrow on a 12-lead ECG, the rhythm is supraventricular tachycardia. Without a prior ECG, the determination of wide versus narrow QRS width is made by examining more than one lead.[3] The specific QRS configuration in a wide-QRS tachycardia can be further analyzed as outlined in Chapter 12 (pages 274 to 279). One useful measurement is the precise duration of the QRS complex; if it is 0.16 second or more, a ventricular origin is strongly suggested, particularly if the patient's normal QRS duration is narrow and there is no preexcitation or class I (and particularly Ic) drug therapy.[1,4] In general, the narrower the QRS duration, the more likely the tachycardia is of a supraventricular origin, although aberration and VT overlap even down to a QRS width of 0.12 second.

The specific QRS configuration during the tachycardia is generally not sufficiently predictive to aid in the localization of the tachycardia, although some patterns are likely to be ventricular (see Chapter 12). The regularity of a tachycardia is variably helpful; sustained tachycardias can be regular regardless of the level of origin. Regularity is helpful if AV dissociation is present or if the atrial rate can be shown to differ from the ventricular rate. In this last instance, if the QRS complex is narrow, the rhythm is accelerated junctional tachycardia, and if wide, VT. A sustained wide-QRS tachycardia that is irregular is most likely atrial flutter or fibrillation with aberration or ventricular preexcitation. Sustained VT or AV junctional reentry tachycardias are usually very regular. Nonsustained VTs, on the other hand, are often irregular. Rapid narrow-QRS tachycardias must be carefully examined for regularity to separate atrial fibrillation from other causes. At a rate of 220 beats per minute, a 0.04-second variability in the RR interval indicates a difference of 30 to 40 beats per minute and strongly suggests atrial fibrillation, whereas with slower rates, a 0.06-second variability may be of no diagnostic significance.[5]

What Is the AV Relationship? (i.e., Association or Is There AV Dissociation?

If the answer to these questions can be obtained, the diagnosis can usually be established. If there is AV dissociation, the arrhythmia is either AV junctional or ventricular tachycardia, depending on the origin of the QRS complex. With rare exceptions, AV junctional reentry tachycardias have a 1:1 AV relationship. On the other hand, when there is a 1:1 AV (or VA) relationship with a wide-QRS tachycardia, it can originate at any of the three levels. If the atrial rate is less than the ventricular rate because of either AV dissociation or retrograde VA block, the localization of the tachycardia is easy and is determined by the QRS width: Narrow-QRS tachycardias reflect an accelerated junctional rhythm, and because AV junctional tachycardias with aberration cannot be diagnosed from the surface ECG (see Chapter

7, page 146), such wide-QRS tachycardias should be considered ventricular until proved otherwise.[6]

What Are the Characteristics of the Tachycardia's Onset, Termination, Interruption, and Response to Interventions?

THE ONSET

The initiating beat usually reliably differentiates supraventricular from ventricular tachycardia. Premature ventricular complexes (PVCs) almost always initiate ventricular tachycardias (Fig. 8–5; see Fig. 8–4), whereas premature atrial complexes (PACs) almost always initiate atrial tachycardias (Fig. 8–6). Atrioventricular junctional reentry tachycardias can be initiated by either PVCs or PACs, but most frequently are initiated by PACs (Fig. 8–6A). A tachycardia initiated by a PAC, therefore, is either atrial or involves the AV junction. Paroxysmal supraventricular tachycardias frequently demonstrate aberration, particularly of the initial beat or beats. The aberration may recur intermittently or remain for the duration of the tachycardia. Any wide-QRS tachycardia initiated by a PAC, therefore, is still considered supraventricular until proved otherwise.

Other features of the initiating beat may

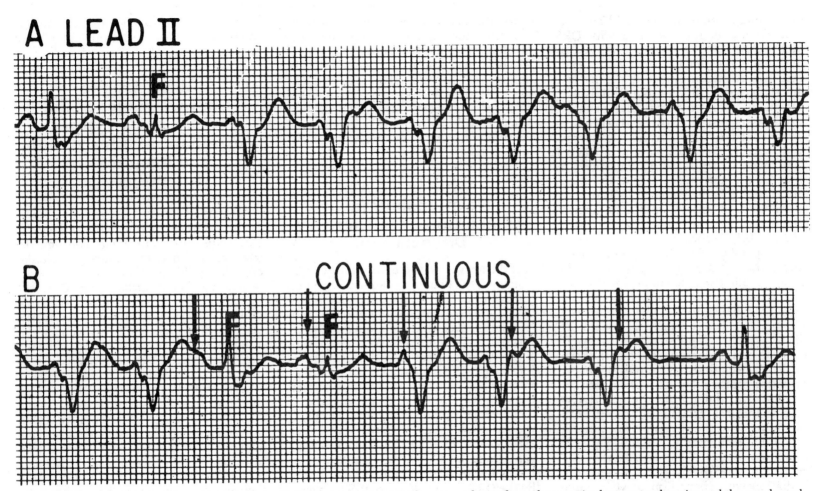

FIGURE 8–5. (*A*) Fusion beats (F), due to a collision between the activation wave fronts from the ventricular pacemaker site and the conducted sinus beats, identify AV dissociation and therefore show that the wide QRS rhythm is ventricular. (*B*) Fusion beats (*F*) continue, and the AV dissociation is more obvious (dissociated P waves are indicated by arrows). Note that fusion beats occur only with an appropriately timed prior P wave.

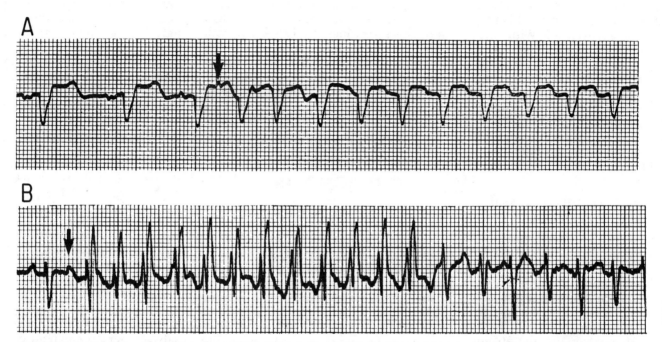

FIGURE 8–6. (*A*) A wide-QRS tachycardia is initiated by a PAC (arrow) and has the same QRS morphologic characteristics as the sinus beats. The rhythm is therefore supraventricular. The most likely differential includes some variety of reentry, either in the atria or AV junction. (*B*) A PAC (arrow) initiates a wide-QRS tachycardia that is irregularly irregular, two features typical of atrial flutter-fibrillation. The rSR′ configuration of the wide-QRS tachycardia is typical of aberration but is not diagnostic. However, the morphologic change in QRS complexes from wide to normal without a pause during the tachycardia is quite typical of aberration. All these features assist in making the correct diagnosis of paroxysmal atrial flutter-fibrillation with initial aberration.

be helpful in the differential diagnosis. With PJT, the initiating PAC usually conducts with a prolonged PR interval and has morphologic characteristics different from those of the tachycardia. With automatic atrial tachycardias, the degree of PR prolongation depends on the prematurity of the inciting P wave and the rate and regularity of the subsequent P waves (i.e., the earlier the P waves, the longer the subsequent PR intervals).[7] In addition, the P-wave morphology is identical throughout the tachycardia, whereas with PJT, the inciting PAC differs from the P waves during the tachycardia.

TERMINATION, INTERRUPTION, AND RESPONSE TO INTERVENTIONS

The characteristics of termination of the tachycardia can also provide useful information.[8] Reentry tachycardias end abruptly, whereas gradual slowing is characteristic of tachycardias that are due to automaticity. If the last beat of a regular tachycardia is a P wave, then the arrhythmia usually originates below the atrium (i.e., is AV junctional or ventricular). A transient interruption with a premature, narrow QRS complex usually identifies atrial capture or fusion and therefore underlying VT (see Fig. 8–5). Termination in response to a vagal maneuver or a drug that directly or indirectly affects AV nodal conduction (such as verapamil, adenosine, β-blockers, acetylcholinesterase inhibitors, or phenylephrine) is most typical

of PJT (both atrioventricular reciprocating tachycardia or atrioventricular nodal reentry). Slowing of the rate in response to these same interventions may reflect sinus slowing or increased AV block with some variety of atrial tachyarrhythmia (commonly, the slowing in AV conduction exposes the atrial activity). These various features are summarized in Figure 8–7.[9]

CLINICAL FACTORS IN THE DIFFERENTIAL DIAGNOSIS

Clinical Setting

Consideration of the clinical setting can help in the differential diagnosis of tachyarrhythmias by indicating the arrhythmia's possible location. For example, a sustained tachyarrhythmia in a patient with a recent myocardial infarction is most likely ventricular, whereas in a young patient with no history of heart disease, a tachycardia is more likely to be supraventricular.

History

The history specifically related to the arrhythmia is also important, particularly regarding the onset, termination, and provoking or relieving factors. Was the onset of the arrhythmia preceded by the development of anginal pain? Was it produced by exercise? Patients who find that self-taught vagal maneuvers such as gagging, neck massage, and deep breathing terminate their tachycardias are most likely suffering from PJT. Syncope should raise the question of ventricular tachycardia or a supraventricular tachycardia with an extremely rapid ventricular response (and, therefore, ventricular preexcitation).

Physical Examination

The physical examination during the tachycardia is discussed in Chapter 3. One of the purposes of the physical examination is to determine the rhythm regularity and the AV relationship during a tachyarrhythmia. A regular tachyarrhythmia with signs of AV dissociation indicates that a wide-QRS tachycardia is ventricular in origin or that a narrow-QRS tachycardia is due to an enhanced pacemaker in the AV junction. As already mentioned, vagal maneuvers such as carotid massage or a Valsalva maneuver can be used to determine if the vagally innervated portions of the heart are affected. The absence of response to vagal maneuvers, however, is not diagnostic of a VT, because the effectiveness of these maneuvers is attenuated or absent in supraventricular tachycardias if the patient is hypotensive, has a high degree of sympathetic tone, or simply has a tachycardia that is poorly responsive to vagal interventions.

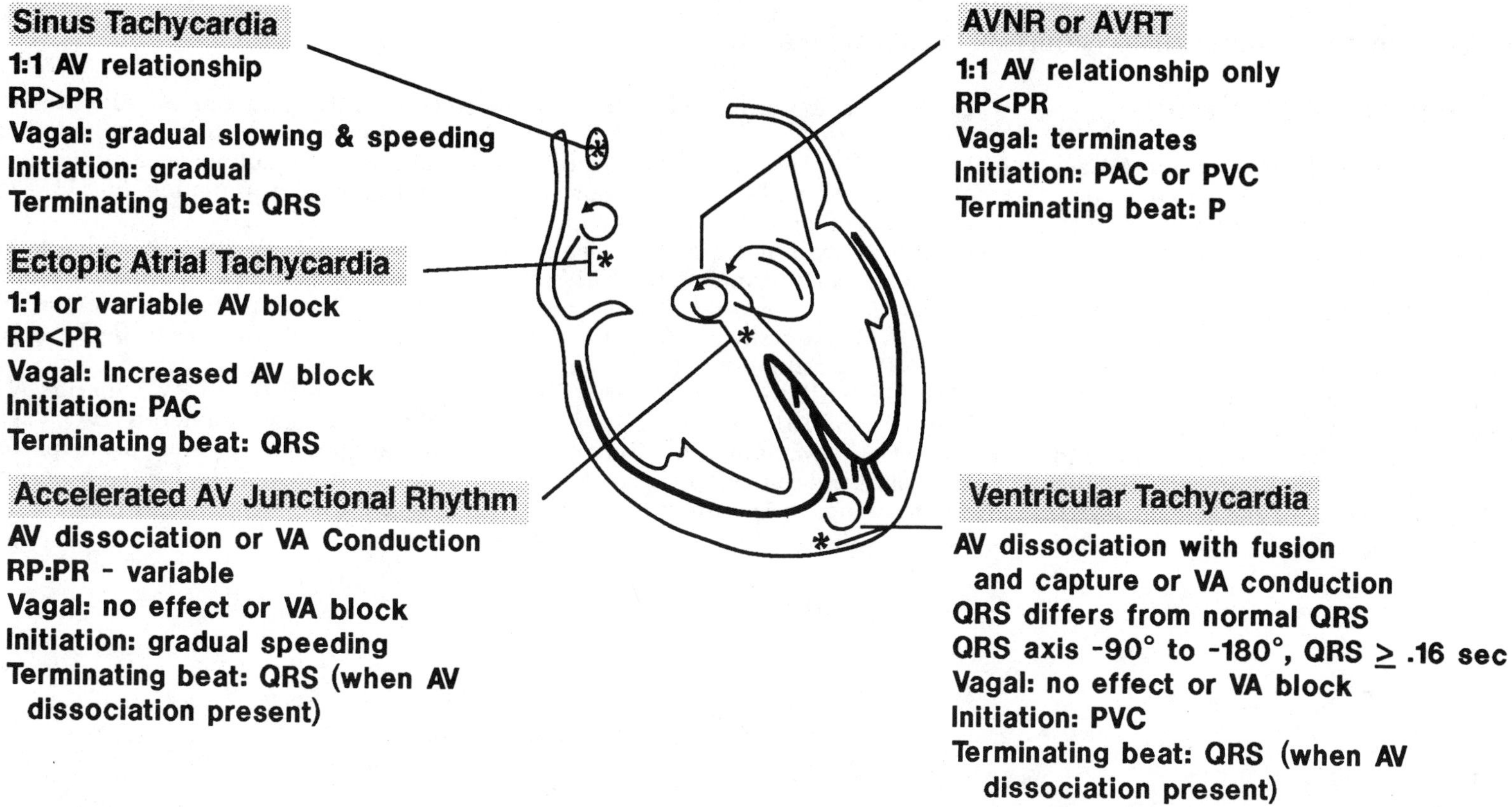

Sinus Tachycardia

1:1 AV relationship
RP>PR
Vagal: gradual slowing & speeding
Initiation: gradual
Terminating beat: QRS

Ectopic Atrial Tachycardia

1:1 or variable AV block
RP<PR
Vagal: Increased AV block
Initiation: PAC
Terminating beat: QRS

Accelerated AV Junctional Rhythm

AV dissociation or VA Conduction
RP:PR - variable
Vagal: no effect or VA block
Initiation: gradual speeding
Terminating beat: QRS (when AV
 dissociation present)

AVNR or AVRT

1:1 AV relationship only
RP<PR
Vagal: terminates
Initiation: PAC or PVC
Terminating beat: P

Ventricular Tachycardia

AV dissociation with fusion
 and capture or VA conduction
QRS differs from normal QRS
QRS axis -90° to -180°, QRS $\geq$ .16 sec
Vagal: no effect or VA block
Initiation: PVC
Terminating beat: QRS (when AV
 dissociation present)

FIGURE 8–7. The key points in the differential diagnosis of tachyarrhythmias: the AV relationship; the relationship between RP and PR intervals; the modes of initiation and termination; and the response to vagal maneuvers. The AV relationship is a central diagnostic factor; AV dissociation identifies a His bundle rhythm (with narrow QRS complex) or a ventricular rhythm (with wide QRS complex). If the AV relationship is 1:1 and the QRS complex is narrow, it may be helpful to analyze the RP interval (measured from any R wave to the next P wave) versus the PR interval (from the *same* P wave to the onset of the next QRS complex). Atrial (particularly sinus) tachycardias have an RP interval that exceeds the PR interval. When the tachycardia stops, analysis of whether the terminating wave form is a P wave or QRS complex is also helpful. A terminating QRS complex typically indicates either atrial tachycardia or ventricular or junctional tachycardia with AV dissociation. A terminating P wave typically signifies paroxysmal AV junctional tachycardia utilizing an accessory pathway (i.e., the tachycardia breaks because of prolonged antegrade conduction through the AV node). With ventriculoatrial (VA) association, however, both junctional and ventricular tachycardia may also end with a P wave. AVNR = atrioventricular nodal reentry; AVRT = atrioventricular reciprocating tachycardia; PVC = premature ventricular complex.

REFERENCES

1. Akhtar M, Shenasa M, Jazayeri M, Caceres J, and Tchou P: Wide QRS complex tachycardia: Reappraisal of a common clinical problem. Ann Intern Med 109:905–912, 1988.
2. Benditt DG, Pritchett ELC, Smith WM, and Gallagher JJ: Ventriculoatrial intervals: Diagnostic use in paroxysmal supraventricular tachycardia. Ann Intern Med 91:161–166, 1979.
3. Kremers MS, Black MH, Wells P, and Solodyna M: Effect of preexisting bundle branch block on the electrocardiographic diagnosis of ventricular tachycardia. Am J Cardiol 62:1208–1212, 1988.
4. Kuchar DL, Thorburn CW, Sammel NL, Garan H, and Ruskin JN: Surface electrocardiographic manifestations of tachyarrhythmias: Clues to diagnosis and mechanism. PACE 11:61–82, 1988.
5. Miles W, Prystowsky EN, Heger J, and Zipes DP: Evaluation of the patient with wide QRS tachycardia. Med Clin North Am 68:1015–1038, 1984.
6. Akhtar M, Mahmud R, Tchou P, Denker S, and Gilbert CJ: Normal electrophysiologic response of the human heart. Cardiol Clin 265:365–386, 1986.
7. Gillette PC and Garson AL: Electrophysiologic and pharmacologic characteristics of automatic ectopic atrial tachycardia. Circulation 56:571–575, 1977.
8. Stewart RB, Bardy GH, and Greene HL: Wide complex tachycardia: Misdiagnosis and outcome after emergent therapy. Ann Intern Med 104:766–771, 1986.
9. Waxman MB, Wald RW, Sharma AD, Huerta F, and Cameron DA: Vagal techniques for termination of paroxysmal supraventricular tachycardia. Am J Cardiol 46:655–664, 1980.

CHAPTER 9

The Nonparoxysmal Atrial Tachycardias

ROBERT A. WAUGH, MD, and
GALEN S. WAGNER, MD

Outline

The sinus node (synonyms are *sino-atrial* [*SA*] *node* and *sinoauricular node*) contains the highest concentration of pacemaking cells, which normally have the fastest rate of diastolic depolarization. The location of the sinus node in the high right atrium explains why normal atrial depolarization produces upright P waves in electrocardiogram (ECG) leads I, II, and aVF. Other potential atrial pacemaking cells are located throughout the atria, particularly in the right atrium and the area surrounding the atrioventricular (AV) node. Under appropriate circumstances, these potential pacemakers can be accelerated and cause clinically apparent tachyarrhythmias.

This chapter discusses those tachycardias that are atrial in origin and, for the most part, reflect accelerated phase-4 diastolic depolarization. Enhanced normal or abnormal automaticity is the basic mechanism that produces nonparoxysmal tachycardias. Where appropriate, triggered automaticity, another potential mechanism, is discussed as well. Table 9–1 summarizes the classification, mechanisms, and important ECG characteristics of these nonparoxysmal or automatic atrial tachyarrhythmias. The junctional or His bundle tachycardias, though "supraventricular" and for the most part due to enhanced automaticity, are not atrial in origin. Chapter 11 discusses them in more detail (see Chapter 11, pages 239 to 240).

CLASSIFICATION

The nonparoxysmal atrial tachycardias are (1) sinus tachycardia, (2) wandering atrial pacemaker, (3) multifocal atrial tachycardia (MAT), and (4) automatic atrial tachycardias. Except for sinus tachycardia, a multiplicity of terms and controversies surround the nomenclature and postulated mechanisms of these various atrial rhythm problems.

Sinus Tachycardia

Sinus tachycardia is the most common nonparoxysmal atrial tachyarrhythmia, but it is neither a "disorder" of automaticity nor even an arrhythmia per se. It is a normal response to physiologic stimulation (Fig. 9–1). Because it is so common and so often related to symptoms such as palpitations, however, it warrants inclusion in the differential diagnosis of many tachyarrhythmias. Thus, it receives independent treatment in this text.

Table 9–1. MECHANISMS AND ECG CHARACTERISTICS OF ATRIAL TACHYCARDIAS

CLASSIFICATION	MECHANISM	RATE RANGE (beats/min)*	ATRIAL MORPHOLOGY	PR INTERVAL	HIGHER-DEGREE BLOCK
Sinus tachycardia	Enhanced normal automaticity	100–220	Discrete, constant	<0.20 sec	No
Wandering atrial pacemaker	Enhanced normal automaticity and/or sinus default	<100	Discrete, variable	Variable	No
Multifocal atrial tachycardia	Enhanced normal, enhanced abnormal, and/or triggered automaticity	>100 but <220	Discrete, variable	Variable, usually <0.2 sec	No
Sustained automatic atrial tachycardia	Enhanced abnormal and/or triggered automaticity	>100 but <220	Discrete, constant	>0.2 sec	Yes

*Rate ranges are a rough guide: a given arrhythmia is not excluded by a higher or lower rate.

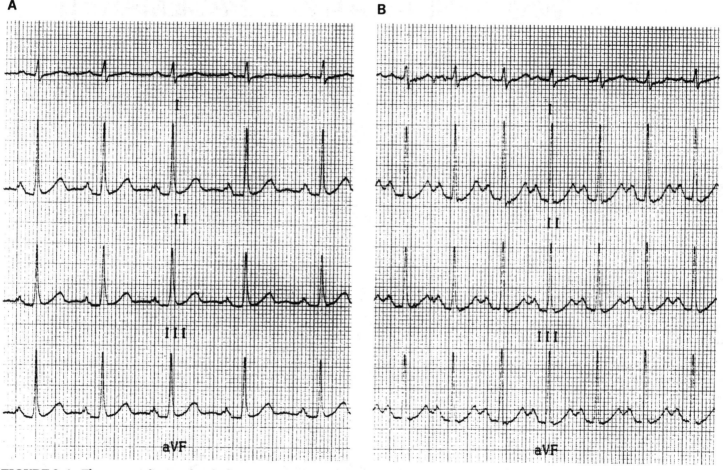

FIGURE 9–1. These recordings, taken before (*A*) and during (*B*) exercise, illustrate the changes in sinus P waves caused by sinus tachycardia. At peak exercise, the P-wave amplitude and peaking increase. Similar P-wave changes can also result from intravenous sympathetic agonists—hence the term, "epinephrine P waves."

WANDERING ATRIAL PACEMAKER

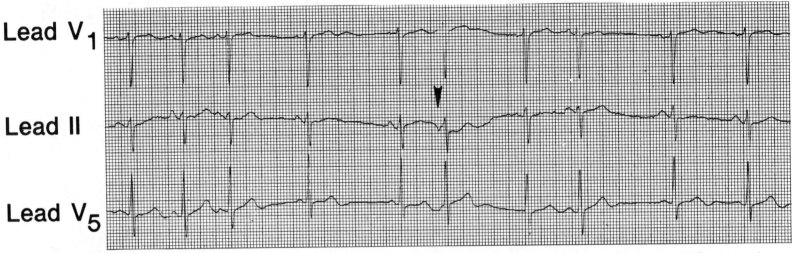

FIGURE 9–2. This example of wandering atrial pacemaker was recorded in an asymptomatic 84-year-old patient. At least three different atrial pacemaker sites are reflected by corresponding morphologic changes in the P wave and changes in the P-P intervals. The variability in the PR interval most likely reflects variability in the distance of the atrial pacemaker site from the atrioventricular (AV) node. The shortest PR interval follows an inverted P wave in lead II (arrowhead), compatible with a low atrial (i.e., perinodal) pacing site. Though not seen here, PR intervals may also vary inversely as a function of the timing of the P wave in relation to the preceding R wave (i.e., short RP intervals reflect recent AV node depolarization with subsequent PR prolongation, and vice versa).

Wandering Atrial Pacemaker

Wandering atrial pacemaker (Fig. 9–2) is a generally accepted term. Frequently added are specifications of where the pacemaker is wandering to (e.g., *wander-ing pacemaker within the sinus node* and *wandering pacemaker from the sinus node to the AV node*). These judgments, based on P-wave morphology, are inexact and bereft of clinical significance.

Wandering atrial pacemaker, by virtue of one component of its definition (rate less than 100 beats per minute), does not fulfill the classic definition of tachycardia (rate greater than 100 beats per minute). On the other hand, tachycardia is a relative term. Except for sinus tachycardia, all automatic atrial rhythms with rates greater than 60 and less than 100 beats per minute are more rapid than an escape rhythm and, therefore, are technically tachycardias (see Chapter 1).

Multifocal Atrial Tachycardia

Multifocal atrial tachycardia (MAT) and *chaotic atrial tachycardia (CAT)* are interchangeable terms. *Multifocal atrial tachycardia* is the term used in this text.

Automatic Atrial Tachycardia

The remaining automatic atrial tachycardias have a variety of names. Some use the term *ectopic atrial tachycardia* to refer interchangeably to all automatic and reentry atrial tachycardias that are not sinus tachycardia, AV junctional reentry tachycardia, or atrial flutter-fibrillation. Indeed, differentiating reentry from automaticity is frequently difficult and the therapy is commonly the same. This chapter discusses the nonparoxysmal (or automatic) pacemaker atrial tachycardias, and Chapter 10 discusses the paroxysmal (or reentry) atrial tachycardias.

LOW ATRIAL SITES

The term *nodal rhythm* typically refers to arrhythmias with negative P waves in ECG leads II, III, and aVF. These P waves may precede (usually by less than 0.12 second), coincide with, or follow the QRS complex. The term *nodal tachycardia* re-fers to similar rhythms with a rate greater than 60 beats per minute. Because there is controversy whether the AV node itself can function as a pacemaker when nonsinus P waves precede the QRS complex (regardless of their morphologic characteristics), the rhythm is considered atrial. Rhythms with normal QRS complexes and no preceding P waves (regardless of whether retrograde ventriculoatrial conduction occurs) are considered junctional (i.e., from the distal AV node–His bundle area) (see Chapter 11, pages 239 to 240).

There are no data to indicate that the diagnosis, therapy, or prognosis of these automatic atrial tachycardias depends on site of origin. The low tachycardias, however, are sufficiently common to merit special attention even though they are grouped generically as automatic atrial tachycardias.

ATRIAL TACHYCARDIA WITH AV BLOCK

Use of the term *paroxysmal atrial tachycardia (PAT) with block* to refer to all atrial tachycardias with AV block (usually second-degree with 2:1 conduction) is misleading and often incorrect. It is erroneous because automatic atrial tachycardias are *non*paroxysmal in onset or offset (although abrupt exit block may simulate the termination of a reentry tachycardia). In addition, whether AV block is present depends on the atrial rate, on autonomic balance, and on whether digitalis is a causative factor. Furthermore, there are *true* paroxysmal atrial tachycardias (e.g., sinus and intra-atrial reentry [see Chapter 10, pages 203 to 206]) that may or may not have AV block. Finally, and again inappropriately, AV junctional reentry tachycardia is often called PAT. This arrhythmia is not primarily atrial and, when AV nodal, also rarely may show block to either the atria or the ventricles. Using the same name for these widely divergent supraventricular tachycardias does little to clarify the issues. The preferred nomenclature is the most specific and least confusing possible—for example, *automatic atrial tachycardia with 2:1 AV block*.

MECHANISMS

As noted in Chapter 1 (page 8), tachycardias can arise from either enhanced normal or abnormal automaticity, and these mechanisms probably account for most pacemaker-induced atrial tachycardias. The discovery of triggered automaticity[1] and the persistent speculation that it may cause a variety of arrhythmias[2,3] have complicated the clinical approach to arrhythmias (see Chapter 1, page 8). Triggered automaticity shows interesting parallels to some clinical arrhythmias, but its clinical importance remains controversial. Until recently, the induction of triggered automaticity has been a laboratory phenomenon requiring nonphysiologic tissue manipulations (e.g., a perfusate sodium concentration of zero). A recent study, however, reported a new calcium channel that is operative under physiologic conditions and that might be responsible for the induction of triggered automaticity during clinical digitalis toxicity.[4] Although this study was not performed in an intact cell, its findings lend credibility to the possible clinical role of triggered automaticity.

If it is proved to be a cause of clinical arrhythmias, triggered automaticity will be a confounding variable in the clinical approach to arrhythmia diagnosis. For example, the appearance of a "burst" of triggered activity (i.e., activity that is abrupt in onset and offset [see Fig. 1–5]) may be difficult to differentiate from a reentry mechanism. Table 9–1 summarizes the mechanisms of the various automatic atrial tachycardias.

Sinus Tachycardia

The sinus node normally has the fastest rate of phase-4 diastolic depolarization, both at rest and with changes in autonomic balance. The sinus node is therefore the dominant pacemaker under widely varying conditions. Sinus tachycardias occur most commonly in response to increased sympathetic tone. They also may reflect withdrawal of parasympathetic tone (e.g., the administration of atropine) either alone or in combination with increased sympathetic tone

(e.g., exercise). Sinus tachycardia is therefore due to enhanced normal automaticity and is a physiologic, not pathologic, response to changes in autonomic balance initiated by a variety of stimuli (see Fig. 9–1).

Wandering Atrial Pacemaker

A wandering atrial pacemaker is due to enhanced automaticity of pacemaker cells from one or more atrial sites that compete with the sinus node. The competing pacemakers may be located anywhere in the atria (including a different area of the sinus node) or in the His bundle. In healthy young adults, this arrhythmia is frequently due to enhanced parasympathetic tone suppressing the sinus node and allowing the emergence of an escape junctional rhythm. In this latter instance, the arrhythmias also might be considered a bradyarrhythmia due to pacemaker failure. In the elderly, the arrhythmia is independent of vagal tone and frequently is sustained. In this age group, it probably reflects degenerative atrial changes related to age and associated instability of the sinus node pacemaker (see Fig. 9–2).

Multifocal Atrial Tachycardia

Multifocal atrial tachycardia is due to the emergence of more than two competing atrial sites at an average rate that qualifies as "tachycardia" (i.e., greater than 100 beats per minute). It frequently occurs during acute respiratory illness, when factors enhancing normal and abnormal automaticity (endogenous and exogenous catecholamines and bronchodilators) are likely to be high. A sensitivity (even without toxic serum levels) to xanthine derivatives also may be an etiologic factor.[5]

A favorable response to verapamil provides circumstantial evidence that calcium-mediated triggered automaticity plays an etiologic role.[2] In addition, isoproterenol induces triggered activity in the atria of laboratory animals.[6] On the other hand, MAT does not occur exclusively with either acute respiratory failure or xanthine-derivative therapy, and verapamil is not always effective.[7] The likelihood that MAT may reflect any of these three mechanisms should be kept in mind.

Automatic Atrial Tachycardias

Atrial pacemaker cells remote from the sinus node (i.e., "ectopic" pacemakers) may become dominant either on a transient basis or on a more more sustained basis, with a rate range similar to that of sinus tachycardia. They reflect a faster rate of phase-4 diastolic depolarization of these sites as compared with that of the SA node. Contributing factors are most often drugs, metabolic influences, enhanced sympathetic tone (in combination with default of the sinus node), or disease processes such as inflammation or ischemia. The basic mechanisms are most likely enhanced normal and abnormal automaticity.

Usually, these automatic atrial arrhythmias begin at rates fast enough to capture and overdrive the sinus node. Slowing of the sinus pacer usually results in an escape (or nonacclerated) rhythm from a lower site. On occasion, a latent, initially slow ectopic atrial pacemaker may emerge and then "warm up" to a faster rate.

Digitalis has a predominantly parasympathetic effect on the normal sinus node, whereas it enhances diastolic depolarization in other pacemaking tissue. This facilitates the emergence of nonsinus pacemaker rhythms, including atrial, AV junctional, and ventricular tachycardias.[8] In the experimental laboratory, digitalis[2] or ouabain[9] can induce triggered automaticity, another possible mechanism for some digitalis-toxic rhythms.

Regardless of the basic mechanism, when stimulation occurs in the atria, a *nonparoxysmal* or automatic atrial tachycardia results. If the dominant effect is in

the His bundle or bundle branches, then accelerated junctional or ventricular arrhythmias result (see Chapter 11, pages 239 to 240, and Chapter 12, pages 264 to 265).

CLINICAL METHODS OF DIAGNOSIS
Sinus Tachycardia

As discussed earlier, sinus tachycardia displays the classic hallmark of enhanced automaticity—a gradual onset and offset (Fig. 9–3). In addition, its P waves are

MCL 1

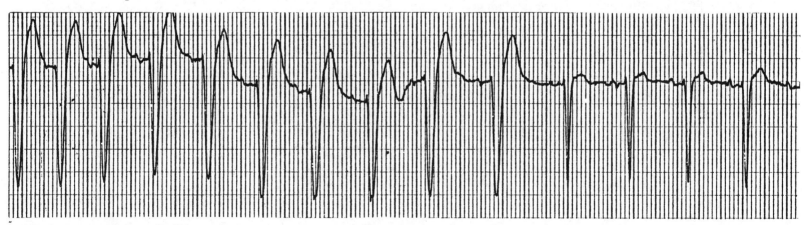

FIGURE 9–3. During exercise, this patient developed a wide-QRS tachycardia at 150 beats per minute, with one apparent P wave before each QRS complex and a PR interval of about 0.12 second. After cessation of exercise, gradual slowing and the clear emergence of one P wave for each QRS complex proved the diagnosis of sinus tachycardia. With slowing, the left bundle branch block also resolved, proving the diagnosis of tachycardia-dependent left bundle branch aberration. (Note the decreased QRS width and the repolarization changes of the last four QRS complexes.)

A

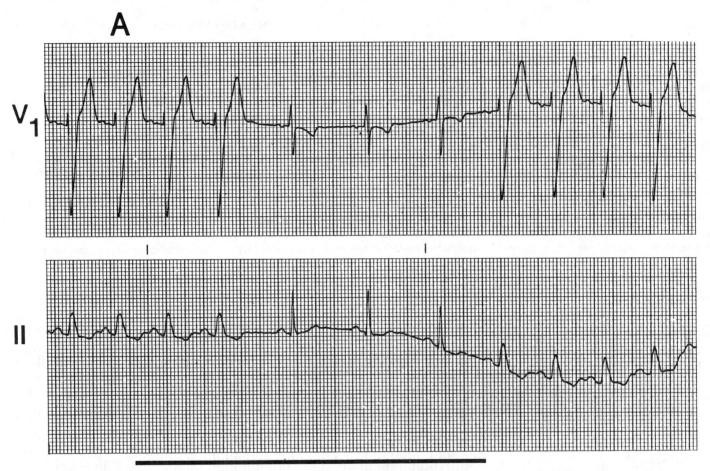

Carotid Sinus Massage

FIGURE 9–4. These two recordings illustrate the use of carotid sinus massage to resolve the differential diagnosis of wide-QRS tachycardias. In both recordings, carotid sinus massage produced two classic features of sinus tachycardia: gradual rate slowing and the emergence of P waves identical to those of sinus rhythm. (*A*) During carotid sinus massage, the QRS complex also transiently narrowed, proving that the wide QRS complex was due to tachycardia-dependent left bundle branch (LBB) aberration.

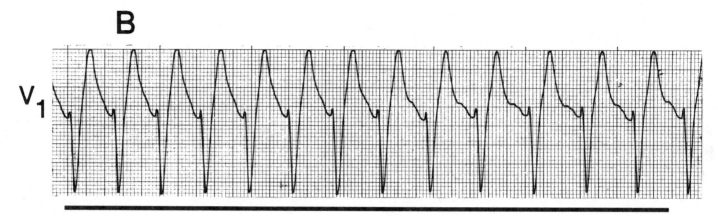

Carotid Sinus Massage

FIGURE 9–4. (*Continued*) (*B*) During carotid sinus massage, the QRS configuration persisted unchanged, proving that the widened QRS complex was due to fixed LBB aberration.

morphologically similar to those of sinus rhythm. A slightly different P-wave configuration, however, does not rule out sinus tachycardia. Increased P-wave peaking, particularly in leads II, III, and aVF (see Fig. 9–1), can occur during sinus tachycardia from both exercise[10] and intravenous catecholamines.[11] This peaking may reflect a shift of the dominant pacemaker within the SA node itself, but a variety of poorly defined factors are probably responsible. The lower rate range for sinus tachycardia is greater than 100 beats per minute. The upper rate for a young healthy subject in response to maximal stimulation (e.g., exercise, intravenous isoproterenol) may exceed 220 beats per minute. The rate in the nonexercising, hospitalized adult rarely exceeds 160 beats per minute. Atrioventricular conduction is 1:1 with a shorter PR interval than during sinus rhythm, because the same factors that accelerate the sinus node also accelerate AV nodal conduction. The QRS complex is that of sinus rhythm unless there is tachycardia-dependent aberrant intraventricular conduction (Fig. 9–4; see Fig. 9–3; Chapter 4, pages 81 to 82; Chapter 7, pages 146 to 154; and Chapter 12, pages 266 to 279).

Wandering Atrial Pacemaker

An atrial rate less than 100 beats per minute with two or more different P-wave configurations defines wandering atrial pacemaker. Sometimes, however, it is difficult to tell whether morphologic differences between waves reflect different sites of origin or atrial fusion beats. Enhanced vagal tone is a common cause for wandering atrial pacemakers that vary in phase with respiration. Pulmonary-mediated reflexes further slow the sinus node and shift the pacemaker to the AV junc-

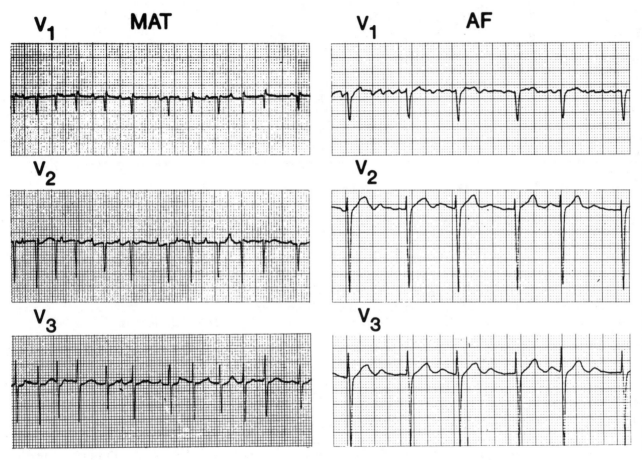

FIGURE 9–5. These simultanous electrocardiographic leads V_1, V_2, and V_3 contrast multifocal atrial tachycardia (MAT) with atrial fibrillation (AF). With MAT, discrete P waves of more than two different morphologic types precede each QRS complex with an overall rate greater than 100 per minute. The PR intervals vary with P-wave prematurity (i.e., there is a reciprocal RP-PR relationship [see Figs. 9–6 and 9–13]); however, even very premature P waves conduct (e.g., the P wave following the third QRS complex in the left-hand portion of the strip), which reflects the high sympathetic tone in this patient with chronic lung disease and acute respiratory failure. With atrial fibrillation, discrete P waves are replaced by a continuously undulating baseline best seen in V_1. Both MAT and atrial fibrillation produce an irregularly irregular ventricular response.

tion. In the elderly, the PP intervals are usually grossly irregular. The PR intervals vary from normal to prolonged, depending on the distance of the various competing sites from the AV node and their prematurity (i.e., the shorter the RP interval, the longer the subsequent PR interval) (see Fig. 9–2).

Multifocal Atrial Tachycardia

An irregularly irregular atrial tachycardia averaging more than 100 beats per minute with more than two different P-wave configurations defines MAT (Fig. 9–5). Atrial rates most often are between 130 and 180 beats per minute, but may exceed 200 beats per minute. The PR intervals vary inversely with the degree of prematurity of the P wave. Very early P waves may block, owing to physiologic refractoriness of the AV node. More typically, the high sympathetic tone of the usual clinical setting helps the AV conduction of even very premature P waves (see Fig. 9–5 and pages 197–198). The QRS configuration is usually similar to that of sinus rhythm, although the irregularity of the rhythm, like atrial fibrillation, produces long and short cycles that favor aberration of the early beats. The differentiation of MAT from atrial fibrillation is important because the two arrhythmias frequently occur in the same clinical settings and even in the same patients. Recognizing the discrete P waves of MAT versus the totally irregular, nondiscrete atrial activity of fibrillation (see Fig. 9–5) is key to the correct diagnosis. When the P waves are diminutive or obscured by ST-T waves, esophageal or intra-atrial monitoring (with or without an intervention to slow the ventricular response) may help.

Automatic Atrial Tachycardias

NONSUSTAINED AUTOMATIC ATRIAL TACHYCARDIAS

Nonsustained automatic atrial tachycardias are most often from 3 to 20 beats per minute with irregular and variable atrial rates (Figs. 9–6 and 9–7). They begin with a premature P wave that differs morphologically from that of sinus rhythm, but the initiating and subsequent P-wave configurations are the same. These tachycardias also show a gradual, though frequently irregular, rate acceleration (or warm-up), typical of a pacemaker mechanism. The rate may be anything that is faster than the sinus rate (rates less than 100 beats per minute are common), and peak rates rarely exceed 180 per minute. The PR intervals vary inversely with P-wave prematurity and rate and vary directly with distance of the ectopic site from the AV node. Their offset also may be gradual, but abrupt termination is common (see Fig. 9–6).

SUSTAINED AUTOMATIC ATRIAL TACHYCARDIAS

Sustained automatic atrial tachycardias are much less common than the nonsustained variety. The atrial rates can reach 220 beats per minute or more in the adult and even higher in children. In children, and to a lesser extent in adults, they show marked temporal rate variability both spontaneously and in response to treatment.

The P-wave characteristics are similar to those of nonsustained automatic atrial tachycardias. At rates under 150 beats per minute, 1:1 AV conduction with first-degree AV block is common. The PR interval varies with the proximity of the ectopic site to the AV node, its prematurity and rate, autonomic AV nodal tone, and whether digitalis or other AV-node–active drugs are present.

Low Atrial Origin. A "low" atrial tachycardia is sufficiently frequent to merit separate consideration. Negative P waves in leads II, III, and aVF precede each QRS complex. The PR interval is usually 0.12 second or less, and the rate range is variable but typically less than 120 beats per minute and regular. A similar rhythm features a PR interval greater than 0.12 second. These rhythms can be

MCL 1

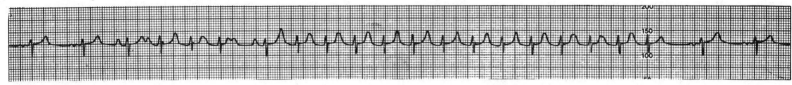

MCL 5

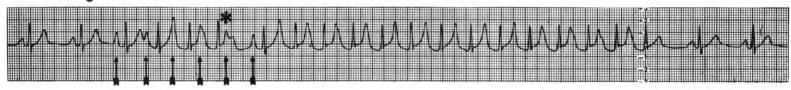

FIGURE 9–6. This nonsustained supraventricular tachycardia was recorded in a 63-year-old woman. Her "palpitations" reflected premature ventricular complexes, and this run of supraventricular tachycardia was asymptomatic. Two sinus beats are followed by an atrial tachycardia whose initial and subsequent P waves were morphologically identical. (The arrows denote the inciting and subsequent five P waves of the tachycardia.) The atrial rate accelerates, is somewhat irregular, and shows variable AV conduction (i.e., there is reciprocal RP-PR variability; one very premature P wave is even nonconducted [asterisk]). The tachycardia then terminates abruptly. A QRS complex is the last complex of the tachycardia. These features are typical of enhanced automaticity (i.e., a nonparoxysmal mechanism) from an "ectopic" atrial focus. The abrupt offset likely reflects exit block from the site of enhanced automaticity. This finding is particularly common in this age group, and the condition rarely produces symptoms, reflects serious heart disease, or requires therapy.

produced by pacing from the ostia and from within the coronary sinus (and presumably, therefore, the left atrium), so that the terms *coronary sinus rhythm* and *left atrial rhythm* are used(see Fig. 9–7).[12]

Automatic atrial tachycardias with monomorphic P waves that are different from sinus P waves and yet not inverted in the inferior ECG leads presumably reflect still other atrial sites of origin.

Digitalis Toxicity. Supraventricular tachycardias with any degree or periodicity of AV block and atrial rates under 220 beats per minute should strongly suggest a digitalis-induced automatic atrial tachycardia (Fig. 9–8).

With atrial tachycardias due to digitalis, the P-wave vector is usually normal (Fig. 9–9, *left*). The P-wave configuration, however, is frequently diminutive and different from that of sinus rhythm.[8] The rate ranges (100 to 220 beats per minute) parallel those of sinus tachycardia and many other supraventricular tachycardias. The PP intervals are usually slightly irregular when slower and more regular when faster. With atrial rates from 130 to 150 beats per minute, AV conduction is frequently 1:1 but with a prolonged PR interval. The significance of the latter finding is frequently missed.

With the administration of more digitalis, faster atrial rates follow, with either type I or fixed second-degree AV block. The block reflects increased AV nodal refractoriness due to both the faster atrial

MCL 1

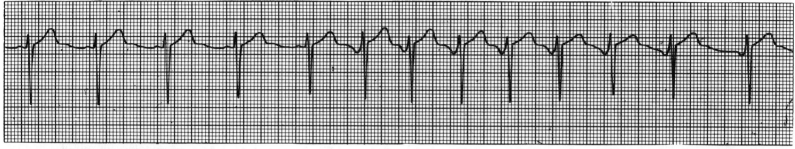

MODIFIED II

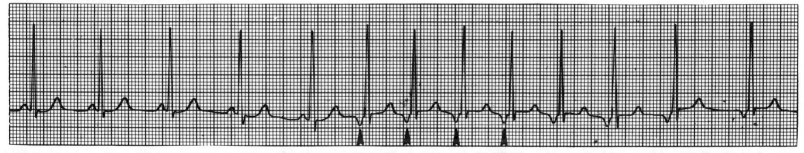

FIGURE 9–7. In this asymptomatic teenager, after five beats of sinus rhythm, a nonparoxysmal (or automatic) focus emerges. The inverted P waves in modified lead II (arrowheads) reflect a low atrial site. Note that this PR interval is not less than 0.12 second, a difference from the usual low atrial "junctional" rhythm, in which the P waves precede the QRS complex by less than 0.12 second. Inverted P waves and this PR interval can be produced by pacing from the coronary sinus ostia or from within them (hence the terms "coronary sinus" and "left atrial" rhythms). In this case, the peak atrial rate only transiently exceeded 100, but even the average rate exceeds the usual escape atrial rate and so is still classified as a tachycardia. Its persistence despite subsequent slowing to a rate less than that of the initial sinus rhythm is due to overdrive suppression of the sinus node.

K⁺ - 3.1 mEq/L: Digoxin Level - 4.6 ng/ml

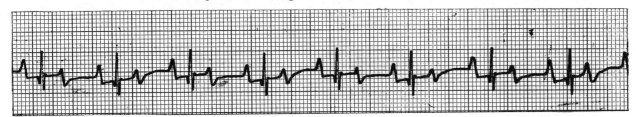

Withheld Digoxin; Replaced Potassium
K⁺ - 4.6 mEq/L: Digoxin Level - 2.2 ng/ml

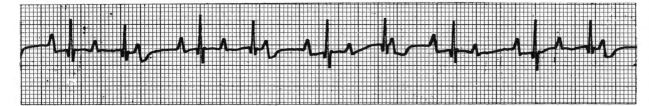

FIGURE 9–8. *(Top)* This patient with an elevated serum digoxin level (4.6 ng/ml) and hypokalemia (3.1 mEq/L) developed an atrial tachycardia (167 beats per minute) with 2:1 AV block. Digoxin therapy was withheld, and the hypokalemia was corrected. *(Bottom)* Twenty-four hours later, potassium and digoxin levels had improved. Although the atrial rate had slowed to 136 beats per minute, 2:1 AV block persisted. This sequence is typical of a digitalis-induced, nonparoxysmal (or automatic) atrial tachycardia. With continued observation and withholding of digoxin therapy, normal sinus rhythm returned 12 hours later.

rate and the direct depressant effect of digitalis.[8] When digitalis toxicity is suspected, serum drug and potassium levels should be measured. With hypokalemia, with or without an elevated serum digitalis level, slowing of the atrial rate or resolution of the tachycardia with either potassium supplementation (carefully avoiding iatrogenic hyperkalemia) or

stopping further digitalis therapy is almost diagnostic of a digitalis-induced automatic atrial tachycardia (see Fig. 9–8).

DIFFERENTIAL DIAGNOSIS

Differentiating sinus tachycardia from automatic atrial tachycardia, atrial flutter, and other atrial or AV junctional tachycardias (with or without AV block) is a com-

mon clinical problem. The following sections discuss this differential diagnosis, including the importance of the atrial rate and morphology, the mode of onset and offset, the status of AV conduction, and the response of the tachyarrhythmia to interventions. Just as with all supraventricular tachycardias, a QRS width of 0.12 second or more adds ventricular tachycardia

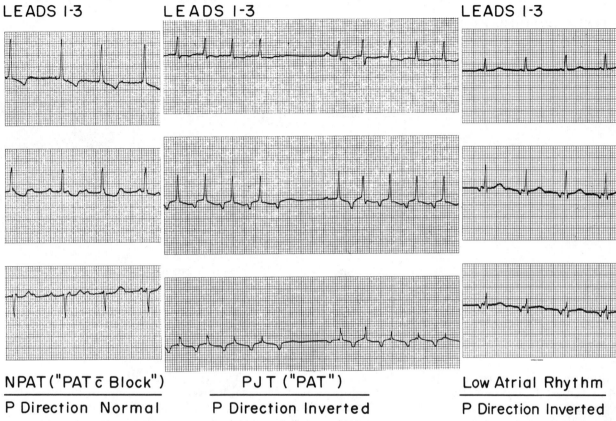

LEADS I-3   **LEADS I-3**   **LEADS I-3**

NPAT ("PAT c̄ Block")   PJT ("PAT")   Low Atrial Rhythm

P Direction Normal   P Direction Inverted   P Direction Inverted

FIGURE 9–9. These three electrocardiographic recordings of simultaneous leads, I, II, and III (1 to 3) show the morphologic differences in P waves with various atrial tachycardias. *(Left)* Atrial tachycardias due to digitalis typically produce P waves that have a relatively normal axis (approximately 90° in this example), compatible with a location high in the right atrium. The P waves of other atrial tachycardias also depend on the site of atrial origin. *(Middle)* With paroxysmal AV junctional tachycardia (PJT), inverted P waves in leads II and III reflect retrograde atrial activation from the area of AV junctional reentry. In this example, PJT was due to retrograde atrial activation via an accessory pathway. (Note the characteristic relatively long RP interval.) With PJT due to atrioventricular nodal reentry, the P waves and QRS complexes are passive participants, and while the "apparent" RP interval tends to be short (most often, the P waves and QRS complexes are simultaneous), the relationships between P waves and QRS complexes can be quite variable. In the midportion of this strip, the PJT ceases briefly, and one sinus P wave occurs, allowing direct comparison of the P waves of sinus rhythm with those of PJT. *(Right)* A low atrial tachycardia (a frequent variety of nonparoxysmal atrial tachycardia [NPAT]) also produces retrograde atrial activation with negative P waves in leads II and III. Note, however, that the atrial rate is much slower than that of PJT. The P waves also precede the QRS complexes by less than 0.12 second, which is consistent with an ectopic atrial focus near the AV node. (Compare with Fig. 9–7.) PAT = paroxysmal atrial tachycardia.

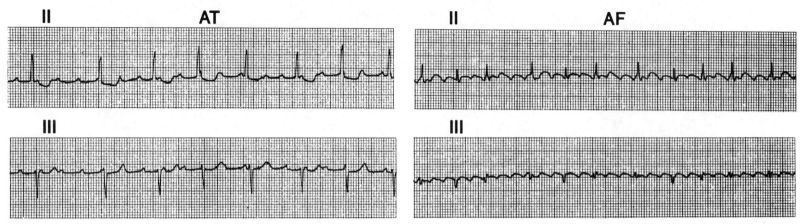

FIGURE 9–10. These two electrocardiograms (ECGs), from different patients, illustrate the utility of atrial morphology in the differential diagnosis of atrial tachycardias. With automatic atrial tachycardia (AT) (atrial rate = 188 beats per minute), there is variable, but predominantly 2:1, AV block. The single atrial focus causes discrete periods of atrial depolarization and repolarization corresponding to the discrete P waves and intervening isoelectric PP intervals. With atrial flutter (AF) (atrial rate = 270 beats per minute), there is variable AV block. The continually reentering atrial wave front corresponds to the typical "sawtooth" atrial electrogram (usually best seen in leads II, III, and aVF). Note the lack of a discrete isoelectric interval separating the repetitive and morphologically constant "F" (or flutter) waves.

to the diagnostic dilemma. (Fig. 9–10; see Figs. 9–3 and 9–4).

Atrial Rate. Although there may be overlap in the rate ranges for these tachyarrhythmias, an accurate measurement of atrial rate can be helpful in the differential diagnosis. For example, atrial rates above 220 beats per minute likely reflect atrial flutter. At slower atrial rates (typically 200 to 220 beats per minute), atrial flutter remains a possibility, especially with hyperkalemia or the use of class Ia or class Ic drugs. (The class Ic drugs, in particular, may be associated with atrial rates well

below 200 beats per minute.) The response of the atrial rate to a vagal intervention is also a helpful differential point; speeding favors atrial flutter (see Chapter 4, page 93, Chapter 10, page 218 and Fig. 10–11).

Morphology, Onset, and Offset of Atrial Activity. With sinus tachycardia, the P-wave morphologic characteristics of the initial and subsequent beats are constant and similar to those of sinus rhythm. With automatic atrial tachycardias, the initiating and subsequent P waves are also morphologically constant

but differ morphologically from those of sinus rhythm. With reentry atrial and AV junctional tachycardias, the initiating P wave differs morphologically from that of the ensuing tachycardia. With automatic atrial tachycardias and intra-atrial and AV junctional reentry tachycardias, the P waves occurring during the tachycardia are discrete (Fig. 9–10, AT). With generalized atrial reentry, a sawtooth pattern of atrial activity is typical (see Fig. 9–10; Chapter 5, page 110 and Fig. 5–2; and Chapter 10, pages 210 to 212 and Fig. 10–1).

The nonparoxysmal nature of sinus tachycardia (see Figs. 9–1, 9–3, and 9–4) and the other pacemaker atrial tachycardias versus the sudden onset and offset of reentry supraventricular tachycardias is also a helpful differential point. Whereas a sudden onset with no warm-up favors reentry, an abrupt offset is less conclusive, because exit block from the pacemaker site is common and mimics termination of reentry.

AV Conduction. Apparent sinus tachycardia with first-degree AV block should always raise the question of automatic (nonsinus) atrial tachycardia with 1:1 AV conduction. Alternatively, missing a second, hidden P wave means missing the diagnosis of atrial flutter or an automatic atrial tachycardia with 2:1 AV block (Figure 9–11).

With all atrial tachycardias, the status of AV conduction depends on several factors. These include the atrial rate, autonomic balance, the presence of digitalis or other AV-node–active drugs, and the underlying "health" of the AV node itself.

Response to an Intervention. If the P-wave morphology and rate, PR relationship, or the onset and offset of the tachycardia cannot be analyzed, then it may be necessary to perform a vagal maneuver (see Chapter 4, pages 73 to 76; Chapter 10, page 218; Chapter 11, pages 251 to 255). Transient rate slowing identifies sinus tachycardia (see Fig. 9–4), abrupt cessation identifies AV junctional reentry (see Fig. 9–9, *middle*), and an increase in the AV block identifies either an automatic atrial tachycardia or atrial reentry (see Fig. 9–11).

Note that with all *intra*-atrial tachycardias, the degree of AV block may increase in response to a vagal maneuver while the basic arrhythmia remains unperturbed. Increased AV block, therefore, is not a helpful differential point. Sinus tachycardia is least likely to exhibit increased AV block in response to enhanced vagal tone; when it does occur, it usually identifies concomitant AV-node disease (Fig. 9–12). Sometimes, esophageal or intra-atrial monitoring, with or without a vagal intervention, may be necessary to identify the atrial rate, its vagal responsiveness, and the AV relationship.

INTERACTION WITH THE AUTONOMIC NERVOUS SYSTEM

The sinus node slows in response to vagal stimulation and speeds back to its original rate once the maneuver ceases (see Fig. 9–4). The rate of automatic atrial tachycardias is not responsive to vagal stimulation. Changes in sympathetic tone, on the other hand, can vary the sinus rate, sometimes dramatically. Whereas automatic atrial tachycardia rates also can vary in response to changes in sympathetic tone, the degree of change is less.

The ability of vagal maneuvers to induce AV block depends on the background sympathetic-parasympathetic balance and the underlying health of the AV node. When sympathetic tone is high (e.g., in the typical setting of sinus tachycardia), a vagal maneuver is unlikely to produce even first-degree AV block. With a diseased AV node (see Fig. 9–12), or with automatic atrial tachycardia, however, carotid sinus massage can increase the degree of AV block. With digitalis-induced automatic atrial tachycardia, the concomitant effects of digitalis and enhanced vagal tone on AV nodal conduction can produce marked increases in AV block. Patients with MAT are typically ill, and the resulting high sympathetic tone typically makes the atrial rate and AV conduction unresponsive to vagal maneuvers.

USE OF INVASIVE ELECTROPHYSIOLOGY

Invasive electrophysiologic studies (EPSs) are usually not necessary in either the diagnosis or treatment of these arrhythmias. On occasion, an esophageal electrogram may be technically inadequate or appear to identify atrial activity that is coincident with or obscured by the QRS complex. In such instances, an intra-atrial recording may reveal the true timing of atrial excitation. Occasionally, sustained atrial tachycardias unrelated to

A.

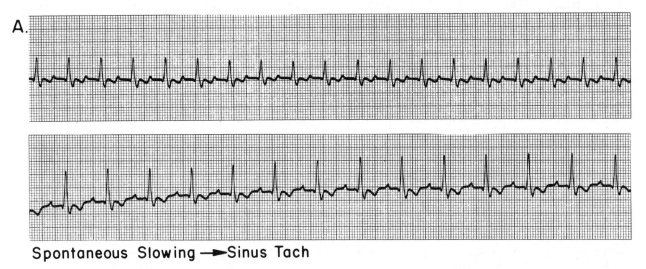

Spontaneous Slowing ➔Sinus Tach

B.

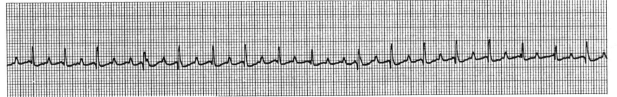

Spontaneous Slowing ➔At Flutter With 2:1 Block

FIGURE 9–11. These ECGs (*A* and *B*), from different patients, show apparent sinus tachycardia (Sinus Tach) and first-degree AV block. This combination should always arouse strong suspicion of either automatic atrial tachycardia with first-degree AV block, or automatic atrial tachycardia or atrial flutter with 2:1 AV conduction (and a second P wave that is not apparent on the ECG). In the bottom strip of (*A*), spontaneous slowing of the atrial rate allows identification of P waves similar morphologically to P waves of this patient's sinus rhythm. This finding proves the unusual occurrence of true sinus tachycardia with first-degree AV block. The bottom strip of (*B*) was recorded shortly after the top strip, during a spontaneous increase in the degree of AV block. It shows an atrial rate of 250 beats per minute with a sawtoothed atrial electrogram. Thus, the rhythm is atrial flutter with 2:1 AV conduction, not sinus tachycardia or automatic atrial tachycardia with first-degree AV block.

CAROTID SINUS MASSAGE

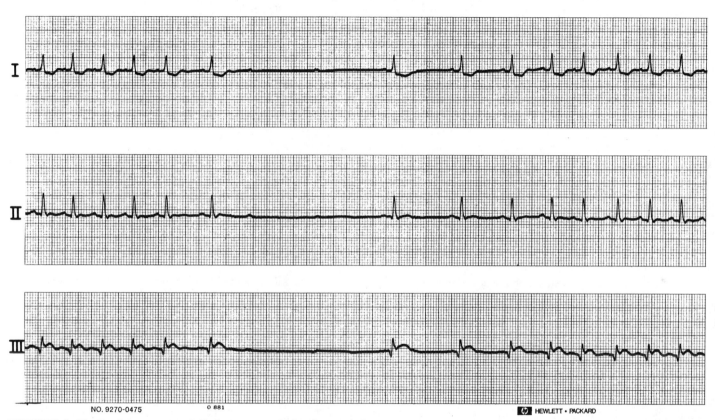

FIGURE 9–12. During an acute inferior myocardial infarction, this patient, who was not receiving digitalis, developed a regular, supraventricular tachycardia at 130 beats per minute with a normal PR interval. With the increased vagal tone of carotid sinus massage, the atrial rate slowed gradually, and the P waves were identical to those of sinus rhythm—two features typical of sinus tachycardia. In this patient, the tachycardia reflected an elevated sympathetic tone related to volume depletion. Carotid sinus massage also produced unexpected second-degree AV block with two nonconducted P waves. This AV block occurred despite increased sympathetic tone because the vagal effects of carotid sinus massage combined with the enhanced parasympathetic tone and ischemia in the AV node that are typical of acute inferior myocardial infarction.

digitalis are unresponsive to noninvasive diagnostic and empiric therapeutic interventions. Low-energy DC shock, esophageal pacing, or more detailed EPS may be necessary to differentiate automaticity from reentry (see Chapter 10, pages 206 to 207). With automatic atrial tachycardias, the rhythm cannot be elicited by atrial pacing but may be induced by the intravenous administration of sympathetic agonists. Premature atrial complexes and atrial pacing may reset and cause transient overdrive of these tachycardias but do not terminate them. For refractory automatic tachycardias, EPS also can test further drug therapy and pinpoint the site of tachycardia preparatory to its ablation or excision. Enthusiasm for the latter approach should be tempered, because the atrial pacemaker sites may be multiple and another can emerge to replace the ablated one.

CLINICAL FEATURES

Table 9–2 summarizes the approaches to management of the nonparoxysmal atrial tachycardias.

Table 9–2. PHARMACOLOGIC MANAGEMENT OF NONPAROXYSMAL (AUTOMATIC) ATRIAL TACHYCARDIAS

ARRHYTHMIA	TO SLOW ATRIAL RATE	TO SLOW VENTRICULAR RATE	TO CONVERT TO NSR
Sinus tachycardia	Treat underlying condition; administer β-blockers.	—	—
Wandering atrial pacemaker	—	—	—
Multifocal atrial tachycardia	Stop β-agonists and theophyllines; correct hypoxia.	Administer verapamil or β-blockers*	Administer verapamil or β-blockers.
Nonsustained atrial tachycardia	Administer verapamil or β-blocker.	—	—
Digitalis-induced atrial tachycardia	—	—	Stop digitalis; correct hypokalemia.
Non–digitalis-induced sustained atrial tachycardia	Administer β-blockers or class Ia or class Ic[†] drugs.	Administer β-blockers, verapamil, or digoxin.	Administer β-blockers or Class Ia or Class Ic[†] drugs

NSR = normal sinus rhythm.

*Digoxin is also frequently given because of the high incidence of associated atrial flutter-fibrillation, not as a method of controlling the ventricular rate during multifocal atrial tachycardia.

[†]Only flecainide is approved for treatment of this arrhythmia and then only in patients "without structural heart disease . . . with disabling symptoms." The use of flecainide or other drugs requires careful consideration but may be indicated in selected patients who have hemodynamically significant tachycardias that are refractory to conventional therapy.

Sinus Tachycardia

PREDISPOSING CLINICAL SETTINGS

An increase in sympathetic activity should produce sinus tachycardia, and when this does not happen, sinus node disease may be present. Sinus tachycardia commonly occurs in response to anxiety, but when patients do not perceive their anxiety, they may seek medical help for a "rapid heartbeat" or "pounding." Exercise is another common, easily recognized cause of sinus tachycardia. In hyperthyroidism, sinus tachycardia (even during sleep) is so usual that its absence (except with concomitant β-blocker therapy) should cast doubt on the diagnosis. Besides all the usual reasons, patients with heart disease may develop sinus tachycardia in response to congestive heart failure. Successful treatment of the failure secondarily diminishes sympathetic tone and leads to slowing of the heart rate.

NATURAL HISTORY

The natural history of sinus tachycardia is that of the underlying cause. In acute myocardial infarction, for example, sinus tachycardia is ominous when it reflects a high sympathetic tone from extensive myocardial damage. Sinus tachycardia usually slows with resolution of the inciting condition, and the slowing is gradual, in contrast to the abrupt termination of reentry tachycardias. At times, sinus tachycardia may persist after resolution of the inciting cause. For example, after exercise, a variable period must pass, depending on general conditioning and ventricular function, before the sinus rate returns to normal. Similarly, some patients develop sinus tachycardia during the early phase of acute myocardial infarction because of pain, anxiety, or ventricular dysfunction that persists after the inciting condition, or conditions, are resolved.

METHODS OF TREATMENT

Usually, treatment of sinus tachycardia itself is rarely indicated. Rather, the emphasis should be on identifying and correcting the underlying condition, such as treatment of infection to resolve fever and adequate analgesia to relieve pain. Treatment of hyperthyroidism normalizes the heart rate, although sometimes concomitant β-blocker therapy may be necessary to blunt the cardiovascular consequences of hyperthyroid storm. With inappropriate sinus tachycardia following myocardial infarction (i.e., no congestive heart failure), treatment with even a small dose of a β-blocker may sometimes cause prompt sinus slowing. With sinus tachycardia due to anxiety, anxiolytic drugs may be tried but are usually unsuccessful in the long term. The emphasis should be on identifying the source of anxiety.

When reassurance fails and patients continue to have intolerable palpitations, β-blocker therapy may blunt the sympathetic effects of anxiety and provide symptomatic relief. Drugs may be given as needed or, with frequent symptoms, continuously. In both situations, the initial dose should be low (e.g., 10 mg of propranolol three to four times per day or as needed). The dose can then be titrated up or down according the patient's response. "Up-regulation" of β-receptors over time may be associated with diminishing effectiveness of a given drug dose. Exercise training to enhance general cardiovascular conditioning and parasympathetic tone is a "physiologic" alternative.

Multifocal Atrial Tachycardia

CLINICAL SETTINGS AND NATURAL HISTORY

Multifocal atrial tachycardia occurs most often in the setting of acute respiratory failure, where hypoxia, hypercarbia, respiratory acidosis, and treatment with bronchodilators such as the xanthine derivatives are common. It also occurs with other conditions such as acute pulmonary embolism, congestive heart failure, coronary artery disease, valvular heart disease, and, rarely, as an isolated finding. It affects patients over a wide age range but is more common beyond the seventh decade. Concomitant digitalis therapy is frequent, although it is not a digitalis-toxic arrhythmia. (A patient may have both digitalis toxicity and MAT without any cause-effect relationship.)

Frequently, MAT reflects the severity of underlying pulmonary disease, respiratory failure, and theophylline levels, as does the associated high mortality rate. Its resolution typically mirrors successful therapy and falling theophylline levels. Any associated hemodynamic deterioration is usually due to the pulmonary disease, although with concomitant left heart disease, the tachycardia may contribute to worsening ventricular function, ischemia, and so forth.

METHODS OF TREATMENT

Treatment of underlying hypokalemia or hypomagnesemia and respiratory failure is a key first step in the management of MAT. The elimination of theophylline and sympathetic-agonist therapy usually resolves the arrhythmia.

The arrhythmia is typically resistant to treatment with the class I antiarrhythmic drugs. Because associated atrial fibrillation is common (occurring in up to 50% of patients), digitalis therapy is common. This drug, however, is ineffective in either converting the rhythm or slowing the ventricular response unless it reaches toxic levels with pathologic AV block. Verapamil (an intravenous 1-mg test dose followed by 4 mg over 5 minutes, and 5 minutes later [as necessary] another 5 mg over 5 minutes) can either terminate the arrhythmia or slow the rate of MAT (Fig. 9–13).[2] On the other hand, verapamil does not always work and metoprolol may be even more effective.[7] β-Blockers are contraindicated in the presence of heart failure or active bronchospasm. With chronic obstructive pulmonary disease, wheezing frequently reflects factors other than bronchospasm, and a number of studies have shown that their use is not associated with a deterioration in pulmonary function.

Automatic Atrial Tachycardias (Including Wandering Atrial Pacemaker)

CLINICAL SETTINGS AND NATURAL HISTORY

Wandering atrial pacemaker occurs in healthy young adults with a high resting parasympathetic tone, and in the elderly, where it is independent of vagal tone. It is usually an asymptomatic, incidental finding of no clinical significance other than to be differentiated from atrial fibrillation with a well-controlled ventricular response.

Occasionally, wandering atrial pacemaker may occur in concert with sinus nodal dysfunction or a tachycardia-bradycardia syndrome. It is most likely a chance occurrence rather than a pathophysiologic phenomenon and reflects the common denominator of increasing age and degenerative changes in atrial tissue.

Automatic atrial tachycardias that are either nonsustained or sustained but at a rate of less than 120 to 150 beats per minute are common. For example, in patients over 60 years of age, the incidence of these tachycardias during ambulatory ECG monitoring exceeds 15%. They arise in a variety of clinical settings and are usually asymptomatic, incidental ECG findings of little or no clinical significance.

Digitalis-induced automatic atrial tachycardias are more common with electrolyte imbalances such as hypokalemia and are therefore more frequent in patients on concomitant diuretic therapy (Fig. 9–8). Toxicity also may reflect an elevated serum digitalis level. During chronic digitalis therapy, the addition of quinidine, verapamil, flecainide, and propafenone also may increase serum digoxin levels. (The converse—that stopping one of these drugs during chronic digoxin therapy may result in a significant fall in serum digoxin levels—is also true.) With the purified digitalis glycosides, there may be no accompanying extracardiac visual or gastrointestinal symptoms of digitalis toxicity.

Digitalis was once a common cause of automatic atrial tachycardia, but in more recent series, its relative frequency as a

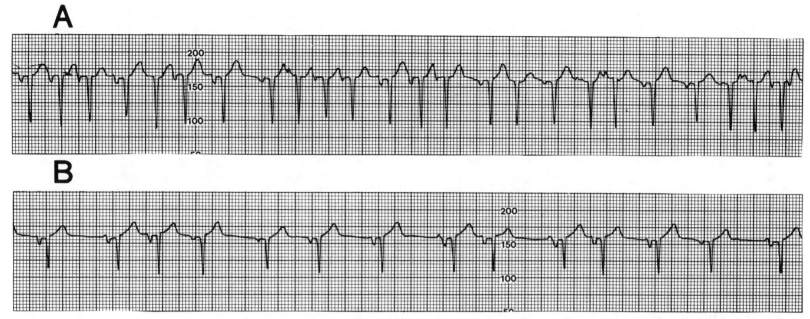

FIGURE 9–13. (*A*) A patient with chronic lung disease receiving theophylline therapy developed MAT. At least three different P-wave configurations occur at a tachycardiac and irregularly irregular rate. There is some reciprocal variability between the RP and PR intervals, but even very premature P waves conduct. (*B*) After intravenous administration of verapamil, the atrial rate slowed, but the varying P-wave configurations persisted.

causal factor has fallen significantly. Reasons for this decline include the more frequent and refined use of digoxin, with its relatively shorter half-life, radioimmunoassay techniques for measuring serum levels, and therapeutic alternatives to "aggressive digitalization."

Non–digitalis-induced sustained automatic atrial tachycardias may occur after open-heart surgery, with myocarditis, and with congestive heart failure from a variety of causes. In general, they are a less frequent clinical problem in adults.

In infants, children, and young adults, non–digitalis-induced automatic atrial tachycardias are more common. They also are more likely to cause clinical problems due to a rapid ventricular rate. With a concomitant congestive cardiomyopathy, the tachycardia may have an etiologic role rather than simply being a secondary manifestation.

METHODS OF TREATMENT

Wandering atrial pacemaker and non-sustained automatic atrial tachycardias do not need treatment.

Digitalis-induced automatic atrial tachycardias resolve gradually on stopping the drug and on correcting serum potassium levels to at least 4 mEq/L (avoiding hyperkalemia, which can cause or potentiate AV block). Catheter manipulation within the right ventricle carries the risk of inducing life-threatening ventricular arrhythmias. Temporary transvenous pacing, therefore, is indicated only if the ventricular rate is inadequate.

Digitalis-induced atrial tachycardia with block may take several days or even longer to resolve. Thus, it is important to consider that *two* abnormalities are present: an accelerated atrial rate and AV block. If either resolves alone, the patient's clinical status may deteriorate. For example, slowing of the atrial rate without resolution of the AV block may slow the ventricular rate. On the other hand, resolution of AV block without slowing the atrium may increase the ventricular rate (see Fig. 9–4). Automatic atrial tachycardias due to digitalis are usually not life-threatening. The potential for ventricular rate changes and the coexistence or emergence of other, even lethal, digitalis-toxic arrhythmias underscore the need for close observation with ECG monitoring during treatment. The use of digoxin antibody fragments is rarely warranted.

In adults, non–digitalis-induced, sustained automatic atrial tachycardias are usually self-limited. When necessary, an empiric regimen or one determined acutely during EPS can be used. Therapy is often identical with that of intra-atrial reentry tachycardia, a fortunate coincidence given the frequent difficulty in differentiating the two arrhythmias. Drugs (e.g., a class Ia or class Ic agent* or a β-blocker) may be used to try to suppress the tachycardia. Alternatively, digoxin combined with either verapamil or a β-blocker may induce AV block and slow the ventricular rate independent of the atrial rate. Experience with other antiarrhythmic drugs is limited, and some (e.g., high-dose amiodarone) have a high incidence of serious side effects. Rarely in adults, and more commonly in children, medical therapy can neither terminate the arrhythmia nor control the ventricular rate. Such patients can develop a tachycardia-induced congestive cardiomyopathy, and catheter or operative ablation of the ectopic focus may be considered. Ventricular dysfunction has improved with successful ablative surgery for a variety of tachyarrhythmias, including automatic atrial tachycardia.[13] Given the potential for lifelong antiarrhythmic drug therapy in children, some experts favor early recourse to operative correction, but this issue remains controversial, particularly because there may be multiple atrial pacemakers.

---

*Of the class Ic drugs, only flecainide is approved for this use by the Food and Drug Administration and then only in patients with structurally normal hearts whose arrhythmia is unresponsive to conventional therapy.

REFERENCES

1. Ferrier GR, Saunders JH, and Mendez C: Cellular mechanism for the generation of ventricular arrhythmias by acetylstrophanthidin. Circ Res 32:600–609, 1973.
2. Levine JH, Michael JR, and Guarnieri T: Treatment of multifocal atrial tachycardia with verapamil. N Engl J Med 312:21–25, 1985.
3. Hordof AJ, Spotnitz A, Mary-Rabine L, Edie RN, and Rosen MR: The cellular electrophysiologic effects of digitalis on human atrial fibers. Circulation 57:223–229, 1978.
4. Hill JA, Coronado R, and Strauss HC: Reconstitution and characterization of a calcium-activated channel from heart. Circ Res 62:411–415, 1988.
5. Levine JH, Michael JR, and Guarnieri T: Multifocal atrial tachycardia: A toxic effect of theophylline. Lancet I:12–14, 1985.
6. Lipsius SL: Triggered rhythms in atrial muscle. J Electrocardiol 20:33–37, 1987.
7. Arsura EL, Lefkin AS, Scher DL, Solar M, and Tessler S: A randomized dou-

ble-blind placebo controlled study of verapamil or metoprolol in multifocal atrial tachycardia. Am J Med 85:519–524, 1988.

8. Lown B, Marcus F, and Levine HD: Digitalis and atrial tachycardia with block. N Engl J Med 260:301–309, 1959.

9. Cranefield PF and Aronson RS: Initiation of sustained rhythmic activity by single propagated action potentials in canine cardiac Purkinje fibers exposed to sodium-free solution or to ouabain. Circ Res 34:477–481, 1974.

10. Bellet S, Eliakim M, Deliyiannis S, and Figallo EM: Radioelectrocardiographic changes during strenuous exercise in normal subjects. Circulation 25:686–694, 1962.

11. Levine HD: Vagal stimulation in the presence of supraventricular mechanisms. In Dreifus LS, Likoff W, and Moyer JH (eds): Mechanisms and Therapy of Cardiac Arrhythmias. Grune & Stratton, New York, 1966, p. 167.

12. Lau SH, Cohen SI, Stein E, Haft J, Rosen KM, and Damato AN: P waves and P loops in coronary sinus and left atrial rhythms. Am Heart J 79:201–214, 1970.

13. Packer DL, Bardy GH, Worley SJ, et al: Tachycardia-induced cardiomyopathy: A reversible form of left ventricular dysfunction. Am J Cardiol 57:563–570, 1986.

CHAPTER 10

The Paroxysmal Atrial Tachycardias

ROBERT A. WAUGH, MD

OUTLINE

The most frequent and clinically important paroxysmal (or reentry) atrial tachyarrhythmia is atrial flutter–fibrillation. In hospitalized populations, it may occur in up to 15% of patients. While other varieties of paroxysmal intra-atrial tachyarrhythmias occur, they are much less frequent and even more rarely cause clinically significant problems.

Clinical descriptions of what was undoubtedly atrial flutter–fibrillation[1] long preceded the development of the ability to study the electrical activity of the heart. Lewis first used electrocardiography in 1909[2] to show that the irregularity of the ventricles was due to fibrillation of the "auricles." Since this initial description, controversy has surrounded postulated mechanisms for this arrhythmia. Even now, the two ends of its spectrum (flutter and fibrillation) are treated as separate, distinct entities in terms of underlying cause, mechanism, and treatment.

Sentinel landmarks in our understanding of this arrhythmia have included the use of quinidine[3] and electrical current[4] for cardioversion and the discovery of its risk for systemic embolization.[5] More recent observations, coincident with invasive electrophysiologic techniques, have included the termination of atrial flutter with atrial pacing,[6,7] the phenomenon of entrainment,[8] and invasive approaches to treatment, including implantable antitachycardia atrial pacing devices,[9]

His bundle ablation and atrial ablation (initially by catheter-delivered electrical current[10,11,12] and more recently by catheter-delivered radiofrequency energy).[13,14]

Given the frequency and clinical significance of this arrhythmia, it is fortunate that there are multiple methods of managing it, including an increasing array of drugs, electrical cardioversion, and various types of pacing, and ablative procedures. This chapter discusses focal and generalized atrial reentry arrhythmias, with the emphasis on the latter more common and significant problem.

CLASSIFICATION
Focal Reentry

Reentry in the sinus node and reentry in other localized areas of atrial tissue make up this subgroup of arrhythmias. Neither type of reentry obligatorily involves the atrioventricular (AV) node; depending on a variety of factors, AV block may or may not be present. These are true examples of *paroxysmal atrial tachycardia (PAT)*, a commonly used term for what is actually an infrequent arrhythmia (see Chapter 9, page 181). *Sinus node reentry tachycardia* and *paroxysmal sinus tachycardia* are synonymous terms. Although *paroxysmal* appropriately implies reentry, *sinus tachycardia* refers to a prototypical pacemaker rhythm. The term *sinus* (or *sinoatrial* [*SA*]) *node reentry tachycardia* is less confusing. Focal atrial reentry tachycardias are also commonly called *atrial tachycardia*, with the reentry mechanism implied. *Intra-atrial reentry tachycardia* is another common term. In clinical practice, the automatic and intra-atrial reentry tachycardias may be difficult to differentiate. Fortunately, their therapy and significance are frequently the same. Grouping these arrhythmias under the term *ectopic atrial tachycardia* is a frequent practice, but the use of terms that identify the site and mechanism, when possible, provides a less confusing nomenclature.

Generalized Reentry

There are clinically significant differences in how atrial flutter and fibrillation behave in terms of ventricular rate and regularity, stability, and response to therapeutic interventions. Despite these differences, it is practical to consider them within the broad spectrum of generalized atrial reentry; certain aspects then become comparable to ventricular flutter–fibrillation (Fig. 10–1; see Chapter 12, page 266). Table 10–1 illustrates the utility of this classification by showing both the

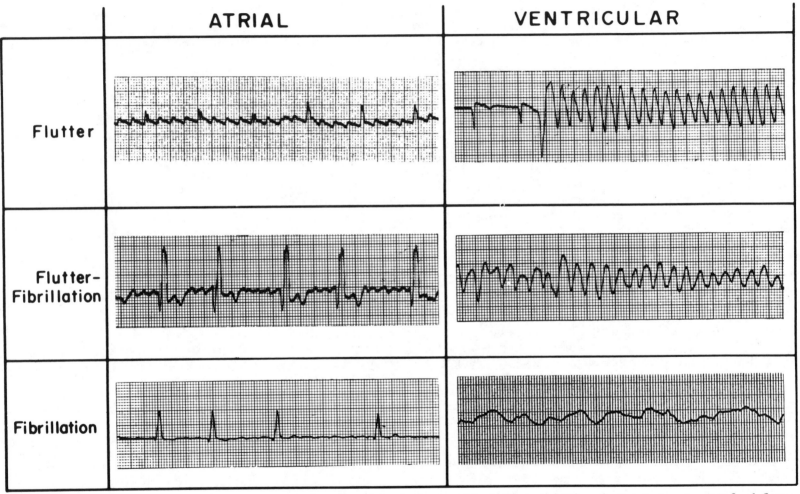

FIGURE 10–1. The analogy between macroreentry in the atria and that in the ventricles is illustrated. When the reentering circuit is fixed, flutter results (top strips).

Table 10–1. SPECTRUM OF ATRIAL FLUTTER–FIBRILLATION

Atrial Rate	200	220		300	400	500+
Ventricular Rate	200	180	150		100	70
Ventricular Regularity	Regular	Regular, regularly irregular	Regular		Irregularly irregular	
Name	Slow flutter		"Classic flutter"	Flutter–fibrillation		Fibrillation
Stability	Unstable					Stable
Effectiveness of Digoxin to ⇑ AV Block*	Ineffective		Difficult to maintain >2:1			More effective
Conversion with DC Shock	Lower energy					Higher energy
Conversion with Atrial Pacing	Easy		Difficult			Impossible

AV = atrioventricular.

*As long as sympathetic AV nodal tone is low.

continuum and the contrasts within the generalized atrial-reentry spectrum.

Two specific subgroups of atrial flutter are *common*, or *type I* (atrial rates less than 320 beats per minute, with the reentry loop generally oriented in the frontal plane), and *uncommon*, or *type II* (atrial rates greater than 320 beats per minute, with the reentry loop generally oriented in the horizontal plane). Recognizing this variability in atrial rate and atrial morphologic characteristics is sometimes helpful both in diagnosis and in management decisions.

It is important to reemphasize that while these unifying features help in understanding this arrhythmia, its behavior at the two ends of the spectrum (flutter versus fibrillation) has significantly different clinical implications, which demand consideration in planning therapeutic interventions.

MECHANISMS

Focal Reentry

These atrial tachycardias are infrequent and their mechanisms have only recently been proved. Earlier investigations postulated the need for a "critical" mass of excitable tissue and for an anatomic obstruction (or circuit) to sustain reentry, which are unlikely conditions in a small mass of atrial tissue. More recent studies, however, have found reentry in a small tissue mass with no focal anatomic obstruction.[15] Other studies have described sinus nodal reentry in isolated tissue preparations and in the intact laboratory animal; in addition, clinical examples of both sinus nodal and intra-atrial reentry or *atrial tachycardia* are well documented.[16,17]

Generalized Reentry

Despite the controversies concerning mechanism, atrial flutter and atrial fibrillation reflect generalized reentry (or macroreentry) within atrial muscle, with flutter and fibrillation representing the two ends of the atrial rate and regularity spectrum (see Table 10–1). The atrial rate with flutter is usually between 250 and 320 beats per minute; in untreated patients, it is usually about 300 beats per minute. As the atrial rate increases above 360 beats per minute, atrial activity typically becomes more irregular (as does the ventricular response) and assumes the appearance of flutter-fibrillation. It may have either some characteristics of both

flutter and fibrillation at a single point in time or change cyclically in appearance between the two. Terms commonly used in this latter situation include *impure flutter, coarse atrial fibrillation*, and *flutter-fibrillation*. As the atrial rate increases even further, discrete regular atrial activity disappears, and the atrial electrogram becomes typical of frank atrial fibrillation (Fig. 10–2). The reentrant pathway in flutter is more constant and predictable, whereas in fibrillation, the reentry circuits may be multiple or are variable and unpredictable. The continuous reentry responsible for both corresponds to the replacement of discrete P waves on the surface electrocardiogram (ECG) by patterns of continuous atrial activity: the classic "sawtooth" pattern (alternating positive and negative waves with no isoelectric interval separating areas of discrete atrial activity) at the flutter end of the spectrum, and more chaotic and irregular undulations at the fibrillation end. Figure 10–3 illustrates the different aspects of the flutter-fibrillation spectrum via a simultaneous recording of an intra-atrial electrogram and surface ECG leads.

CLINICAL METHODS OF DIAGNOSIS

Several ECG features are important in differential diagnosis. These include how

the arrhythmia starts and stops, the atrial rate, the P-wave morphologic characteristics (of both the initiating beat and the beats occurring during the tachycardia), and the pattern of AV conduction. Concomitant clinical features or the response to an intervention may provide additional key information. As with other supraventricular tachycardias, a wide QRS complex requires expanding the differential diagnosis to include ventricular tachycardia. Table 10–2 summarizes the important ECG features of the reentry atrial tachycardias.

Focal Reentry

With these tachycardias, the onset is abrupt and typically follows a premature P wave that differs morphologically from that of either the baseline rhythm or the subsequent sustained tachycardia. The P waves of sinus node reentry tachycardia are similar to those of sinus rhythm, whereas the P waves of intra-atrial tachycardia differ from those of sinus rhythm. The P wave for a given run is monomorphic but can vary depending on the atrial reentry site. The typical atrial rates are 150 to 220 beats per minute (sinus node reentry is usually less than 180 beats per minute). At the more rapid rates, particularly with 1:1 AV conduction, assessing P-

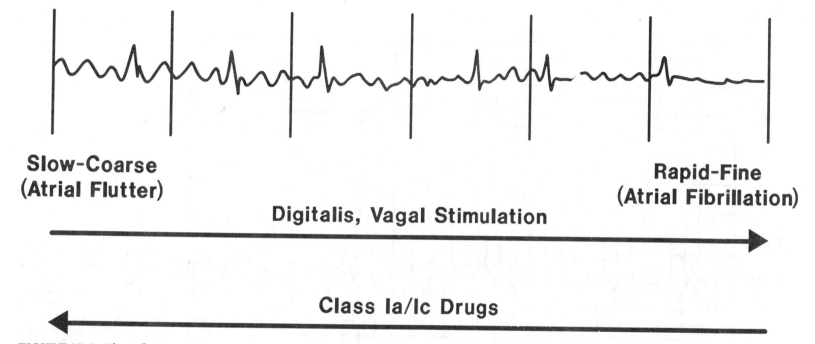

**Slow-Coarse
(Atrial Flutter)**

**Rapid-Fine
(Atrial Fibrillation)**

Digitalis, Vagal Stimulation

Class Ia/Ic Drugs

FIGURE 10–2. The influence of drugs and autonomic tone on the rate and regularity of atrial reentry. The pathognomonic response of flutter to either vagal stimulation or digitalis is atrial rate speeding (i.e., flutter becomes fibrillation). The reverse occurs with the class Ia or class Ic drugs.

wave morphologic characteristics becomes difficult because of superimposition of P waves on the preceding ST-T waves. The PR interval can vary, but at rest with high parasympathetic tone, first- and second-degree AV block are common. Both types of focal atrial reentry tachycardias also may end abruptly, either spontaneously (rarely following a spontaneous premature atrial beat), or more predictably with atrial pacing or transthoracic cardioversion. The rich autonomic innervation of the sinus node probably explains why sinus node reentry sometimes stops in response to enhanced vagal tone. In general, vagal interventions are not helpful in differentiating automaticity from atrial reentry, as both types of tachycardia usually continue unabated while the degree of AV block increases.

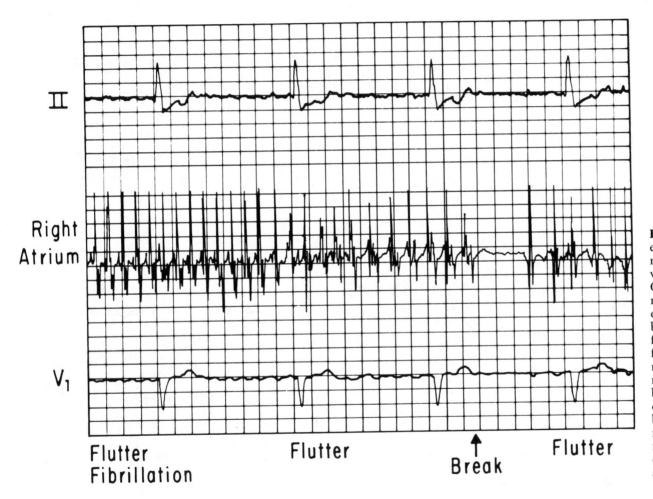

FIGURE 10–3. An atrial electrogram (right atrium) is recorded simultaneously with surface leads II and V_1. On the left, the extremely rapid and regular atrial reentry rate is at the boundary between unusually fast atrial flutter and fibrillation (i.e., flutter-fibrillation). In the middle of the strip, the atrial reentry rate remains regular but slows toward more typical flutter just before it breaks suddenly. On the right, after the first spontaneous atrial beat, reentry recurs with the appearance of atrial flutter.

Table 10–2. THE PAROXYSMAL OR REENTRY ATRIAL TACHYCARDIAS

ARRHYTHMIA	RATE RANGE (beats/min)*	ATRIAL MORPHOLOGY	VENTRICULAR RESPONSE
Sinus node reentry tachycardia	120–180	Discrete and regular (similar to sinus P waves)	Some degree of AV block depending on autonomic tone
Atrial reentry tachycardia	120–220	Discrete and regular (different from sinus P waves)	Some degree of AV block depending on autonomic tone
Atrial flutter	220–340†	Sawtooth configuration and regular	2:1 AV block common; less block with enhanced sympathetic tone and preexcitation
Atrial fibrillation	>340	Nondiscrete and irregular	Some degree of AV block; less block with enhanced sympathetic tone and preexcitation

AV = atrioventricular.

*These rate ranges are meant as a rough guide: A given arrhythmia is not excluded by virtue of a higher or lower rate.

†Rates below 220 beats/min are particularly common with class Ic drug therapy.

Generalized Reentry

ONSET AND OFFSET

Generalized reentry tachycardias begin abruptly following premature atrial activation, usually from a premature atrial complex (PAC) (Fig. 10–4), and more rarely from premature ventricular complexes (PVCs) with retrograde atrial capture. The latter is particularly likely with preexcitation, as retrograde conduction via the accessory pathway facilitates early atrial activation. Termination, occurring either spontaneously or in response to drugs or electrical cardioversion, is also abrupt (see Fig. 10–4). These particular features help differentiate atrial flutter–fibrillation from pacemaker-induced atrial tachycardias but do not differentiate among various atrial reentry tachycardias. Termination in response to a vagal intervention is much more typical of AV junctional reentry than of atrial flutter–fibrillation.

ATRIAL ACTIVITY

The key to the diagnosis of atrial flutter–fibrillation is in the identification of the rate and morphology of atrial activity. These features are usually discernible on a rhythm strip or a 12-lead ECG (noting particularly leads II and V_1).

Atrial Rate. Accurate measurement of the atrial rate may give the diagnosis. For example, simply determining that the atrial rate is greater than 220 beats per minute makes atrial flutter most likely (Fig. 10–5*A*).

The differential diagnosis among various atrial tachycardias becomes more difficult with atrial rates around 200 to 220 beats per minute, at which range there is maximum rate overlap among the various supraventricular tachycardias (see Fig. 10–5*B*). Atrial flutter rarely slows to this degree spontaneously but often does so in response to class Ia or class Ic drugs. Hyperkalemia is a rare cause for similar degrees of slowing. On the other hand, these atrial rates are within the upper range of sinus tachycardia (due to exercise or iso-

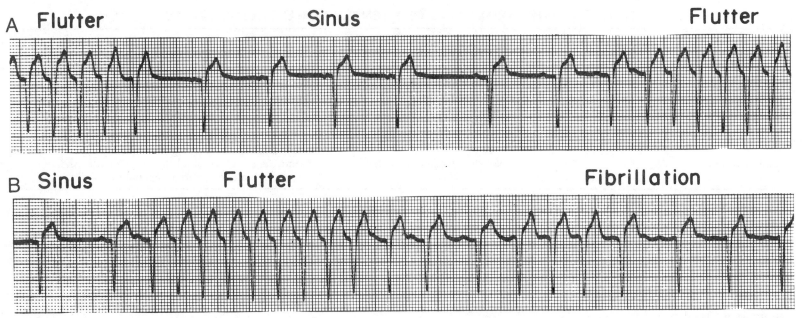

FIGURE 10–4. The typical features of atrial flutter–fibrillation, including initiation by premature atrial complexes (PACs), sudden spontaneous termination, and variability in ventricular rate and regularity, are depicted in these strips from the same patient. (*A*) The sudden cessation or break in this rapid supraventricular tachycardia makes a reentrant (or paroxysmal) mechanism most likely. An escape atrial rhythm continues until another PAC reinitiates reentry supraventricular tachycardia. (*B*) The ventricular rate of the tachycardia (again, initiated by a PAC) varies from rapid and relatively regular to slower and irregularly irregular. Thus, it is reasonable to assume that the basic problem is atrial flutter–fibrillation and that (*A*) reflects one end of the spectrum: atrial flutter.

proterenol) or automatic atrial tachycardias and are common with paroxysmal AV junctional tachycardia (PJT). (See Chapter 11.)

Atrial Morphology. The most helpful point in the differential diagnosis of these slower tachycardias is atrial morphology. A sawtooth pattern in any lead identifies atrial flutter regardless of the atrial rate (see Fig. 10–5*B*), whereas discrete P waves in all leads suggest automatic atrial tachycardia. *Very* slow atrial flutter (less than 200 beats per minute) may mimic an automatic atrial tachycardia with discrete P waves and intervening isoelectric intervals. In these cases, a careful review of drug therapy and corresponding serial ECGs may be helpful.

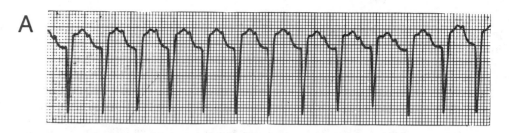

During Carotid Sinus Massage

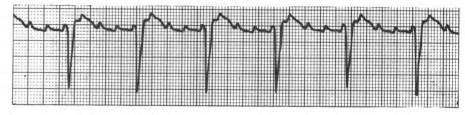

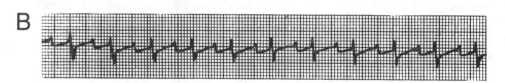

During Carotid Sinus Massage

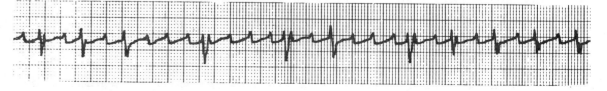

FIGURE 10–5. (*A*) In the top strip, a wide-QRS tachycardia at 135 beats per minute appears to show a P wave preceding each QRS complex with a top normal to slightly prolonged PR interval suggesting sinus tachycardia with first-degree atrioventricular (AV) block and aberration. Carotid sinus massage increases the degree of AV block, unmasks atrial activity at 270 beats per minute, and proves atrial flutter with 2:1 AV conduction. (*B*) In the top strip, a narrow-QRS tachycardia at 115 beats per minute shows one apparent P wave for each QRS complex, with a PR interval of 0.22 second, suggesting sinus tachycardia with first-degree AV block. Carotid sinus massage induces AV block and unmasks a regular atrial rate of 230 beats per minute. The differential diagnosis includes automatic atrial tachycardia and atrial reentry (focal and generalized [i.e., flutter]). The typical "sawtooth" atrial electrogram identifies regular, generalized atrial reentry (i.e., atrial flutter). In retrospect, a hint of superimposed flutter waves can be seen in the top strip of (*B*). Note, for example, the S wave of the second QRS complex.

The ECG leads that display atrial activity to the best advantage depend on the atrial arrhythmia (see Figs. 5–2 and 9–10). With common atrial flutter, leads II, III, and aVF are most likely to be oriented in the plane of the reentering wave front and display the typical sawtooth pattern. Lead V_1 is least likely to show it because a portion of the reentering wave front is likely to be isoelectric to the anterior precordium. In lead V_1, therefore, even classic atrial flutter may show apparently discrete P waves followed by an isoelectric interval, falsely suggesting an automatic or focal atrial reentry tachycardia. On the other hand, lead V_1 is most likely to show the totally irregular baseline of atrial fibrillation or the sawtooth pattern of type II flutter. Note that even with a very careful analysis, "fine" atrial fibrillation may masquerade as atrial asystole.

Sometimes the various rhythm strips and standard 12-lead ECG do not show P-wave activity satisfactorily. In these cases, an intervention to slow the ventricular rate (see Chapter 4, pages 79, 88 to 96, and 96 to 101, and Table 4–1) or the use of specialized ECG recordings may be tried. The latter include Lewis leads (exploring the right precordium using the right- and left-arm ECG leads) or esophageal and atrial leads (see Chapter 5, pages 110 to 116). Often, a simple autonomic intervention may be used, or intravenous adenosine, verapamil, or edrophonium chloride suffices, provided the patient is hemodynamically stable (Fig. 10–6; see Fig. 10–5).

THE VENTRICULAR RESPONSE

Regularity and Rate. With flutter, the ventricular response may be regular or regularly irregular, but during uncomplicated atrial fibrillation it is always irregularly irregular (see Table 10–1). Even without a precise definition of atrial activity, an irregularly irregular ventricular response with a morphologically constant QRS complex makes atrial fibrillation most likely. The standard ECG usually identifies multifocal atrial tachycardia (MAT), which mimics atrial fibrillation (Fig. 10–7; see Chapter 9, pages 186 and 197 to 198, and Figs. 9–5 and 9–13). The atrial flutter rate is typically 300 beats per minute and the AV conduction is 2:1. Thus, any regular supraventricular tachycardia at 150 beats per minute (even without definitively characterizing atrial activity) is likely to be atrial flutter (Fig. 10–8).

AV Block. Atrioventricular block is atypical with sinus tachycardia and PJT. Its presence, therefore, should suggest either atrial flutter, an automatic atrial tachycardia, or the rare PAT due to focal atrial reentry. With untreated atrial flutter, AV conduction is usually 2:1 but may be as rapid as 1:1 or quite slow (Fig. 10–9). Interestingly, the ratio of AV conduction often displays even periodicity (i.e., 1:1, 2:1, 4:1, and so forth), although other ratios may occur, particularly with treatment or atrial rates less than 220 to 240 beats per minute.

Increased AV block in response to a vagal intervention is usual with all intra-atrial tachycardias and does not differentiate among them. Any resulting definitive characterization of atrial activity, however, may help (see Figs. 10–5 and 10–6).

Concomitant Clinical Findings. Flutter is more likely when digitalis therapy is not part of the clinical situation, because automatic atrial tachycardias are still typically digitalis-induced. Unfortunately, many patients with this differential diagnosis are also receiving digitalis, and its presence, therefore, is not as helpful. Even serum digitalis levels may be misleading. Elevated levels with or without typical clinical features of digitalis toxicity may coexist with atrial flutter, even when the drug has not caused the arrhythmia.

Coexistent conditions associated with increased atrial pressure or size (e.g., mitral valve disease, left ventricular failure, and chronic obstructive pulmonary disease) favor the likelihood of atrial flutter–fibrillation. Any of these factors, in addition to the added stress of a surgical operation, also favor atrial flutter–fibrillation (see pages 221 to 224).

WIDE-QRS TACHYCARDIA

Wide QRS complexes during any tachycardia require differentiating aberration from ventricular ectopy (see Chapter 7,

Carotid Sinus Massage

LEAD V₁

LEAD V₅

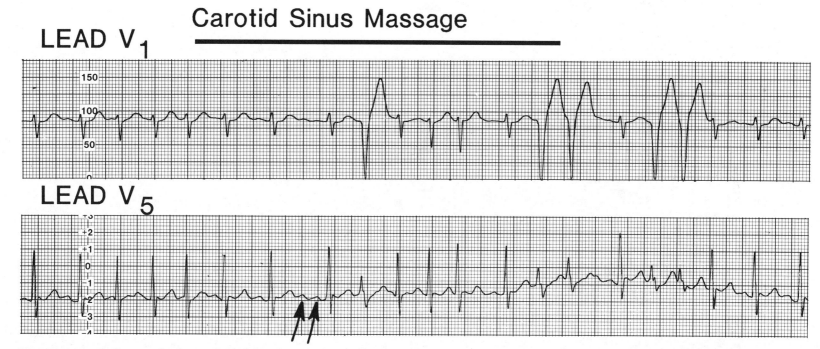

FIGURE 10–6. The use of enhanced vagal tone to unmask atrial activity. This electrocardiogram (ECG), from a patient complaining of a rapid heartbeat, shows a rapid, slightly irregular supraventricular tachycardia with some QRS complexes preceded by what appear to be P waves that are morphologically variable (e.g., the left-hand portion of this strip). During carotid sinus massage, AV nodal block increases sufficiently to reveal "coarse" atrial fibrillation waves (arrows in lead V_5). The slowing is also associated with the emergence of wide-QRS beats and couplets showing features typical of aberration (note the "long-cycle, short-cycle" patterns and the absence of relative pauses after the wide beats). (See also Fig. 10–10.)

pages 146 to 154, and Chapter 12, pages 268 to 279). Wide beats (either in isolation or in runs) are frequent during atrial fibrillation, particularly with a rapid ventricular response (Fig 10–10; see Fig. 10–6). The resulting combination of long and short cycles and fast heart rate favors aberration. That is, beats terminating short cycles after a prior long cycle are very likely to encounter refractoriness in some portion of the ventricular conduction system, which leads to aberration. The tendency of aberration to persist, once it is established, further enhances mimicry of ventricular tachycardia (see Fig. 10–10). The differential diagnosis is usually not too difficult, and the same hints for differentiating the origin of

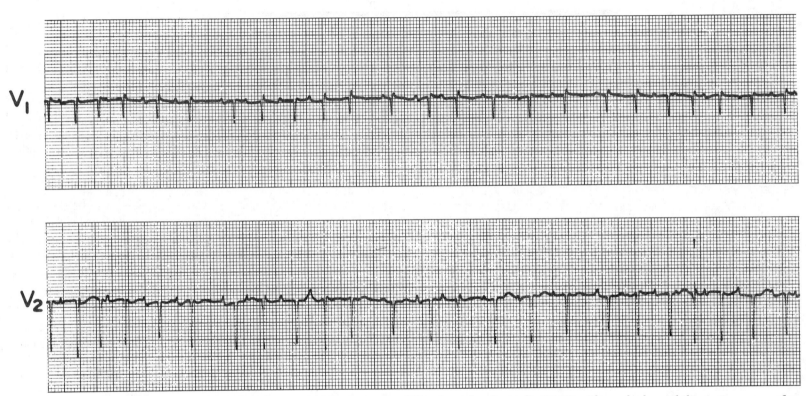

FIGURE 10–7. Simultaneous leads V_1 and V_2 show typical features of multifocal atrial tachycardia (MAT) with marked variability in P-wave configuration, rate, and regularity. While this irregularly irregular rhythm may mimic atrial fibrillation clinically, the ECG reveals discrete P waves preceding most QRS complexes, thus presenting a distinct contrast to atrial fibrillation, which lacks discrete P waves. The PR interval varies with P-wave prematurity (i.e., the RP and subsequent PR intervals vary reciprocally). In this patient with respiratory failure and high adrenergic tone, even very premature P waves conduct.

A

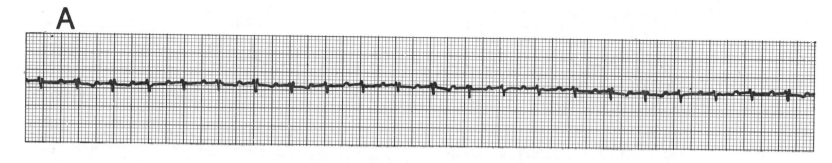

B

Carotid Sinus Massage

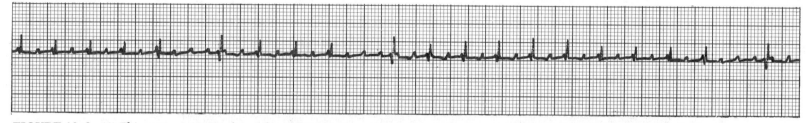

FIGURE 10–8. (*A*) This narrow-QRS tachycardia at 150 beats per minute has one apparent P wave for each QRS complex and suggests sinus tachycardia. This rate, however, is so characteristic that it should always suggest atrial flutter with 2:1 conduction. (*B*) Carotid sinus massage unmasks atrial activity at 300 beats per minute and proves atrial flutter even without the typical sawtooth configuration in this lead. Both strips are lead V_1.

premature wide beats during sinus rhythm can be applied here (Chapter 7, pages 146 to 154). There are additional points, unique to atrial fibrillation, that strongly favor aberration. These include:

- Wide-QRS runs that are irregularly irregular at a rate similar to the adjacent atrial fibrillation (i.e., the run's periodicity and rate are similar to the surrounding atrial fibrillation)
- No relative pauses following the runs (i.e., there is no evidence of concealed retrograde conduction into the AV node)

- An occurrence only during periods of rapid AV conduction (i.e., ventricular tachycardia is more likely to emerge during slower heart rates)
- A variable coupling interval between the normal and wide beats (i.e., fixed coupling is more likely with ventricular ectopy)

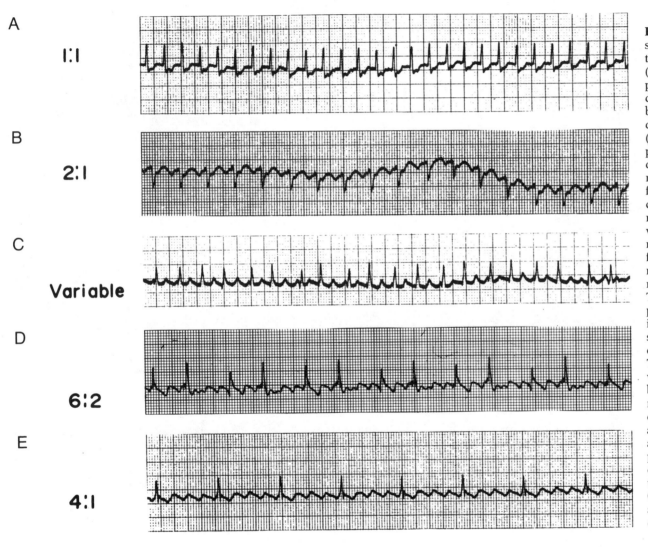

A
1:1

B
2:1

C
Variable

D
6:2

E
4:1

FIGURE 10–9. These ECGs show the various AV conduction patterns of atrial flutter. (*A*) The atrial rate is 215 beats per minute with 1:1 AV conduction. (Flutter was proved by a sawtooth atrial pattern during a vagal maneuver.) (*B*) The atrial rate is 300 beats per minute with 2:1 AV conduction. Note the constant relationship between the flutter waves and the QRS complexes. (*C*) The atrial rate is 330 beats per minute with a variable ventricular response. Note the typical flutter waves during the period of increased AV block near the end of the strip. (*D*) The atrial rate is 300 beats per minute with a regularly irregular ventricular response (six flutter waves for every two QRS complexes). The resulting "bigeminal" ventricular response possibly reflects Wenckebach periodicity at two different levels in the AV node. (*E*) The atrial and ventricular rates are about 260 and 65 beats per minute, respectively. The constant relationship between the flutter waves and QRS complexes proves AV association with 4:1 AV conduction.

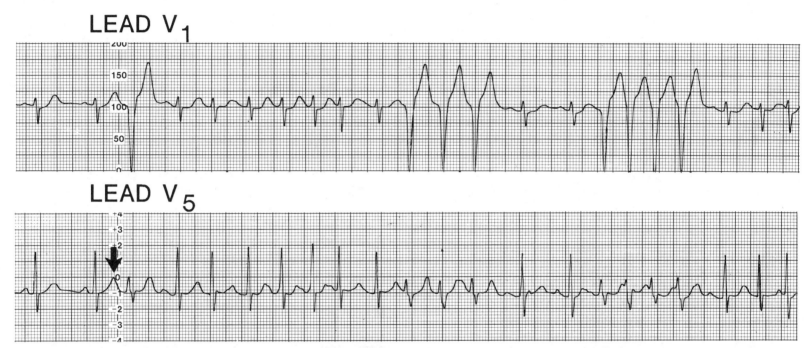

FIGURE 10–10. In this patient (same as in Fig. 10–6), two beats of sinus rhythm are followed by an aberrated PAC (note the distorted T wave from a superimposed P wave [arrow in lead V_5]. During the ensuing supraventricular tachycardia, there are runs of nonsustained wide-QRS tachycardia that show a number of features typical of aberration, including morphologic characteristics identical to those of the aberrated PAC; a long-cycle, short-cycle pattern; the absence of relative pauses after the runs; and rates similar to the rate of the adjacent supraventricular tachycardia (in this case, atrial fibrillation). When runs of wide-QRS tachycardia are seen *only* during concomitant supraventricular tachycardia, aberration is by far the most likely diagnosis.

- Wide beats showing variable width within the same morphologic family
- With intermittent atrial fibrillation, the presence of wide QRS runs *only* in the setting of atrial fibrillation.

(See Chapter 7, pages 146 to 154, and Chapter 12, pages 268 to 279, regarding the differential diagnosis of wide-QRS beats).

INTERACTION WITH THE AUTONOMIC NERVOUS SYSTEM

The autonomic nervous system may affect atrial reentry by stopping it, by changing its rate or the degree of AV block, or by providing a milieu that allows it to occur.

Sinus node reentry is most likely to stop in response to vagal maneuvers. The occasional termination of atrial flutter during a vagal maneuver is likely a chance occurrence. It is less likely a cholinergic effect on the atrium, where conduction speeds more than the refractory period shortens, thus breaking the reentry circuit. This cholinergic effect of speeding intra-atrial conduction may be reflected in the atrial rate (e.g., atrial flutter speeds [Fig. 10–11*A*] and may even reach atrial fibrillation rates [Fig. 10–11*B*]). Because cholinergically mediated atrial rate speeding identifies atrial flutter, it can be an important observation in the differential diagnosis of atrial tachycardias with rates in the range of 200 to 220 beats per minute.

Although enhanced vagal tone only rarely terminates generalized atrial reentry, it can contribute to its initiation. In the experimental animal, for example, atrial fibrillation induced by rapid atrial pacing alone rapidly reverts to sinus rhythm with cessation of pacing. When combined with vagal stimulation, such pacing-induced atrial fibrillation continues, despite cessation of pacing, for as long as the vagal stimulation continues. This may have a clinical counterpart, in that some patients experience paroxysmal atrial fibrillation when vagal tone is highest (i.e., at rest, after meals, or in the early morning hours).

Lastly, the autonomic nervous system can influence the arrhythmia through its indirect and direct effects on AV nodal conduction. Acetylcholine indirectly slows the ventricular response to generalized atrial reentry by speeding the atrial rate and by increasing concealed conduction into the AV node and its refractoriness (Fig. 10–12). With all atrial tachycardias, enhanced parasympathetic tone also can slow the ventricular response by directly prolonging AV nodal conduction time (see Fig. 10–11*A* and 10–12). On the other hand, an increase in sympathetic tone enhances AV nodal conduction and the ventricular rate. Alterations in autonomic balance and the resulting changes in ventricular rate can be important in the symptomatic manifestations of these tachycardias.

USE OF INVASIVE ELECTROPHYSIOLOGY

Focal Reentry

Invasive electrophysiologic techniques are rarely necessary with these arrhythmias but can be used to prove the diagnosis and test antiarrhythmic drug therapy. The efficacy of programmed stimulation in terminating the tachycardia may be tested as a baseline procedure preparatory to drug trials or implantation of an antitachycardia pacemaker. In exceedingly rare instances, an incessant tachycardia refractory to therapy may require invasive electrophysiologic studies to localize the site of reentry preparatory to catheter or operative ablation or excision.

Generalized Reentry

Invasive electrophysiology is also seldom necessary in the diagnosis or management of atrial flutter–fibrillation. On occasion, when the rate and regularity of the atrial rhythm are in question, esophageal or intravascular recordings of atrial activity can be extremely helpful (see Figs. 5–4 and 5–5). When the arrhythmia

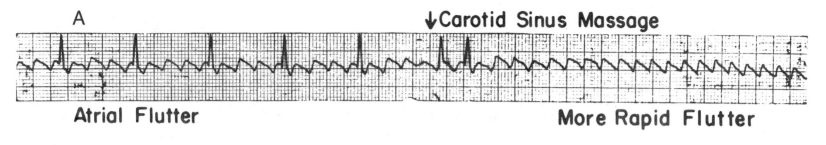

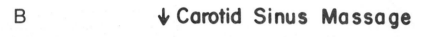

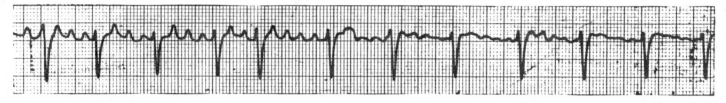

FIGURE 10–11. (*A*) The speeding of this atrial flutter from 300 to 330 beats per minute during carotid sinus massage may reflect an acetylcholine-induced speeding of atrial muscle conduction from enhanced vagal tone. The combination of the direct effect of increased vagal tone on the AV node and the indirect effect of an increased atrial rate increasing concealed conduction into the AV node, and thereby increasing refractoriness, contributes to a dramatic increase in the degree of AV block. (*B*) The left-hand portion of the ECG shows coarse atrial fibrillation (or "impure" atrial flutter). With the enhanced vagal tone of carotid sinus massage, the reentry rate speeds to frank atrial fibrillation. An accompanying decrease in the ventricular rate cannot be documented in this short rhythm strip.

is at the flutter end of the spectrum and particularly with atrial rates under 300 per minute, atrial pacing can effect cardioversion of some varieties of atrial flutter (see Chapter 16, pages 410 to 419).

With atrial flutter–fibrillation and ventricular preexcitation, a detailed electrophysiologic study is mandatory to find the minimum refractory period of the accessory pathway during the arrhythmia and

in response to various drugs. In addition, radiofrequency ablation of a portion of the right atrium shows promise as a method for preventing recurrences of atrial flutter.[14] A fifth use for invasive elec-

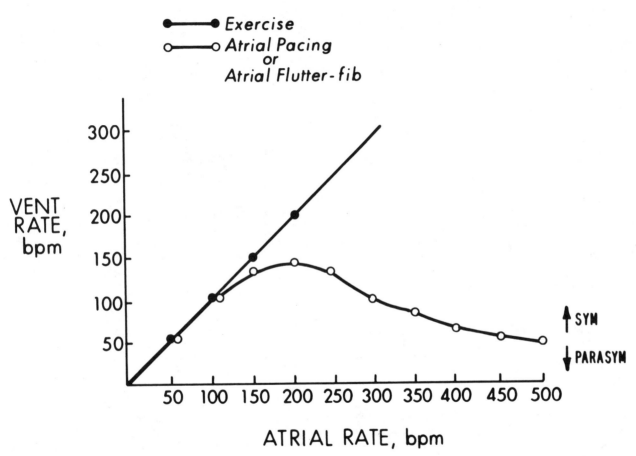

FIGURE 10–12. The line of identity (solid circles) identifies the typical 1:1 AV relationship of increases in atrial rate mediated through exercise or adrenergic stimulation. With atrial rate increases from other mechanisms (e.g., atrial pacing or atrial flutter–fibrillation [open circles]), a 1:1 AV relationship pertains for the lower rates, but when atrial rates exceed approximately 150 beats per minute, AV nodal block typically occurs. At any given atrial rate, increased sympathetic tone (SYM) can facilitate AV conduction, or increased parasympathetic tone (PARASYM) can impair it. VENT = ventricular.

trophysiology is to resolve the question of aberration versus ectopy for wide QRS complexes whose diagnosis is not clear from other criteria (see pages 212 to 218). This differential diagnosis is more difficult when wide beats occur during atrial flutter. For example, with flutter and an early wide QRS complex following each narrow complex, the differential diagnosis resides between atrial flutter with ventricular bigeminy and atrial flutter with alternating 4:1 and 2:1 AV conduction and aberration of the early complexes. Finding a His bundle spike before the wide QRS complex readily resolves the issue (see Chapter 6, page 125).

CLINICAL FEATURES

Focal Reentry

PREDISPOSING CLINICAL SETTINGS

Like PJT, focal reentry tachycardias may occur with no underlying organic heart disease. In other instances, atrial dilation or fibrosis may facilitate the reentry circuit. Reported series are small and subject to recruitment biases, making it difficult to assess the relationship between these arrhythmias and associated heart disease. Underlying heart disease may facilitate arrhythmia recognition without a cause-effect relationship per se. For example, the tachycardia may precipitate a bout of angina pectoris.

NATURAL HISTORY

The natural history of these tachycardias is usually that of any underlying heart disease. In otherwise normal subjects, they do not appear to have additive prognostic significance. When incessant, they may rarely cause congestive heart failure due to a tachycardia-induced cardiomyopathy.

METHODS OF TREATMENT

The cornerstone of initial therapy is reassurance about the generally benign nature of the arrhythmia. If the tachycardia is infrequent and has no significant hemodynamic consequences, treatment is not necessary. For patients requiring therapy, Table 10–3 summarizes various options, depending on whether the goal is to slow the rate or to restore sinus rhythm.

With sinus node reentry, instruction in performing vagal maneuvers may be all that is necessary. Pharmacologic therapy parallels the outline for automatic atrial tachycardias (see Chapter 9, pages 197 to 200), and it is frequently empiric, beginning with the least toxic drug, digoxin. If necessary, a class Ia drug may be added to attempt prophylaxis against recurrence of the arrhythmia. Alternatively, drugs may be used to induce some degree of AV block and diminish symptoms by slowing the ventricular rate. The class Ic drugs may be considered for highly symptomatic patients without structural heart

disease whose arrythmias are refractory to conventional therapy.

Generalized Reentry

PREDISPOSING CLINICAL SETTINGS

In contrast to focal atrial reentry, atrial flutter–fibrillation, particularly if sustained or recurrent, usually occurs in association with organic heart disease. Chronic atrial dilation resulting from ventricular or AV valve dysfunction is the rule.

Acute atrial stresses such as pulmonary embolism or acute mitral regurgitation, while less probable causes, can produce atrial flutter–fibrillation. The arrhythmia becomes increasingly frequent as the acute process becomes chronic. In all clinical settings, increasing age is an important additional risk factor for the arrhythmia. In any age group, but particularly in the elderly, it frequently causes symptomatic deterioration.

Ventricular Dysfunction. Atrial fibrillation in the setting of left-sided heart failure is common. While the cause of the failure may be multifactorial, it always involves an increased left atrial pressure resulting in left atrial dilation. The increased left atrial pressure may stem from either systolic dysfunction or diastolic dysfunction with reduced left ventricular compliance. For example, atrial flutter–fibrillation during acute myocardial infarc-

Table 10–3. TREATMENT OF REENTRY ATRIAL TACHYCARDIAS

ARRHYTHMIA	TO SLOW ATRIAL RATE	TO SLOW VENTRICULAR RATE	TO CONVERT TO NSR	TO MAINTAIN NSR
Sinus node and atrial reentry tachycardia	—	Digoxin, verapamil, β-blockers,	Class Ia or class Ic*, atrial pacing, ? β-blockers DC cardioversion	Class Ia or class Ic*, ? digoxin
Regular generalized atrial reentry (atrial flutter)	Rarely class Ia or class Ic*†	Digoxin plus verapamil, diltiazem, or β-blockers‡	Digoxin, class Ia or class Ic*, atrial pacing, DC cardioversion, ? β-blockers	Class Ia or class Ic*, amiodarone* I, RF atrial ablation
Irregular generalized atrial reentry (atrial fibrillation)	—	Digoxin plus verapamil, diltiazem, or β-blockers	Digoxin, class Ia or class Ic*, DC cardioversion, ? β-blockers	Class Ia or class Ic*, amiodarone* I, atrial surgery

NSR = normal sinus rhythm.

*Of these drugs, only flecainide is approved by the Food and Drug Administration for treatment of supraventricular tachycardias in patients without structural heart disease and with disabling symptoms.

†The usual goal is abolition of the arrhythmia. Rarely, the atrial rate can be slowed so that the usual 2:1 AV block, in combination with an AV-node–blocking drug, allows improved ventricular rate control.

‡With stable atrial flutter, maintenance of reasonable degrees of atrioventricular (AV) block can prove quite difficult with these drugs, either alone or in combination.

tion is common, with an incidence of up to 15%. Its presence typically reflects extensive infarction and elevated left ventricular filling pressure. Sometimes, atrial infarction may be a factor. With concomitant mitral apparatus dysfunction, mitral regurgitation is an additional atrial stress. It may be an early clue to eventual clinical heart failure. Another frequent clinical setting is chronic obstructive lung disease with respiratory failure. The attendant hypoxia, hypercarbia, right ventricular failure, and tricuspid regurgitation combine to produce parallel pathologic changes in the right side of the heart, with right atrial enlargement.

AV Valve Dysfunction. Atrial flutter–fibrillation occurs frequently with both rheumatic and nonrheumatic mitral valve disease and can be the initial clinical manifestation of valve dysfunction. It occurs at some point in the clinical course of up to 85% of patients with significant mitral regurgitation and is only slightly less common with mitral stenosis.

Atrial flutter–fibrillation is common with hypertrophic obstructive cardiomyopathy, where mitral regurgitation and markedly reduced left ventricular compliance combine to cause left atrial enlargement. In any patient, this arrhythmia merits a careful evaluation for underlying mitral valve disease.

Perioperative State. Perioperative atrial flutter–fibrillation is common. With cardiac surgery, direct manipulation of the heart is an obvious factor. With any surgery, the depressant effect of most general anesthetics on ventricular function also plays a role. Inhaled anesthetics inhibit lung ciliary function and promote the accumulation of pulmonary secretions, adding to the perioperative oxygenation and acid-base problems. The depression of the cough reflex and any postoperative chest or abdominal pain that inhibits voluntary coughing also contribute to the problem. Perioperative fluid overload constitutes another atrial stress. The increase in heart disease related to age (e.g., coronary artery disease) provides a backdrop for all perioperative stresses. Anesthesia and perioperative drugs further complicate the picture by producing amnesia or analgesia and the loss of symptomatic clues to perioperative myocardial infarction. Serial ECGs and CK-MB enzyme levels in such instances are frequently helpful. In the perioperative setting, atrial flutter–fibrillation is often repetitive, and all factors are important in planning therapeutic interventions.

In the preceding clinical settings, the common denominator on both sides of the heart is atrial distention that, with chronicity, causes atrial myofiber hypertrophy and fibrosis.

Toxic or Metabolic Factors. Advanced hyperthyroidism is likely to be associated with atrial fibrillation. In the elderly patient with so-called apathetic hyperthyroidism, it may the one clinical clue to the diagnosis. Although this condition might be considered an example of the arrhythmia with no associated heart disease, it occurs only in older patients with advanced hyperthyroidism and associated "high-output" heart failure. Concomitant hypertensive and coronary heart disease are frequent cofactors.

The myocardial depressant effects of alcohol, particularly when it is consumed in excess, can cause a variety of acute arrhythmias, including atrial fibrillation. Atrial fibrillation in association with binge drinking is one type of "holiday heart syndrome." The arrhythmia usually converts to sinus rhythm with abstinence and falling alcohol levels. Sometimes, atrial fibrillation reflects a combination of the stress of acute alcohol intoxication and underlying ventricular dysfunction due to alcoholic cardiomyopathy.

Sinus Node Dysfunction. Atrial flutter-fibrillation is a typical component of sinus node dysfunction (see Chapter 13, pages 305 to 307). Both conditions are more common in the older population. The arrhythmia frequently worsens the symptomatic manifestations of underlying coronary artery disease or left ventricular failure from a variety of causes. On occasion, associated heart disease is minor, and the major symptoms stem from the arrhythmias. Older patients also typically have more atrial and conduction system fibrosis. These factors potentiate both atrial flutter–fibrillation and, with its termination, unstable atrial pacemakers (with periods of sinus arrest or atrial asystole) and slow or absent junctional (His) escape pacers. In the older age group, cerebral hypoperfusion with presyncope and syncope may occur during the tachycardia or the posttachycardia bradyarrhythmias. Drugs given for recurrent atrial flutter–fibrillation (e.g., digoxin, class Ia or class Ic agents, amiodarone, and calcium blockers or β-blockers) can depress escape pacers and potentiate posttachycardia bradyarrhythmias.

Acute Pericarditis and Chronic Pericardial Constriction. Intuitively, one might expect atrial flutter–fibrillation and other atrial arrhythmias to be common during acute pericarditis. Except for sinus tachycardia related to fever, pain, and anxiety, however, atrial arrhythmias are unusual. When generalized atrial reentry occurs, it usually is brief, is at the fibrillation end of the spectrum, and implies associated underlying heart disease or pericardial constriction.[18] Correction of chronic constriction is usually not associated with the ability to restore sinus rhythm. This finding likely reflects the typical long duration of the arrhythmia before surgery.

Lone Atrial Fibrillation. In a small patient subset, atrial fibrillation occurs as an isolated finding. With chronicity, chest x-ray and echo indices of mild left atrial enlargement occur but with no stigmata of atrioventricular valvular disease,* ventricular dysfunction, or metabolic derangement. *Lone atrial fibrillation* refers to the condition of patients in this subgroup.

Natural History

The natural history of atrial flutter–fibrillation generally mirrors that of the underlying primary process. The arrhythmia's presence should suggest an advanced stage of disease, and its spontaneous disappearance usually reflects successful management. Initially, the clinician may alter the presence of atrial flutter–fibrillation by either pharmacologic or electrical ablation. In later stages, it may be necessary to "live with" this tachycardia and aim therapy at controlling the ventricular rate. On occasion, the arrhythmia can have independent prognostic significance because of its relation

---

*Most series predate Doppler ultrasonography.

to systemic embolization or to significant hemodynamic or electrical instability.

Embolization. Atrial fibrillation causes stasis of intra-atrial blood flow, increasing the likelihood of thrombus formation with pulmonary or systemic embolization. This adds independent prognostic significance that extends across all clinical syndromes.[4] Atrial flutter, with its more organized atrial contraction, may pose less risk for stasis and embolization. Atrial flutter, however, is less common than atrial fibrillation, and its risk for embolization is not as well characterized. Generalized atrial reentry sometimes travels the spectrum of rate and regularity. The more "impure" the flutter or the longer the periods of intermixed atrial fibrillation, the higher is the risk of embolization.

Embolization is most likely when the arrhythmia occurs with heart failure, cardiomyopathy, or mitral valve disease, particularly mitral stenosis. Patients under 60 years of age with "lone" atrial fibrillation are at the lowest risk for embolization. With chronicity, embolization is distressingly common in all clinical settings, with occasionally devastating consequences, including death or severe residual disability. With acute atrial fibrillation, embolization may occur at the onset of the arrhythmia, during the arrhythmia, with termination, and even up to several

days following termination of the arrhythmia. The risk of embolization is significantly less with recurrent atrial fibrillation. With chronic atrial fibrillation, embolization is most frequent during the first year, although it may occur at any time, even after years of apparent clinical stability. In all clinical situations, the cumulative risk of embolization relates directly to chronicity, patient age, and severity of underlying disease.

Hemodynamic or Electrical Instability. In some clinical circumstances, the arrhythmia may combine with features of the underlying disease process to produce serious consequences such as syncope, sudden death, or catastrophic heart failure. These events may have additive prognostic significance.

Patients with a rapidly conducting AV node or accessory pathway typically have a rapid ventricular response to atrial tachyarrhythmias. The ventricles may be activated so rapidly that a drop in cardiac output or ventricular fibrillation ensues, leading to syncope or sudden death. With mitral stenosis, the loss of atrial systole combined with a rapid heart rate can produce a marked elevation in left atrial pressure with catastrophic pulmonary edema. With myocardial infarction and atrial fibrillation, the prognosis is most closely related to the extent of myocardial damage. On occasion, however, the tachycardia and loss of atrial systole may combine to increase infarct size or further compromise the hemodynamic balance.

METHODS OF TREATMENT

General Principles. Treatment of atrial flutter–fibrillation depends (1) on the clinical setting; (2) on its clinical consequences; (3) on whether it is acute, recurrent, or chronic (and, if chronic, on its duration); and (4) on whether it is at the flutter or the fibrillation end of the spectrum. Patients with concomitant ventricular preexcitation form a small subgroup with unique therapeutic implications. Left atrial size determined by echocardiography is another, more controversial factor.

An analysis of these factors usually determines whether to tolerate the arrhythmia and control the ventricular rate or to attempt to restore and maintain sinus rhythm. For example, cardioversion of transient episodes of repetitive perioperative atrial flutter–fibrillation serves little purpose. Initial therapy should be directed at stabilizing the patient by correcting any hypotension, heart failure, and electrolyte imbalance. Digitalis in combination with verapamil, with diltiazem, or with a β-blocker may be administered to slow the ventricular response. A class Ia drug (e.g., intravenous procainamide) may be used if the goal is to restore sinus rhythm or to prevent recurrences of the arrhythmia. With chronic atrial fibrillation (duration of 1 year or more), the likelihood of successful cardioversion or maintenance of subsequent sinus rhythm is small. Similarly, the larger the left atrium, the less likely is long-term sinus rhythm. An echocardiographic left atrial diameter greater than 4.5 cm reportedly predicts less successful long-term sinus rhythm.[19] These data, however, are from a selected series of patients (mitral valve disease and hypertrophic cardiomyopathy), and left atrial size is not an absolute guideline for cardioversion. Some patients with atrial diameters greater than 4.5 cm may maintain sinus rhythm for prolonged periods following cardioversion, whereas others with smaller atria may not.

When underlying heart disease is severe and irreversible, it is usually best to treat the underlying disease and accept the arrhythmia while controlling the ventricular rate. When the atrial fibrillation is due to mitral valve disease, on the other hand, careful consideration should be given to operative valve repair or replacement. If the patient is not a surgical candidate, one trial of cardioversion (chemical or electrical) is probably reasonable. Table 10–3 summarizes treatment strategies according to whether the goal is establishing a slower ventricular rate or restoring sinus rhythm.

Acute Anticoagulation Therapy. Whether to anticoagulate before attempting cardioversion is an important initial decision that should be independent of the decision of whether to select drug therapy or countershock as the means of cardioversion. With arrhythmias of recent onset (less than 3 days) not associated with prior embolization, mitral valve disease, cardiomyopathy, or congestive heart failure, the risk of embolization with cardioversion is low. When any of these factors are present, at least 3 weeks of warfarin therapy may prevent new thrombi from forming, while any thrombi already present stabilize or resolve. Whether transesophageal echo imaging of the atria to "exclude atrial thrombi"[20] will help further refine decisions for anticoagulation awaits further investigation.

With prior embolization, more intensive warfarin therapy may be necessary (i.e., prothrombin time ratios of 1.5 to 2.0 times control, using the rabbit brain thromboplastin assay commonly available in the United States). In lower-risk subgroups, prothrombin time ratios of 1.2 to 1.5 times control are recommended.[21] Some patients with an indication for anticoagulation revert to sinus rhythm before 3 weeks of therapy can be effected. In such instances, the clinician can only hope for the best. After cardioversion, warfarin should be continued for a month or so until the stability of sinus rhythm is known. When the risk for embolization with recurrent atrial fibrillation is high (e.g., prior embolization, mitral valve disease), a longer period of postcardioversion anticoagulation therapy may be warranted.

Digitalis Therapy. The time-honored role of digitalis in the treatment of atrial fibrillation is being increasingly questioned. At doubt are its efficacy in restoring sinus rhythm acutely, maintaining it chronically, and controlling the ventricular response with chronic or recurrent atrial fibrillation. Not withstanding these doubts, however, it remains a very commonly used drug.

In the acute situation, 0.5 mg of digoxin is the recommended initial dose and agent (it is contraindicated in patients with ventricular preexcitation). Intravenous administration provides the most predictable pharmacokinetics. Two additional doses of 0.25 mg 2 to 4 hours apart may be given, depending on the ventricular response. Sinus rhythm typically follows in some patients, although whether this represents chance or a cause-effect relationship is debatable. One double-blind, placebo-controlled trial showed no difference between digoxin and placebo in the rate of return to sinus rhythm.[22] With heart failure and even without cardioversion, improved hemodynamics may lower sympathetic tone and further help in rate control. When sympathetic tone remains high, digoxin alone is usually ineffective in controlling the ventricular rate.

For chronic prophylaxis, digoxin is the cheapest, safest, and most convenient antiarrhythmic drug. It is also the least effective drug and may sometimes even potentiate atrial fibrillation (its vagally mediated indirect effects on atrial tissue may be profibrillatory). Quinidine and, to a lesser degree, verapamil, flecainide, and propafenone may raise the serum digoxin concentration and precipitate toxicity (see Chapter 15).

Class Ia and Class Ic Drugs and Amiodarone. The following discussion concentrates primarily on the class Ia drugs; however, the utility of the class Ic drugs and amiodarone in restoring and maintaining sinus rhythm is at least comparable, and may even be superior, to that of the class Ia drugs. Of the class Ic drugs and amiodarone, only flecainide has Food and Drug Administration (FDA) approval for the treatment of patients with atrial flutter–fibrillation. The risk of ventricular proarrhythmia in these patients (particularly when left ventricular function is normal) is likely small but is an important and currently unsettled issue.

These drugs can directly cause cardioversion to sinus rhythm. When hypotension is not present, they can be used when immediate electrical cardioversion is either unsuccessful or contraindicated. They all can increase the ventricular response if slowing the atrial reentry rate results in less concealed AV nodal conduction and reduces the degree of AV nodal

block (Fig. 10–13A). Quinidine has the added problem of having vagolytic and α-blocking properties. The latter cause vasodilation and an increased sympathetic tone; these effects can accelerate AV nodal conduction. Thus, a patient with an atrial rate of 300 beats per minute and 2:1 AV conduction with a ventricular rate of 150 beats per minute may be well compensated. A class Ia or class Ic drug may cause acute deterioration if the atrial rate slows to 220 beats per minute and AV conduction increases to 1:1 (see Table 10–1). This has resulted in the widespread axiom that, except when there is preexcitation (Fig. 10–13B), digitalization (or at least administration of a drug that decreases AV nodal conduction) should be accomplished before giving class I agents. This is particularly true when the baseline rhythm is atrial flutter with a rapid ventricular response, as in Figure 10–13A.

With concomitant dysfunction of the sinus node, these drugs can exacerbate posttachycardia bradycardias by depressing all escape pacemakers. Permanent pacing may be necessary to treat the bradycardias and allow the use of appropriate drugs to control the atrial flutter–fibrillation. In some patients, on the other hand, a class I drug may control the tachycardia with no significant exacerbation of the bradycardia.

With unstable patients, parenteral drug administration is mandatory. The class Ia and class Ic drugs (except for procain-

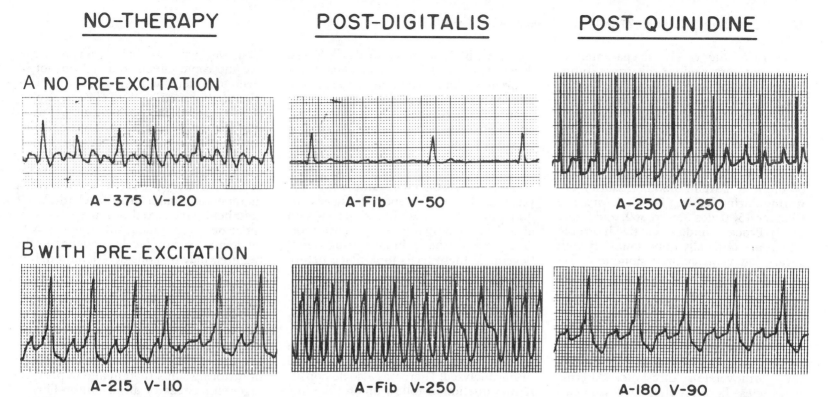

A NO PRE-EXCITATION

A-375 V-120   A-Fib V-50   A-250 V-250

B WITH PRE-EXCITATION

A-215 V-110   A-Fib V-250   A-180 V-90

FIGURE 10–13. These sequences show the variability in ventricular rate that may occur in response to digitalis versus the class Ia and class Ic drugs in the absence (*A*) and presence (*B*) of ventricular preexcitation. (*A, left*) With neither preexcitation nor therapy, atrial flutter–fibrillation at a rate of 375 beats per minute is associated with a ventricular response of around 120 beats per minute. (*A, middle*) Digitalis directly increases the atrial rate and indirectly (by means of enhanced vagal tone) slows AV nodal conduction. The combination of both factors markedly slows the ventricular response. (*A, right*) Quinidine therapy slows the atrial rate and decreases concealed AV nodal conduction. In addition, quinidine is vagolytic and has weak α-blocking properties, two factors which enhance sympathetic tone. All three factors facilitate AV nodal conduction and the ventricular rate. (Note the occasional 1:1 AV conduction.)

(*B, left*) With ventricular preexcitation and no therapy, atrial flutter is still associated with predominantly 2:1 AV conduction. (*B, middle*) Digitalis increases the atrial rate and, with no AV nodal protection, markedly accelerates the ventricular response, owing to rapid conduction over the accessory pathway. The fully preexcited supraventricular complexes are widened, are very rapid, and often may degenerate to, or suggest, malignant ventricular tachyarrhythmias. (*B, right*) The class Ia and class Ic drugs (e.g., quinidine) slow the atrial rate (to 180 beats per minute in this patient) and the conduction over the accessory pathway. The AV conduction remained 2:1, producing a ventricular rate of 90 beats per minute.

amide) are either rarely used parenterally or are not approved for this route. Intravenous procainamide, therefore, is the drug of choice and, if given slowly, is hemodynamically well tolerated. To initiate and sustain a therapeutic level, the patient should be loaded over a 30-minute period, either by a continuous intravenous infusion or by intermittent injections of 20 to 50 mg/min. Careful blood pressure monitoring during loading is mandatory (see Chapter 15, pages 359 to 360, and Table 15–2). Procainamide's negative inotropic effects are clinically important only with severe left ventricular dysfunction. Following unsuccessful countershock, or with repetitive atrial fibrillation, procainamide may directly cause cardioversion and enhance the likelihood of maintaining sinus rhythm following induced or spontaneous reversions. It also enhances the success of countershock by lowering the cardioversion threshold. Alternatively, class Ia drugs after successful cardioversion may prevent recurrent atrial flutter–fibrillation. Indeed, a meta-analysis of six randomized, controlled trials comparing chronic quinidine therapy with no antiarrhythmic drug therapy (other than digitalis) in maintaining sinus rhythm following cardioversion (with atrial fibrillation duration of 3 days or more) showed that quinidine therapy significantly enhanced the likelihood of maintaining sinus rhythm for at least 1 year (50% in the quinidine group compared with 25% in controls).[23] These drugs, however, all have a significant risk of proarrhythmia (see Chapter 15, pages 353 to 354), even when given for supraventricular arrhythmias. Quinidine therapy reportedly carries the highest risk for torsades de pointes (although this apparent increased risk may relate simply to quinidine being the most widely studied of the class Ia drugs). The same meta-analysis that showed therapeutic efficacy for quinidine in maintaining sinus rhythm also showed an increased all-cause mortality rate in the quinidine subgroup.[23] Several of these trials took place before discovery of the quinidine-digoxin interaction, and digitalis toxicity, however unlikely, could have been a confounding variable. In addition, although underlying diagnoses were somewhat evenly distributed between the quinidine and placebo groups, disease severity was uncontrolled or not analyzed. There was also no consistent evaluation or follow-up of quinidine levels, ECG changes, or serum potassium and magnesium levels. This study appropriately raises questions concerning the safety of chronic quinidine therapy (and by inference, all class I drugs); additional clinical research is needed.

About 50% of the episodes of torsades occur within the first 48 hours of initiating therapy. This risk probably justifies hospitalization with monitoring while such drugs are administered for the first time (see also Chapter 12, pages 264 and 288 to 289). Disopyramide has significant negative inotropic effects and should not be given to patients with significant left ventricular dysfunction. With chronic use, all class Ia agents have a high incidence of side effects (mainly gastrointestinal) that lead to discontinuation of therapy.

When the arrhythmia recurs during class Ia therapy, the dosage and frequency of the regimen should be evaluated. A therapeutic trough drug level (drawn 1 hour before the next dose) suggests recurrence despite an adequate regimen. With inadequate serum levels, a change in the regimen may be considered, although in some clinical series, no relationship between serum drug levels and the maintenance of sinus rhythm could be proved.

There is less experience with the class Ic agents than with class Ia agents, but the former appear to be as effective as, or even more effective than, the latter, both in restoring sinus rhythm and in preventing recurrences of atrial flutter–fibrillation. Only flecainide has FDA approval for the management of this arrhythmia and even then only in patients without structural heart disease. The use of class Ic drugs in carefully selected patients with significant symptoms may be warranted, particularly if other drugs have failed. Although these drugs directly slow AV nodal conduction, this effect may be variable. As with the class Ia drugs, the concomitant use of an AV-node–active drug can prevent a paradoxical increase in the ventricular response, particularly when the baseline rhythm is atrial flutter. Flecainide and propafenone are also significantly negatively inotropic. These drug characteristics require careful patient selection, low initial drug doses, and careful follow-up observations of rhythm status.

Amiodarone is effective in preventing recurrent atrial fibrillation, and low-dose regimens (e.g., from 200 mg daily to as infrequently as two to three times per week) can be tried. Whether this reduced drug dosage can reduce the long-term dermatologic, liver, endocrine, and pulmonary toxicity, or whether toxicity relates to the total cumulative dose, remains unproven. There is no question that the lower-dose regimens are clinically well tolerated. Again, its use in this setting should be carefully considered (see Chapter 15, pages 382 to 384). Its low risk of ventricular proarrhythmia may afford the drug unique advantages when used in the setting of structural heart disease.

Chronic Anticoagulation Therapy.
With chronic atrial fibrillation, the risk of embolic stroke requires consideration of long-term anticoagulation. The hemorrhagic complications of anticoagulant therapy warrant a healthy respect, but in certain situations, the benefits outweigh the risks and the guidelines iterated for acute anticoagulation apply to the chronic state (pages 225–226). The lower risks of less aggressive anticoagulation become even more important over the long term. For example, with proximal leg vein thrombosis, less intense long-term warfarin therapy reduces the risk of hemorrhage while sustaining efficacy in preventing pulmonary embolization.[24] Several randomized, controlled trials in patients with nonvalvular atrial fibrillation compared less aggressive warfarin therapy with placebo. They reported striking reductions in the incidence of strokes and a low risk of hemorrhagic complications.[25-27] Any patient with embolization, atrial fibrillation, and no contraindication to anticoagulation, however, should have long-term warfarin therapy with prothrombin time ratios 1.5 to 2.0 times those of controls. The role of aspirin as an anticoagulant in this setting is unclear. In one study, low-dose aspirin (75 mg/day) was ineffective in reducing strokes.[25] In another trial, a higher dose of aspirin (325 mg/day) significantly reduced their incidence.[27] The limb of this latter study comparing aspirin with warfarin is currently ongoing.

β-Blockers, Verapamil, and Diltiazem.
In acute cases of arrhythmia, parenteral β-blockers or verapamil can be used to increase the degree of AV block if the patient is not hypotensive and if cardioversion is contraindicated or unsuccessful. In some instances, β-blockers may also result in sinus rhythm. Even with no reversion to sinus rhythm, the decreased heart rate usually counterbalances any negative inotropic effects of the drug. In patients with questionable ventricular function, it is best to proceed very slowly with small intravenous doses of either verapamil or a short-acting β-blocker such as esmolol. In patients with ventricular dysfunction, verapamil may be better tolerated than β-blockers. The negative inotropic effects of verapamil are typically counterbalanced by systemic arteriolar vasodilation, but congestive heart failure can still occur. When electrical cardioversion follows either β-blocker or verapamil therapy, 0.5 mg of atropine administered intravenously may help the emergence of a stable pacemaker.

Occasionally, hypotension following intravenous administration of verapamil results from arteriolar vasodilation in combination with compromised ventricular function and the negative inotropic effects of the drug. This is particularly likely in patients with atrial flutter–fibrillation and ventricular preexcitation. Besides systemic arteriolar vasodilation and heightened sympathetic tone, verapamil blocks AV nodal conduction. This results in less concealed retrograde conduction into the accessory pathway, with enhanced antegrade conduction, which further contributes to hemodynamic collapse. In these patients, synchronized electrical cardioversion is the initial treatment of choice for atrial fibrillation (see Chapter 17, pages 415 to 416), with intravenous procainamide a second-line approach. Verapamil-induced hypotension can be reversed with intravenous calcium chloride[28,29] or conventional vasopressors.

With chronic atrial fibrillation and normal AV conduction, a disproportionately rapid increase in exercise heart rate is the rule with digoxin therapy alone, even with therapeutic drug levels. Oral verapamil, diltiazem, or β-blockers may help in heart-rate control during rest and exercise. In younger patients with well-maintained ventricular function, even monotherapy with one of these calcium blockers was more effective than digoxin in controlling the ventricular rate. Diltiazem carries the added advantage of not elevating the serum digoxin level. In patients with poor ventricular function, verapamil or diltiazem may be tried in preference to β-blockers but can still worsen congestive heart failure.

Ventricular Preexcitation. Digitalis therapy is contraindicated when atrial flutter–fibrillation occurs in combination with ventricular preexcitation (see Fig. 10–13). With a rapidly conducting accessory pathway, the protection of the AV node against a rapid ventricular response is lost, and the faster the atrial rate is, the faster the ventricular response. Digitalis worsens the situation because it can further increase the ventricular rate by three separate mechanisms: (1) It shortens refractory periods and speeds conduction in atrial tissue, resulting in an even faster atrial reentry rate; (2) accessory pathways usually behave like atrial tissue and the shortened refractory periods may accelerate conduction to the ventricles; and (3) like verapamil, digitalis blocks conduction through the AV node with less concealed retrograde conduction into the accessory pathway, facilitating its antegrade conduction (see Fig. 10–13B). The institution of digitalis therapy in patients with a fast accessory pathway and atrial fibrillation is one presumed mechanism for precipitating sudden death.[30]

The mere presence of a delta wave, however, does not predict that atrial fibrillation, a rapid ventricular response, or acceleration of accessory conduction will occur. The incidence of atrial flutter–fibrillation is far from 100%; it has been reported in up to 25% of symptomatic patients with preexcitation. In some patients, furthermore, the refractory period of the accessory pathway is long enough to prevent a rapid ventricular response to atrial reentry. In addition, digitalis may not significantly accelerate conduction over the accessory pathway.[31] In any patient with ventricular preexcitation and atrial fibrillation, however, it is wise to avoid digitalis therapy unless or until its effects on the accessory pathway can be carefully documented. As a corollary, when a patient with ventricular preexcitation gives a history of palpitations and syncope, paroxysmal atrial flutter–fibrillation should be suspected and digitalis therapy avoided.

The class Ia and class Ic drugs, on the other hand, slow conduction in atrial tissue and the accessory pathway; both effects slow the ventricular response (see Fig. 10–13B). With a stable patient, intravenous procainamide may be the drug of choice. For chronic therapy, rather than choosing a class I drug empirically, clinicians should have patients undergo a detailed electrophysiologic study to define the characteristics of the accessory pathway and guide therapy.

Subgroups by Clinical and Hemodynamic Parameters. All of the preceding considerations are important in planning, initiating, or maintaining therapy, but immediate decisions need to be based primarily on whether the arrhythmia is acute, chronic, or recurrent, and on whether the patient is clinically stable or unstable. A discussion of the various therapeutic options in four subgroups based on these descriptors follows.

ACUTE ONSET: UNSTABLE. In the acute situation with an unstable patient, the arrhythmia is likely to be contributing to the instability of some hemodynamic or other clinical parameter. For example, during acute myocardial infarction, atrial flutter–fibrillation with a rapid ventricular response is clinically unstable. This is true even when there is no pain and the blood pressure is well maintained, because a rapid ventricular rate can increase myocardial oxygen consumption and infarct size. With mitral stenosis, acute atrial fibrillation can result in fulminant pulmonary edema. With atrial fibrillation and a very rapid ventricular response, significant hypotension may occur. In these situations, it is critical to restore sinus rhythm immediately or to slow the ventricular response rapidly. With associated hypotension, early pharmacologic support of the blood pressure is important and may be a prerequisite before other measures can succeed.

When quick control of rapid heart rate is paramount, therefore, the only question is whether to proceed with electrical cardioversion, with drug therapy to slow the heart rate or restore sinus rhythm, or with some combination. In unstable clinical situations, intravenous digoxin is generally slow, unreliable, and of questionable efficacy. Aggressive digitalization also increases the risk of both digoxin toxicity and significant ventricular arrhythmias should subsequent electrical shock become necessary. Intravenous procainamide is frequently effective in restoring sinus rhythm, but its effectiveness is far from 100%, and loading takes time.

The treatment of choice for atrial flutter–fibrillation with an unstable clinical situation, therefore, is electrical cardioversion (see Chapter 17, pages 415 to 416). With a conscious patient, even in an unstable situation, there is usually time for appropriate analgesia and anesthesia of the patient. With atrial flutter, low energies (e.g., 10 to 25 joules) may result in successful cardioversion. With atrial rates

less than 300 beats per minute, atrial pacing (via the esophageal or an intravascular route) is an option. With atrial fibrillation, atrial pacing is ineffective, and reversion to sinus rhythm usually requires energies of 50 to 100 J or more. One common sequence is to begin at 100 J (or, for a repeated cardioversion, at whatever energy level was successful previously) and proceed systematically, as required, to 200 J and 360–400 J of stored energy (see Tables 10–1 and 10–3). An intervening 300-J shock is an optional step if done rapidly and without the need for additional anesthesia.

Failures may be due to either (1) no termination of atrial reentry, or (2) prompt recurrence of the arrhythmia after successful cardioversion. Differentiating these two possibilities requires observing the rhythm immediately following the transthoracic shock. It is helpful to use equipment that prevents or rapidly dissipates any shock-induced charging of circuits and electrodes. This allows a rapid return of the ECG signal for immediate arrhythmia analysis. If no "break" can be documented, higher energies, improved techniques, or ancillary pharmacologic treatment (such as the addition of intravenous procainamide) may be tried. If cardioversion occurred but was transient, repeated electrical shocks are contraindicated. Rather, efforts should be aimed at correcting the factors contributing to the instability of sinus rhythm, such as hypo-

tension, heart failure, hypoxia, acidosis, and electrolyte imbalance. Intravenous procainamide may restore sinus rhythm itself or enhance the success of a second attempt at electrical cardioversion (see Chapter 15, pages 359 to 360). In the short term and particularly with atrial fibrillation, there is little risk of significantly increasing the ventricular response, and concomitant loading with digitalis is rarely necessary.

ACUTE ONSET: STABLE. In the acute situation with a stable patient, one has more flexibility in choosing among the therapeutic options. The previously cited guidelines concerning anticoagulation should be considered first. Management of the underlying acute problem often results in spontaneous reversion to sinus rhythm. If additional therapy is needed, the treatment of choice is pharmacologic, to restore sinus rhythm or the control of ventricular rate. Despite controversies concerning its efficacy, digoxin is still a favored initial drug, particularly with any concomitant heart failure.

If the arrhythmia persists after control of the underlying disease process and digitalization, the choice is between additional pharmacologic therapy and countershock. Pharmacologic maneuvers may be aimed at accepting the atrial arrhythmia and controlling the ventricular rate (e.g., adding β-blockers or verapamil). Alternatively, drugs may be used to attempt cardioversion (e.g., a class Ia drug [see

Chapter 15, pages 358, 360, and 361), either alone or in concert with subsequent electrical cardioversion. With slower atrial flutter (rates less than 300 per minute and the slower the better), atrial pacing via either an esophageal or intra-atrial electrode may also effect cardioversion.

CHRONIC ATRIAL FLUTTER–FIBRILLATION Even with "new" patients, it is usually possible to date the onset of the arrhythmia and define its chronicity. Simple techniques such as reviewing the patient's medical history may provide valuable chronologic clues. This review should include dates of significant changes in symptomatic status or medications and the use of other treatments. Although patients may not know the technical names of various cardiac procedures, most can give a coherent history of and describe what it is like to undergo transthoracic cardioversion or esophageal pacing. Obtaining prior ECGs and medical records and doing the "Bell test" (calling the patient's prior physician or clinic) may prove invaluable.

For arrhythmias with a duration of less than 1 year, one attempt at cardioversion can be considered, depending on the clinical circumstances. For example, a rare patient with severe left ventricular dysfunction may become much more symptomatic with the onset of atrial fibrillation. When symptoms persist despite adequate control of the ventricular rate,

they may reflect the loss of the contribution to stroke volume of coordinated atrial systole, resulting in a lower cardiac output. Vigorous efforts to restore and maintain sinus rhythm, including low-dose amiodarone therapy, may be indicated.

When atrial fibrillation has been present for more than 1 year, the restoration or maintenance of sinus rhythm is less likely, and despite the hemodynamic situation (at least with our current pharmacologic armamentarium), it is probably best to accept the arrhythmia and direct therapy at controlling the ventricular rate and the causes of any associated hemodynamic instability.

Accomplishing optimal ventricular rate control is particularly difficult with chronic atrial flutter as compared with atrial fibrillation. With the latter, the more rapid atrial rates cause more concealed conduction into the AV node, increase AV nodal refractoriness, and result in a slower ventricular response, particularly with the addition of an AV-node–active drug (Fig. 10–14; see Fig. 10–12). With atrial flutter, however, particularly when the reentry rate does not speed in response to digoxin, large doses may be required to control the ventricular response, resulting in a greater risk of toxicity. Even with adequate control of resting heart rate, minimal activity (e.g., simply standing up) frequently increases AV conduction to 2:1 or less, with a re-

sulting abrupt increase in the ventricular rate. Additional therapeutic options might include repeated cardioversion with or without additional pharmacologic therapy such as a class Ia drug (or, under some circumstances, even a class Ic drug or amiodarone). Often, concomitant ventricular dysfunction limits the use of many of these drugs as well as of verapamil and the β-blockers.

RECURRENT ATRIAL FLUTTER–FIBRILLATION. For patients reverting to sinus rhythm after a first episode or for those experiencing recurrences, the question of posttachycardia drug "prophylaxis" against further episodes frequently arises. For example, paroxysmal atrial fibrillation in patients with hypertrophic cardiomyopathy is typically poorly tolerated. The loss of atrial systole in this setting may cause a precipitous drop in stroke volume and cardiac output. In addition, the shortened diastolic filling period of the tachycardia further diminishes stroke volume. The tachycardia itself has positive inotropic effects. These factors all aggravate both the gradient and the mitral regurgitation and may produce marked symptomatic deterioration.

Just as with the chronic arrhythmia (perhaps even more so), patients with recurrent bouts of paroxysmal atrial flutter–fibrillation frequently have a debilitatingly rapid ventricular response despite treatment with a variety of drugs. With recurrent atrial flutter, symptoms are par-

FIGURE 10–14. (*A*) Pre-digitalis, atrial flutter at 310 beats per minute produces either a regular (left-hand portion) or regularly irregular (right-hand portion) ventricular response. After digitalization, the atrial rate has increased significantly, reflecting movement of the reentry rate or regularity from the flutter end of the spectrum to the fibrillation end. The concomitant slowing of the ventricular response reflects slowed AV nodal conduction from both the direct and vagally mediated indirect effects of digitalis on the AV node, as well as increased concealed AV nodal conduction from the digitalis-induced speeding of the atrial rate. Evidence of this effect is particularly dramatic in the right-hand portion of the strip, where the atrial rate becomes extremely rapid. (*B*) This ECG shows a digitalized patient in atrial fibrillation before the administration of quinidine, a class Ia drug. Note the rapid, irregularly irregular atrial rhythm and ventricular response. Quinidine directly slows and regularizes conduction over the atrial reentry circuit (i.e., the arrhythmia moves to the flutter end of the spectrum). The next-to-last beat in the strip is due to transient reversion to sinus rhythm.

A Pre-Digitalis

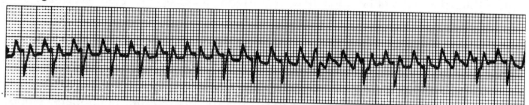

Post-Digitalis

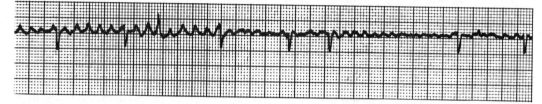

B On Digitalis, Pre-Quinidine

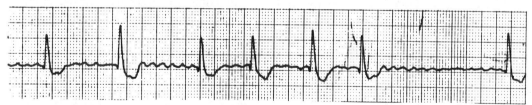

Post-Quinidine

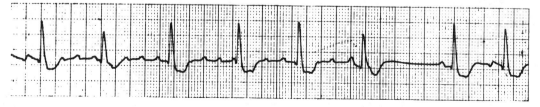

ticularly likely to relate to the difficulty in controlling the ventricular rate. Just as with chronic atrial flutter, the rapid rate may persist despite the combination of digitalis and verapamil or β-blocker therapy (see Table 10–3). The cost and potential mortality or morbidity of currently available antiarrhythmic drugs dictate that the risk-benefit ratios of any treatment regimen be carefully considered.

Recurrence Rates. Up to two thirds of patients experiencing their first episode of atrial flutter–fibrillation do not experience a recurrence in the ensuing year. Drug selection and aggressiveness of therapy, therefore, hinge on several variables, including the hemodynamic consequences of the arrhythmia, the presence of remediable contributing factors, and the occurrence of embolization. For example, with ventricular preexcitation and cardiovascular collapse, even a remote chance of a second episode may be intolerable. An electrophysiologic evaluation with either catheter ablation, or even surgical ablation, of the accessory pathway may be a preferable option. Similarly, with associated embolization, attempts to maintain sinus rhythm and anticoagulation therapy should be aggressive, even though no trial, to date, has addressed whether attempts at achieving and maintaining sinus rhythm lessen the incidence of stroke.

Perioperative atrial flutter–fibrillation with noncardiac surgery, on the other hand, frequently relates to the transient stress of iatrogenic fluid overload. The acutely successful regimen can usually be safely stopped as the patient successfully convalesces (i.e., after the removal of the major intravenous and enteral lines). Similarly, with transient arrhythmias related to other acute remediable stresses, such as hyperthyroidism, pulmonary embolism, or pneumonia, chronic suppressive therapy should be avoided unless the arrhythmia recurs. With cardiac surgery, on the other hand, particularly with associated left ventricular or mitral valve dysfunction, the arrhythmia is often more recurrent. Continuation of the acutely successful regimen for several months postoperatively or even indefinitely may be reasonable. Similarly, with nonremediable underlying factors (e.g., severe left ventricular dysfunction or inoperable mitral valve disease), recurrence is more likely, and a trial of prophylaxis may be warranted.

In some patients, the cause of the arrhythmia is enigmatic or controversial. An example of the latter might be the occurrence of the arrhythmia with trivial mitral regurgitation or with "echocardiographic" mitral valve prolapse and no mitral regurgitation. If the arrhythmia is not associated with embolization or severe symptoms, a trial of further observation to document the "natural history" might be warranted before undertaking chronic drug therapy. With an infrequent arrhythmia (e.g., occurring once or twice a year), the inconvenience of a rare event without drug therapy may more than counterbalance the heavy burden of daily drug therapy. A natural history study may be most valid when the cause of the arrhythmia is obscure, as illustrated by a Duke intern who experienced a bout of atrial fibrillation. Chronic fatigue was the only apparent risk factor. Two doses of oral digitalis 3 hours apart were given, and within 6 hours he reverted to sinus rhythm. No further digitalis was given, and to date (40 years later), the arrhythmia has not recurred.

Chronic Pharmacologic Therapy. With frequent or poorly tolerated recurrences of the arrhythmia, drug therapy to prevent or to limit the duration of the recurrences may be indicated. This decision should take into account issues such as efficacy and the risks of morbidity and mortality.

As previously discussed, the efficacy of chronic digitalis therapy in maintaining sinus rhythm or controlling the rapid ventricular rate of recurrences is questionable (see page 232). The class Ia or class Ic drugs and amiodarone are more effective than digitalis at maintaining sinus rhythm but carry a higher risk for proarrhythmia, significant morbidity, and possibly even mortality (see pages 226 to 229). In addition, because of their potential for increasing the ventricular rate by means of significant atrial rate slowing or other direct or indirect effects on facilitating AV nodal conduction (see Fig. 10–13A), they should always be used in combination with drugs that slow AV nodal conduction. With adequate ventricular function, verapamil, diltiazem, and β-blockers are useful in helping to control the ventricular response.

In patients with hypertrophic cardiomyopathy and poorly tolerated paroxysmal atrial fibrillation, disopyramide can be considered. Amiodarone therapy is also effective, and the use of this potentially toxic compound may be justified when conventional therapy fails. A salutary effect on the hemodynamic consequences of atrial fibrillation also may follow surgical relief of obstruction. The data, however, are insufficient to recommend surgery for managing recurrent atrial fibrillation in this clinical setting.

Rather than long-term, continuous drug prophylaxis, depending on clinical circumstances, the drug may be given as needed for each recurrence. For example, 1000 to 1250 mg of oral procainamide may be given and followed by 750 mg 1 to 2 hours later as necessary. Alternatively, the regimen may be tailored to the individual patient, for example, a bedtime dose may be given to a patient with a nocturnal arrhythmia. Sometimes therapy with a class I drug may be the culprit when it does not completely suppress recurrences *and* moves them toward the flutter end of the spectrum, with consequent difficulty in ventricular rate control. Stopping the drug may allow chronic, stable atrial fibrillation to develop, with commensurately easier control of ventricular rate.

Nonpharmacologic Therapy. Following cardioversion, atrial pacing can theoretically maintain an adequate atrial rate, suppress atrial ectopy, and thus prevent recurrent atrial fibrillation. The efficacy of atrial pacing to prevent recurrent atrial fibrillation is unproven, however, and a multicenter trial is currently underway to address this question. With recurrent atrial flutter, a radio-frequency–responsive pacemaker and atrial leads in combination with a hand-held transmitter placed over the receiver or pacer can effect rapid atrial pacing and either entrainment of the atrial flutter (usually with subsequent reversion to sinus rhythm when pacing ceases) or atrial fibrillation (usually transient and followed by sinus rhythm).[9] Some newer antitachycardia pacemakers can accomplish the same result with totally self-contained circuitry. The device interrogates the arrhythmia and then delivers pacing impulses at predetermined or programmable intervals, sequences, and strengths.[32] In selected patients, the induction of AV block by use of a catheter technique[10–13] or open-heart surgery,[33] with permanent ventricular pacing, may be considered (see Chapter 17, pages 422 to 424). In highly selected patients, open surgical procedures with either cryoablation or incisions of key atrial sites have either stopped the arrhythmias or successfully isolated fibrillating atrial tissue from the SA and AV nodes. In the latter instance, chronotropic competence of sinus node function and the integrity of conduction of the sinus impulse to the AV node may be preserved.[34,35] Radiofrequency catheter ablation techniques in the right atrium of patients with atrial flutter show great promise of a similar or better efficacy in maintaining sinus rhythm with much less acute morbidity/mortality.[14] The question of whether a short-term gain in sinus rhythm is being traded for future misery with subsequent recurrences of a variety of arrhythmias awaits long-term follow-up of larger numbers of patients.

REFERENCES

1. Sommerbrodt J: Ueber Allorhythmie und Arhythmie des Herzens und deren Uraschen. Dtsch Archiv für Klin Med 19:392–423, 1877.
2. Lewis T: Auricular fibrillation and its relationship to clinical irregularity of the heart. Heart 1:306–372, 1909.
3. Parkinson J and Campbell M: The quinidine treatment of auricular fibrillation. Q J Med 22:281–303, 1929.
4. Lown B, Amarasingham R, and Newman J: New methods for terminating cardiac arrhythmias. Use of synchro-

nized capacitor discharge. JAMA 182:548–555, 1962.

5. Sawyer CG, Bolin LB, Stevens EL, Daniel LB Jr, O'Neill NC, and Hayes DM: Atrial fibrillation: Its etiology, treatment and association with embolization. South Med J 51:84–93, 1958.

6. Lister JW, Cohen LS, Bernstein WH, and Samet P: Treatment of supraventricular tachycardias by rapid atrial stimulation. Circulation 38:1044–1059, 1968.

7. Kerr CR, Gallagher JJ, Smith W, et al: The induction of atrial flutter and fibrillation and the termination of atrial flutter with esophageal pacing. PACE 6:60–72, 1983.

8. Waldo AL, MacLean WAH, Karp RB, Kouchoukos NT, and James TN: Entrainment and interruption of atrial flutter with atrial pacing: Studies in man following open heart surgery. Circulation 56:737–745, 1977.

9. Kahn A, Morris JJ, and Citron P: Patient-initiated rapid atrial pacing to manage supraventricular tachycardia. Am J Cardiol 38:200–204, 1976.

10. Gallagher JJ, Svenson RH, Kasell JH, et al: Catheter technique for closed-chest ablation of the atrioventricular conduction system. N Engl J Med 306:194–200, 1982.

11. Scheinman MM, Morady F, Hess DS, and Gonzalez R: Catheter-induced ablation of the atrioventricular junction to control refractory supraventricular arrhythmias. JAMA 248:851–855, 1982.

12. Saoudi N, Atallah G, Kirkorian G, and Touboul P: Catheter ablation of the atrial myocardium in human type I atrial flutter. Circulation 81:762–771, 1989.

13. Langberg JJ, Chin MC, Rosenqvist M, et al: Catheter ablation of the atrioventricular junction with radiofrequency energy. Circulation 80:1527–1535, 1989.

14. Feld GK, Fleck RP, Chen P-S, et al: Radiofrequency catheter ablation for the treatment of human type I atrial flutter. Circulation 86:1233–1240, 1992.

15. Allessie MA, Bonke FIM, and Schopman FJG: Circus movement in rabbit atrial muscle as a mechanism of tachycardia. Circ Res 41:9–18, 1977.

16. Weisfogel GM, Batsford WP, Paulay KL, et al: Sinus node re-entrant tachycardia in man. Am Heart J 90:295–304, 1975.

17. Wu D, Amat-y-Leon F, Denes P, Dhingra RC, Pietras RJ, and Rosen KM: Demonstration of sustained sinus and atrial reentry as a mechanism of paroxysmal supraventricular tachycardia. Circulation 51:234–243, 1975.

18. Spodick DH: Arrhythmias during acute pericarditis. A prospective study of 100 consecutive cases. JAMA 235:39–41, 1976.

19. Henry WL, Morganroth J, Pearlman AS, et al: Relation between echocardiographically determined left atrial size and atrial fibrillation. Circulation 53:273–279, 1976.

20. Manning WJ, Silverman DI, Gordon SPF, Krumholz HM, and Douglas PS: Cardioversion from atrial fibrillation without prolonged anticoagulation with use of transesophageal echocardiography to exclude the presence of atrial thrombi. N Engl J Med 328:750–755, 1993.

21. Dunn M, Alexander J, de Silva R, and Hildner F: Antithrombotic therapy in atrial fibrillation. Chest 89:68S–74S, 1986.

22. Falk RH, Knowlton AA, Bernard SA, Gotlieb NE, and Battinelli NJ: Digoxin for converting recent-onset atrial fibrillation to sinus rhythm. Ann Intern Med 106:503–506, 1987.

23. Coplen SE, Antman EM, Berlin JA, Hewitt P, and Chalmers TC: Efficacy and safety of quinidine therapy for maintenance of sinus rhythm after cardioversion: A meta-analysis of randomized control trials. Circulation 82:1106–1116, 1990.

24. Hull R, Hirsh J, Jay R, et al: Different intensities of oral anticoagulant therapy in the treatment of proximal-vein thrombosis. N Engl J Med 307:1676–1681, 1982.

25. Petersen P, Godtfredsen J, Boysen G, Andersen ED, and Andersen B: Placebo-controlled, randomised trial of warfarin and aspirin for prevention of thromboembolic complications in

chronic atrial fibrillation: The Copenhagen AFASAK study. Lancet 1:175–179, 1989.

26. The BAATAF Investigators: The effect of low-dose warfarin on the risk of stroke in patients with nonrheumatic atrial fibrillation. N Engl J Med 323:1505–1511, 1990.

27. The SPAFS Investigators: Preliminary report of the stroke prevention in atrial fibrillation study. N Engl J Med 322:863–868, 1990.

28. Perkins CM: Serious verapamil poisoning: Treatment with intravenous calcium gluconate. Br Med J 2:1127, 1978.

29. Morris DL and Goldschlager N: Calcium infusion for reversal of adverse effects of intravenous verapamil. JAMA 249:3212–3213, 1983.

30. Wellens HJJ and Durrer D: Wolff-Parkinson-White syndrome and atrial fibrillation. Relation between refractory period of the accessory pathway and ventricular rate during atrial fibrillation. Am J Cardiol 34:777–782, 1974.

31. Sellers TD, Bashore TM, and Gallagher JJ: Digitalis in the preexcitation syndrome: Analysis during atrial fibrillation. Circulation 56:260–267, 1977.

32. Spurrell RAJ, Nathan AW, Bexton RS, Hellestrand KJ, Nappholz T, and Camm AJ: Implantable automatic scanning pacemaker for termination of supraventricular tachycardia. Am J Cardiol 49:753–760, 1982.

33. Giannelli S Jr, Ayres SM, Gromprecht RF, Conklin EF, and Kennedy RJ: Therapeutic surgical division of the human conduction system. JAMA 199:155–160, 1967.

34. Guiradon GM, Klein GM, Sharma AD, and Yee R: Surgical alternatives for supraventricular tachycardia. Am J Cardiol 64:92J–96J, 1989.

35. Cox JL, Boineau JP, Schuessler RB, et al: Successful surgical treatment of atrial fibrillation: Review and clinical update. JAMA 266:1976–1980, 1991.

CHAPTER 11

Atrioventricular Junctional Tachycardias

BARRY W. RAMO, MD

Outline

The atrioventricular (AV) junction is the area of the heart containing the AV node and the His bundle. In the rarely occurring ventricular preexcitation syndromes, the accessory pathway (or pathways) is included in this designation. The tachycardias arising in this region, particularly those due to reentry, have long been studied. The propagation of impulses from the atrium to the ventricle and back to produce echo beats was identified as the basic mechanism in reentry tachycardias early in this century, and this mechanism has been used to explain a broad variety of tachyarrhythmias and bradyarrhythmias. The description by Moe and colleagues[1] of dual AV nodal pathways led the way for the electrophysiologic understanding of AV nodal reentry and its induction in the clinical electrophysiology laboratory.[2] Extensive study of preexcitation syndromes that serve as the anatomic substrate for reentrant arrhythmias not only have led to cures for this particular reentrant arrhythmia, but also have provided a general background for the study of ventricular arrhythmias.

This chapter discusses the tachycardias arising in the AV junction that are due to reentry and enhanced automaticity.

CLASSIFICATION

The classification of premature beats in Chapters 1 and 7 and of tachyarrhythmias

in Chapter 8 outlines the three distinct anatomic sites of origin: the atria, the AV junction, and the ventricles. Figure 11–1 notes the major tachycardias arising in the AV junction.

One tachycardia arising within the AV junction is due to enhanced automaticity in the distal AV node–His bundle and is termed *accelerated junctional rhythm*, or *nonparoxysmal junctional tachycardia (NPJT)* (Fig. 11–2).

The other AV junctional tachycardias are reentrant and are referred to collectively as *paroxysmal junctional tachycardia (PJT)*. Two distinct varieties of PJT exist: those tachycardias due to micro reentry entirely within the AV node (atrioventricular nodal reentry [AVNR]) and those due to "macroreentry," with the AV node and normal infranodal conducting system forming one limb of the tachycardia circuit, and an accessory pathway forming the other (atrioventricular reciprocating tachycardia [AVRT]) (Fig. 11–3; see Chapter 1, page 15). The term *paroxysmal atrial tachycardia (PAT)* is used by clinicians to describe a variety of reentrant and pacemaker supraventricular tachycardias, but it is most frequently used to refer to *AV junctional reentry tachycardias*. As our knowledge of arrhythmias has increased, it has become clear that the term "PAT" is a misnomer for the latter group and should be dropped; these tachycardias are actually AV junctional in location and do not primarily involve the atria.

MECHANISMS

Enhanced Automaticity

Accelerated AV junctional tachycardias are commonly caused by enhanced automaticity in the His bundle. Earlier investigations called into doubt the existence of spontaneous phase-4 depolarization within the AV node and, hence, its role as a potential pacemaker.[3] More recent studies, however, have reopened the question of pacemaker activity within the AV node, particularly in the region of its "junction" with the His bundle. The distinction between where the AV node ends and the His bundle begins, either anatomically or physiologically, is controversial, but this question need not be resolved to diagnose and manage junctional arrhythmias effectively. I have found it helpful conceptually to consider arrhythmias with inverted P waves that precede the QRS complexes in the inferior leads to be *low atrial* (see Chapter 9, page 181), and those with no preceding P waves but with a supraventricular QRS configuration to be *AV junctional*. To try to distinguish between those arising somewhere in the "distal" AV node and those arising in the His bundle is impractical and lacks any clinical significance. I therefore consider tachycardias due to enhanced automaticity in the His bundle or distal AV node collectively to be *accelerated AV junctional tachycardias*.

These junctional tachycardias tend to change rate gradually and, once present,

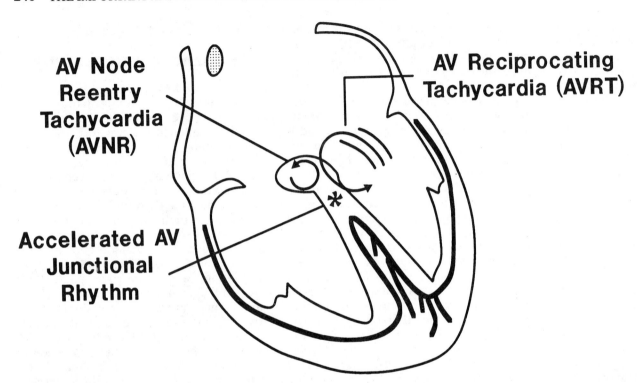

AV Node Reentry Tachycardia (AVNR)

AV Reciprocating Tachycardia (AVRT)

Accelerated AV Junctional Rhythm

FIGURE 11-1. Atrioventricular (AV) junctional tachycardias may be due to reentry or to enhanced pacemaker activity. The reentrant arrhythmias are either microreentry, that is, entirely within the AV node (atrioventricular nodal reentry [AVNR]), or macroreentry, that is involving the normal conduction system and an accessory pathway (atrioventricular reciprocating tachycardia [AVRT]). These two arrhythmias are referred to collectively as *paroxysmal junctional tachycardias (PJT)*. Accelerated pacemaker activity in the AV junction (AV node–His bundle) results in a narrow-QRS tachycardia with or without AV dissociation.

tend to persist. Common causes of such enhanced pacemaker activity are digitalis excess, inferior infarction, myocarditis, and mitral valve replacement; all are exacerbated by hypokalemia. The same conditions that provoke enhanced AV junctional automaticity also can slow AV nodal conduction and facilitate AV dissociation or variable ventriculoatrial (VA) conduction when the retrograde impulses are blocked in the dysfunctional AV node

(see Fig. 11–2). The rate of this tachycardia seldom exceeds 130 beats per minute. These rhythms do not respond to cardioversion and change rate very little in response to autonomic interventions.

Reentry

GENERAL PRINCIPLES

Reentry tachycardias in the AV junction develop in two distinct anatomic substrates that have in common dual path-

ways (the A or α pathway and the B or β pathway) within the AV junction (see Fig. 11–3). On the one hand, the dual pathways are entirely within the AV node and may be more distinct physiologically than anatomically. On the other hand, the dual pathways involve the normal conduction system as one limb and an accessory pathway, separate from the AV node, as the other limb. The latter creates a circuit with anatomically and physiologically dis-

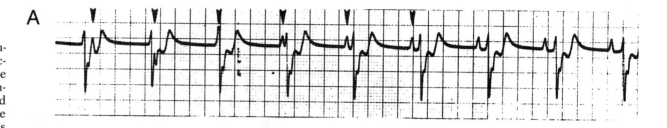

FIGURE 11–2. These examples of accelerated AV junctional rhythms illustrate the two types of AV relationship—dissociation (A) and association with retrograde conduction (B). Arrowheads indicate the atrial activity in both examples. In (A), on the right, a P wave precedes each QRS complex by less than 0.20 second, suggesting that sinus rhythm might be present; on the left, however, the same RR interval occurs with a varying PR interval and proves that no AV association is present. In (B), the RR and PR intervals are constant, as is typical of AV association, which in this case is due to ventriculoatrial (VA) conduction with atrial capture by the junctional focus (i.e., VA association). These rhythms are considered tachycardias because the rates of the junctional pacemakers are faster than the normal AV junctional escape rate.

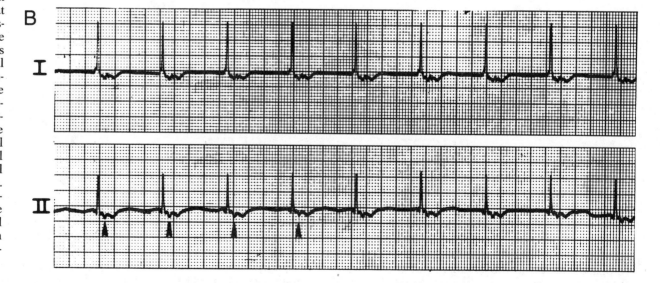

AV NODE REENTRY

AV RECIPROCATING TACHYCARDIA

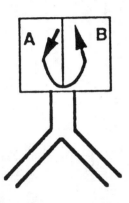

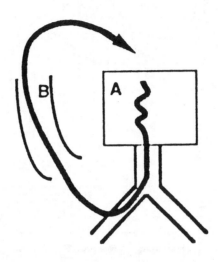

PATHWAY
A
B

RECOVERY TIME
SHORT
LONG

CONDUCTION VELOCITY
SLOW
FAST

FIGURE 11–3. The characteristics of the two functional pathways in AVNR and AVRT. During most reentry tachycardias, the impulse travels antegrade over pathway A to the ventricles and retrograde over pathway B to the atria. The accessory pathway behaves much like the B pathway in the AV node. Recovery time is the time it takes for an area to repolarize sufficiently to conduct an impulse. Conduction velocity is the speed of conduction through the reentrant pathway.

tinct pathways (see Chapter 1, pages 15 to 18).

Paroxysmal junctional tachycardia develops because the electrical impulse is able to reenter or recycle either within the AV node or by using both the AV node and the accessory AV pathway. In patients with the physiologic or anatomic substrate for either AVNR or AVRT, the differing electrophysiologic characteristics of the two pathways allow PJT to develop. The A pathway usually has a short recovery time and a slow conduction velocity, whereas the B pathway has a longer recovery time and a rapid conduction velocity (see Fig. 11–3). During sinus rhythm in patients with AVNR, antegrade movement of the impulse occurs principally through the B pathway (faster conduction velocity) to the ventricles. Because the A pathway is also partially activated, no reentry occurs. The B pathway involves longer recovery than the A pathway, however, so that a premature atrial beat is likely to find the B pathway not recovered (or refractory) and initiate an antegrade impulse in the slower A pathway. If this impulse traverses the A pathway and finds a B pathway that has recovered, it can initiate reentry by traveling retrograde in the B pathway. Such reentry may occur for just one beat, producing a premature atrial complex (PAC), or it may be sustained and cause a tachycardia (Fig. 11–4). Thus, during PJT, the A pathway is used for antegrade conduction, and the B pathway, for retrograde conduction.

Accessory pathways usually are electrophysiologically similar to the B pathway, so reentrant rhythms in ventricular preexcitation typically use the AV node and distal conducting system (the A pathway) as the antegrade limb, and the QRS complex is normal. Because the accessory (B) pathway functions as the retrograde limb, it will be "concealed" or not apparent on the surface electrocardiogram (ECG) during AVRT (Fig. 11–5). Tachycardias using these directions of conduction in the accessory pathway and AV node–His-Purkinje system are termed *orthodromic*. With both varieties of AV junctional reentry, the reentry loop persists as long as the electrical impulse encounters recep-

tive or repolarized cells. When the impulse reaches the His bundle, it spreads in an antegrade direction through the ventricles. When it reaches atrial muscle, it spreads in a retrograde direction through the atria. These patterns of activation result in retrograde P waves alternating with antegrade QRS complexes.

A characteristic feature of PJTs is the 1:1 relationship between atrial and ventricular activity. In the case of the AVRT, the atria and ventricles are essential limbs of the tachycardia circuit and a 1:1 AV relationship is obligatory. In AVNR, the tachycardia circuit is totally contained within the AV node, and 1:1 AV conduction is also the rule; 2:1 conduction to either the atria or the ventricles occurs but is rare.

In PJT, the P waves can theoretically have any temporal relationship to the QRS complexes, depending on the conduction times from the reentry site to the atria versus the ventricles. Most of the time, the P waves occur during or shortly after the QRS complex, because retrograde conduction to the atria is normally slower than antegrade conduction to the ventricles. The retrograde conduction times to the atria (or RP intervals) are usually different in the two varieties of PJT, and their measurement may be helpful in the differential diagnosis of the two tachycardias. The RP intervals are usually shorter in AVNR as compared with AVRT, because the distance from the reentry site

to the atria is shorter in AVNR. The P waves tend to be buried within the QRS complex or, at the latest, in its terminal portion. With orthodromic AVRT due to a Kent bundle, activation of at least a portion of the ventricle before the accessory pathway is engaged is an obligatory condition of the reentry circuit. This longer pathway to retrograde atrial activation is responsible for a longer RP interval; with AVRT, the retrograde P waves appear at the earliest in the terminal portion of the QRS complex, and more commonly are in the ST segment following it. In both varieties of PJT, the RP interval nearly always is shorter than the PR interval (the interval from the retrograde P to the next QRS complex), so that the RP:PR ratio is less than 1.0 (see Fig. 11–4). Rarely, the retrograde RP interval during PJT may be extremely prolonged, with a shorter PR interval and an RP:PR ratio greater than 1.0. Although these "long-RP" tachycardias constitute only about 1% to 2% of the PJTs at tertiary care facilities, they are important, because when they are due to an accessory pathway (with slow decremental retrograde conduction), they tend to be incessant or "permanent" (hence, one of their names: *permanent junctional reciprocating tachycardia*). About 60% of long-RP tachycardias are due to a concealed accessory pathway (usually paraseptal, in the area of the AV node), and about 40% are due to atypical AVNR, wherein antegrade conduction occurs via the fast B

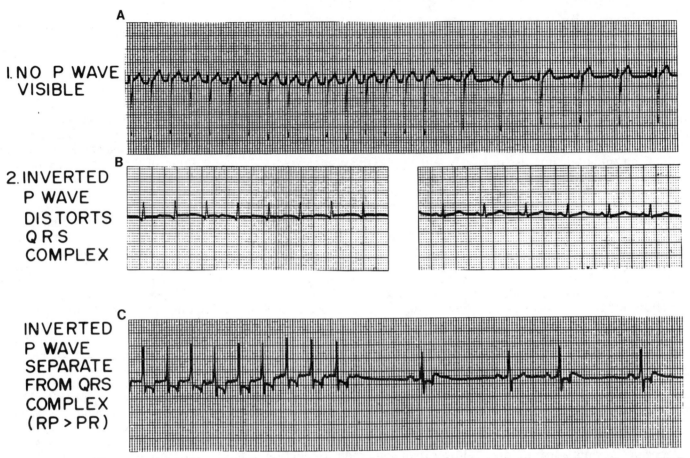

A

1. NO P WAVE VISIBLE

B

2. INVERTED P WAVE DISTORTS QRS COMPLEX

C

INVERTED P WAVE SEPARATE FROM QRS COMPLEX (RP > PR)

FIGURE 11–4. These examples of PJT illustrate the three characteristic associated P-wave patterns: no apparent P waves (*A*); P waves distorting the QRS complex (*B*); and P waves following the QRS complex (*C*). In (*A*), no evidence of atrial activity is visible during the PJT, but a typical P-wave pattern is apparent during sinus rhythm (right). In (*B*), a P wave deforms the onset of the QRS complex during the tachycardia (left); no such deformity is present during sinus rhythm (right). In (*C*), discrete P waves follow each QRS complex during PJT (left) and are also apparent as blocked premature atrial complexes (PACs) during sinus rhythm (right). The PACs are actually AV junctional echo beats due to retrograde conduction through an accessory pathway and are potentially the first beat of AVRT.

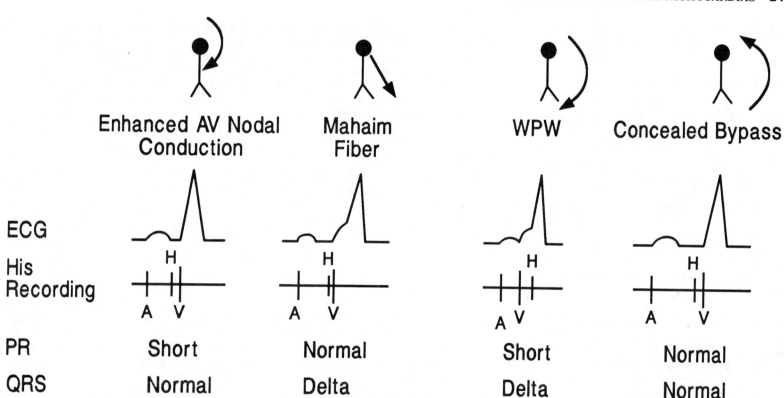

FIGURE 11–5. The common types of accessory pathways (preexcitation) are illustrated (*top*), with the corresponding typical electrocardiogram (ECG) and His recording immediately beneath. The His recording displays atrial activity (A), His activity (H), and ventricular activity (V). Enhanced AV nodal conduction (curved arrow, extreme left panel) may not be due to an anatomic accessory pathway, but behaves as if all or part of the AV node is bypassed. Nodoventricular (or Mahaim) fibers connect the distal AV node or His bundle with the right ventricle or, rarely, the right bundle. The most common preexcitation is the Wolff-Parkinson-White (WPW) variety; the accessory pathway may be manifest (short PR interval and delta wave on the surface ECG) or concealed (no evidence of an accessory pathway on the surface ECG). With the WPW pattern and a manifest accessory pathway, the ventricular activity (V) precedes His activity (H); thus, "preexcitation" of the ventricle occurs. With enhanced AV nodal conduction, the A-H interval is shortened because the AV nodal conduction is more rapid. With a concealed bypass tract (extreme right panel), antegrade conduction is not altered.

pathway and retrograde conduction via the slow A pathway, with the latter accounting for the long RP interval.[4]

VARIETIES OF PREEXCITATION

The term *preexcitation* is defined as activation of a cardiac chamber via a pathway other than the AV node–His Purkinje system (that is, an accessory pathway). An accessory pathway's presence can be inferred when an atrial impulse depolarizes all or part of the ventricle earlier than would be expected from an antegrade impulse traversing the normal, specialized conduction system (see Fig. 11–5). Preexcitation is also defined by retrograde conduction over an accessory pathway; it can be inferred when a ventricular impulse depolarizes the atria sooner than would be expected from an impulse traversing the normal, specialized conduction system in a reverse or retrograde direction. Clinical examples of these two varieties of preexcitation are a manifest accessory pathway producing a delta wave on the surface ECG, and a concealed bypass tract that conducts only in the retrograde direction (Fig. 11–6).

Wolff-Parkinson-White Syndrome.
Wolff-Parkinson-White Syndrome is the classic variant of preexcitation and also the most common. In this syndrome, an accessory pathway of atrial tissue (or Kent bundle) connects the atria and ventricles in an area remote from the AV node. The pathway (or pathways) may occur almost anywhere in the circumference of either the tricuspid or mitral annuli, including the interventricular septum. The surface ECG preexcitation patterns typically reflect the variable underlying anatomy of location or the connections subtended by these accessory pathways, or both (Fig. 11–7). These pathways most frequently occur anteriorly on the right side of the heart (region V) and posteriorly on the left side (region II). The surface ECG patterns corresponding to these two locations are the antiquated type B and type A patterns, respectively, as described in the older literature. The term *Wolff-Parkinson-White (WPW) syndrome* is reserved for patients who have the characteristic ECG, with a PR interval of less than 0.12 second and QRS prolongation with slurring of the initial portion of the QRS complex (delta wave), and symptoms due to AVRT. Wolff-Parkinson-White syndrome also implies that the accessory pathway is a Kent bundle, a bridge of atrial tissue electrically connecting the atria and ventricles. The impulse partially or completely bypasses the normal AV node (hence the short PR interval) and engages the ventricle through the accessory pathway (hence the delta wave reflecting conduction through ventricular myocardium) (see Fig. 11–7).

Lown-Ganong-Levine Syndrome.
The ECG pattern in Lown-Ganong-Levine syndrome consists of a short PR interval with no delta wave and occurs in association with paroxysms of rapid heart action. A putative relationship exists between the short PR interval and the tachycardias (see Fig. 11–7).[5] The cause of the short PR interval has been subject to speculation, with explanations ranging from a fast (but anatomically normal) AV node, to an accessory pathway connecting the atria directly to the distal AV node or His bundle via atrio-nodal or atrio-His fibers. Evidence is mounting, however, that the short PR interval is due to enhanced AV nodal conduction, and that these patients do not have a predisposition to reentrant arrhythmias. The characteristic feature found at electrophysiologic testing is rapid conduction of atrial impulses, with a 1:1 AV relationship at rates of 300 beats per minute or greater. The major risk to these patients, as to those with WPW syndrome, comes from this potential for rapid AV conduction with atrial flutter and fibrillation. Unlike patients with accessory pathways, however, these patients do not have a propensity to AV junctional reentrant rhythms.

Mahaim Fibers.
Nodoventricular pathways, or *Mahaim fibers*, are rare variants of ventricular preexcitation that result in a delta wave (preexcitation of the ventricle) but a normal PR interval. The atrial impulse traverses at least a portion of the AV node (hence the likelihood of a normal PR interval) and enters a bypass tract, which can insert into either the right ventricle or the right bundle. Reciprocating tachycardias can occur with ante-

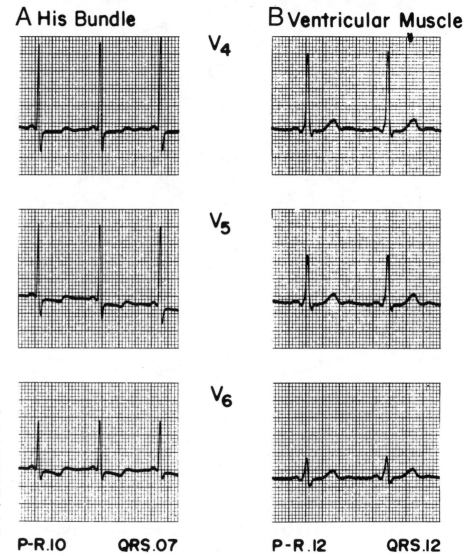

A His Bundle   V₄   **B Ventricular Muscle**

V₅

V₆

P-R .10   QRS .07   P-R .12   QRS .12

FIGURE 11–6. (*A*) This short PR interval (0.10 second) may reflect fast AV nodal conduction and become clinically manifest only during atrial tachycardias that result in rapid AV conduction and ventricular rate. (*B*) Ventricular preexcitation (WPW syndrome) is shown with a PR interval less than 0.12 second, QRS prolongation to 0.12 second, and a slurred initial upstroke of the QRS complex, the delta wave. The appearance of the middle and late portions of the QRS complex are closer to normal, indicating activation of most of the ventricular muscle through normal His–bundle-branch conduction. The entire QRS complex is actually a "fusion" beat.

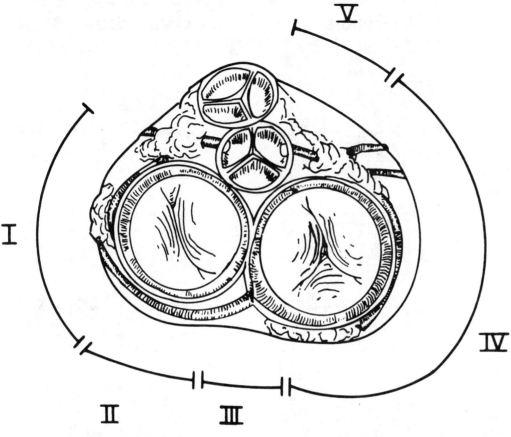

Region	Negative Delta Wave	QRS Axis in Frontal Plane	R>S
I	I and/or aVL	Normal	V_1-V_3
II	III and aVF	-75 to +75	V_1
III	III and aVF	0 to -90	V_2-V_4
IV	aVR	Normal	V_3-V_5
V	V_1 and V_2	Normal	V_3-V_5

FIGURE 11–7. This cross-sectional diagram of the heart at the level of the mitral and tricuspid annuli is subdivided into five anatomic regions: I, left lateral wall; II, left posterior free wall; III, posterior septal and paraseptal; IV, right free wall; and V, anteroseptal and right anterior paraseptal. The table shows the electrocardiographic patterns seen in patients with accessory pathways in these regions. (From Lindsay BD, et al: Concordance of distinguishing electrocardiographic features during sinus rhythm with the location of accessory pathways in the Wolff-Parkinson-White syndrome. Am J Cardiol 59:1093–1102, 1987, with permission.)

grade conduction, usually through the accessory pathway, and with retrograde conduction through the His bundle–AV node. A wide-QRS tachycardia, with either a 1:1 VA relationship or AV dissociation, may be present. Because these pathways always enter the right ventricle or bundle, the QRS complex has a left bundle branch block configuration. The degree of preexcitation depends on the balance between the speed of conduction over the accessory pathway and that over the AV node and His-Purkinje system. Because the latter speed can be quite variable, the degree of preexcitation can vary, with no delta wave on some occasions and fully developed ventricular preexcitation on others.

CLINICAL METHODS OF DIAGNOSIS

The diagnosis of a PJT is based on the presence of a regular, narrow-QRS tachycardia with a 1:1 AV relationship that begins abruptly following a premature beat (usually atrial) and ends abruptly, either spontaneously or in response to an autonomic maneuver or intravenous drug such as adenosine or verapamil. The differential diagnosis of a regular, narrow-QRS tachycardia in the range of 120 to 250 beats per minute was outlined in Chapter 8. In addition to the two varieties of PJT (AVNR and AVRT), the differential diagnosis may include sinus tachycardia, ec-

topic atrial tachycardia, or atrial flutter (Fig. 11–8), as well as an accelerated junctional rhythm.

The diagnosis can be established by answering the following questions:

- *What are the atria doing?* The answer to this question is key to the diagnosis. If it is possible to demonstrate that the atrial rate is slower than the ventricular rate, then the arrhythmia must not originate in the atrium. If there is a 1:1 AV (or VA) relationship, then the arrhythmia may be either atrial or AV junctional in origin. If P waves are visible, consideration of their morphologic features and timing is helpful. In PJT, the P waves are abnormal in axis (retrograde) and the RP interval is usually less than the PR interval. The shortest RP intervals occur in AVNR, and the P wave is usually buried in the QRS complex or superimposed on its terminal portion. Atrioventricular reciprocating tachycardia generally has a longer RP interval, and the retrograde P wave is usually in the ST segment (see Fig. 11–4). When an accurate RP interval can be measured (which frequently requires an esophageal or intra-atrial lead), an interval less than 70 milliseconds is typical of AVNR; an interval of 120 milliseconds or more is typical of AVRT. With ectopic atrial tachycardia, the P waves are usually normal in axis but altered morphologically as compared with sinus P waves. The P waves in ectopic atrial tachycardia are accompa-

nied by either first- or second-degree AV block and by slight irregularities in rate, as compared with the usual metronome-like regularity of established PJT. In atrial flutter, observation of an inferiorly oriented ECG lead (II, III, or aVF) usually reveals the absence of discrete P waves and a continually undulating baseline (see Fig. 11–8).

- *What are the ventricles doing?* In general, AV junctional tachycardias show a narrow QRS complex because the antegrade impulse depolarizes the ventricles, using the same pathway as the normal sinus impulse. A wide QRS complex may result, however, if there is a preexisting bundle branch block or if aberration related to tachycardia develops. More rarely, AVRT occurs with antegrade conduction via the accessory pathway and retrograde conduction via the His–AV node pathway (*antidromic AVRT*). The difficulty in diagnosing AV junctional beats with aberration and a QRS duration of 0.12 second or longer was discussed in Chapters 1 and 8; the same difficulty holds for AV junctional tachycardias with wide QRS complexes. For the most part, this diagnosis cannot be made outside of the electrophysiology laboratory except when a tachycardia converts from a wide- to a narrow-QRS tachycardia during a single paroxysm. Calling a wide-QRS tachycardia "AV junctional with aberration" because the patient is hemodynamically stable is wrong and can lead to serious

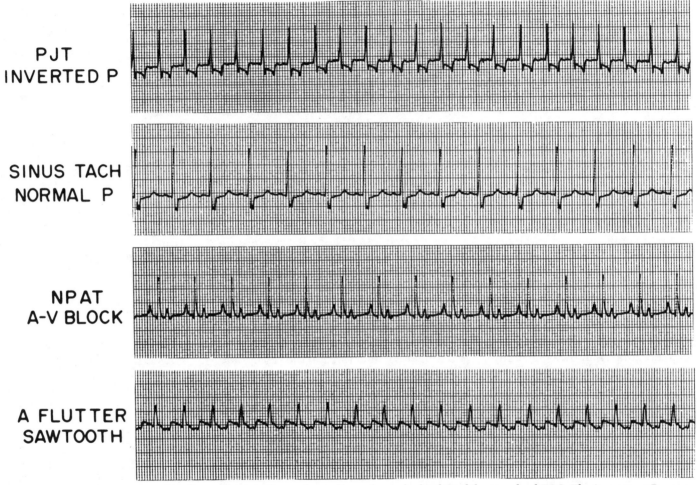

FIGURE 11–8. Four examples of supraventricular tachycardia as shown by lead II of the standard ECG. The important P-wave characteristics relating to differential diagnosis are indicated. A FLUTTER = atrial flutter; A-V = atrioventricular; NPAT = non-paroxysmal or automatic atrial tachycardia; P = P wave; PJT = paroxysmal junctional tachycardia; TACH = tachycardia.

errors in treatment, as when intravenous administration of verapamil results in profound hypotension.

- *What is the AV relationship?* The AV relationship remains constant in PJT even when the rate slows. Atrioventricular dissociation with a narrow-QRS tachycardia suggests that the tachycardia is an accelerated AV junctional rhythm, or that it is ventricular tachycardia with the actual width of the QRS complex becoming apparent only if other leads are examined (see Fig. 1–14).
- *What are the characteristics of the tachycardia's onset, termination, interruption, and response to interventions?* Observing the onset and termination of the tachycardia is helpful in making the diagnosis. Atrioventricular reciprocating tachycardia and AVNR can be initiated with either a PAC or a premature ventricular complex (PVC) or, more rarely, simply an increase in the sinus rate (Fig. 11–9). When a PAC starts a reentry tachycardia, the initiating P wave and the P waves during the tachycardia are different morphologically because they usually originate from different locations. With ectopic atrial tachycardia, on the other hand, the P wave of the first beat and of the beats that follow are usually the same morphologically (see Fig. 9–9). With reentry, the initiating PAC wave conducts through the AV node with a long PR interval, allowing exposure of two potential pathways and initiation of reentry (see Fig. 11–3). If the last sequence in a narrow-QRS tachycardia is a QRS complex followed by a P wave, an intra-atrial tachycardia is excluded, and PJT is much more likely, although this does not differentiate AVNR from AVRT. If the last sequence is a QRS complex without a subsequent P wave, then either an intra-atrial tachycardia or PJT is possible. Normalization of the QRS complex during a tachycardia with an increase in tachycardia rate is virtually diagnostic of AVRT and identifies the accessory pathway as being on the same side as the intraventricular conduction disturbance (Fig. 11–10). With the loss of aberration and an accessory pathway on the same side, the route taken to reach the accessory pathway shortens, with consequent speeding of the tachycardia rate. When the accessory pathway and site of aberration are on opposite sides, loss of aberration does not shorten the reentry circuit, and there is no speeding of the tachycardia rate. Absence of speeding with loss of aberration, however, although compatible with AVRT, is not pathognomonic; the same phenomenon can occur with other tachycardias, such as AVNR and atrial flutter. Alterations in QRS configuration during the tachycardia strongly suggest AVRT but are also seen with AVNR. If a definite diagnosis cannot be made from the foregoing observations, a vagal maneuver may be required, with or without an esophageal or intra-atrial recording (see Chapters 4 and 5).

INTERACTION WITH THE AUTONOMIC NERVOUS SYSTEM

Because the AV node is involved in the reentrant pathway that causes the tachycardia in both AVRT and AVNR, alterations in sympathetic-parasympathetic balance within the AV node can markedly affect whether the tachycardia continues at a different rate or is terminated. Continuation of the tachycardia requires that the impulse continuously encounter receptive tissue. An increase in vagal activity slows conduction and prolongs refractoriness in the AV node. If slowing of conduction predominates, the tachycardia continues but at a slower rate; if prolongation of refractoriness predominates, the tachycardia abruptly breaks (see Figs. 4–20 and 4–21). Clinically, AVRT and AVNR rarely exhibit only a rate slowing during a vagal maneuver. Much more commonly, any rate slowing is slight and occurs just before the arrhythmia stops abruptly (Fig. 11–11).

On the other hand, enhancement of sympathetic activity in the AV node speeds conduction and shortens refractoriness. It thus can either speed the tachycardia, if the shortening of refractoriness predominates, or break the tachycardia, if

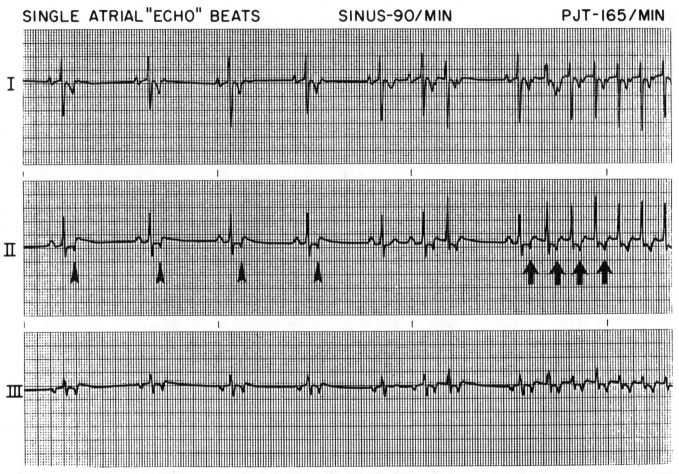

Figure 11–9. In simultaneous leads I, II, and III, retrograde P waves follow each of the first four QRS complexes (arrowheads) and are atrial "echo" beats due to retrograde conduction via a second pathway to the atria. The sinus rate then increases to 90 beats per minute, and a "one-beat" run of paroxysmal junctional tachycardia (PJT) is followed by a sustained run at 165 beats per minute. Retrograde P waves again follow each QRS complex (arrows), with an RP interval of approximately 0.12 second, indicating that this PJT is most likely using a concealed accessory pathway and is an example of AVRT.

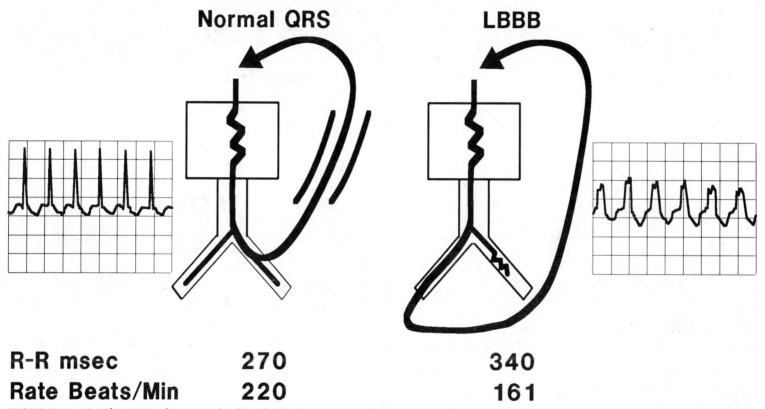

FIGURE 11–10. The ECGs show standard lead I during PJT. Conduction reverted from normal (ECG on left) to left bundle branch block (LBBB) (ECG on right), with associated slowing of the tachycardia. This sequence is illustrated in the diagram and is pathognomonic of AVRT, with the accessory pathway ipsilateral to the site of aberration.

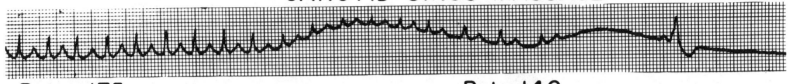

CAROTID SINUS MASSAGE

Rate-175   Rate-140

CAROTID SINUS MASSAGE

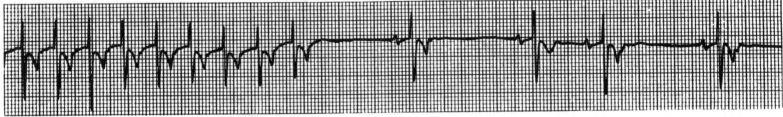

Rate-165   Rate-150

FIGURE 11-11. (*Top*) The atrial rate slows by 35 beats per minute during carotid sinus massage, followed by abrupt breaking of the tachycardia. No discrete P waves are visible during the PJT. A delta wave is apparent during the escape beat, indicating that even though no P waves could be identified in the terminal portion of the QRS complex or the ST segment during the tachycardia, the pattern most likely represented AVRT. (Note: Some patients with accessory pathways may also have AVNR.) (*Bottom*) The atrial rate slows by 15 beats per minute during carotid sinus massage, followed by abrupt breaking of the tachycardia. P waves follow each QRS complex, but no delta wave is present.

the speeding of conduction predominates. Because of the danger inherent in speeding tachycardias, however, parasympathetic rather than sympathetic enhancement is employed clinically in efforts to terminate these arrhythmias. Acceleration of AV node recovery by administration of atropine or catecholamines can also allow the tachycardia to be initiated, as in the initiation of PJT during exercise. If speeding of antegrade conduction occurs without affecting retrograde conduction, an impulse can traverse the AV node via the B pathway and then reenter the AV node via the A pathway because of its rapid recovery. The AV node is usually the weak link in AVNR and AVRT, and catecholamine stimulation may make it more suited to sustain an arrhythmia. Chapter 4 presents further examples of the interaction between PJT and changes in the autonomic nervous system induced by various bedside autonomic maneuvers.

USE OF INVASIVE ELECTROPHYSIOLOGY

Electrophysiologic study (EPS) is useful in evaluating selected patients with PJT (see Chapter 6). The use of EPS should be reserved for patients whose arrhythmias have not lent themselves to diagnosis using standard noninvasive techniques, for patients with arrhythmias refractory to conventional therapy, and for patients with hemodynamically significant arrhythmias in whom empiric therapy might be dangerous. The ability to localize the accessory pathway and measure its baseline and drug-related functional characteristics through EPS can be important in determining the type of pharmacologic or nonpharmacologic interventions most likely to treat the arrhythmia successfully (Table 11–1).

The precise diagnosis can be accomplished with EPS because PJT is easily induced, and once induced, AVRT can be differentiated from AVNR by observing certain characteristics of the arrhythmia. In general, AVNR has a very short retrograde conduction time, and in mapping the pattern of atrial activation, the earliest site of the activation is in the area of the AV node. In patients with AVRT, however, the RP interval is longer. More important, the sequence of atrial activation is different from that of AVNR; the site of the atrial insertion of the accessory pathway is the earliest site of activation. If a left-lateral-wall bypass tract is involved, the atrial electrogram shows that area to be the earliest site activated. The atrial map, therefore, serves as a guide for localizing the

Table 11–1. ELECTROPHYSIOLOGIC STUDIES IN AV JUNCTIONAL TACHYCARDIAS

1. Establish the correct diagnosis differentiating:
   a. Intra-atrial from AV junctional tachycardias
   b. AVNR from AVRT
2. Observe the hemodynamic significance of paroxysmal junctional tachycardia and atrial fibrillation.
3. Provide therapy:
   a. Evaluation of the efficacy of medical therapy in:
      (1) Patients refractory to conventional therapy
      (2) Patients in whom empiric therapy might be dangerous
   b. Evaluation of the patient before and after:
      (1) Antitachycardia pacemaker insertion
      (2) Accessory pathway–His bundle ablation

AV = atrioventricular; AVNR = atrioventricular nodal reentry; AVRT = atrioventricular reciprocating tachycardia.

pathway as well as for establishing the differential diagnosis. Rarely, an accessory pathway may insert into the interventricular septum near the AV node and produce an atrial activation pattern similar to that produced by AVNR. In this setting, when premature ventricular beats are induced at precisely the time the His bundle is refractory, evidence of earlier-than-expected atrial activity confirms the presence of a second or accessory pathway.

Patients with PJT may be refractory to conventional therapy, and EPS provides a means for testing alternative therapies. Most patients with asymptomatic ventricular preexcitation do not have inducible AVRT in the electrophysiologic laboratory, but even asymptomatic patients who have responsibilities that may affect the lives of others (e.g., airline pilots) are sometimes candidates for EPS to determine their risk for sudden death when atrial fibrillation is induced.

Electrophysiologic study also may be helpful in patients who are at risk for sudden death and in whom empiric therapy might be dangerous. This problem is more commonly encountered in patients with ventricular arrhythmias but may occur in patients with AVRT. More specifically, patients with WPW syndrome who experience presyncope or significant lightheadedness, syncope, or prior cardiac arrest, or who are being considered for digitalis therapy can benefit from EPS. In this group, EPS is used to measure the refractory period of the accessory pathway during atrial fibrillation, because most deaths from WPW syndrome are due to a rapid, uncontrolled ventricular response to atrial fibrillation. The mode of induction, the hemodynamic consequences, the mode of termination, and the response to treatment of the arrhythmia can be determined. For life-threatening arrhythmias, such EPS-guided therapy is a more desirable alternative than empirically guided therapy, in which success is often trusted to luck. With the increasing variety of pharmacologic and non-pharmacologic methods of treatment including catheter-based radiofrequency ablation, the localization of these pathways and the measurement of their functional significance through EPS become ever more important.

CLINICAL FEATURES

Predisposing Clinical Settings

Atrioventricular nodal reentry and AVRT are most commonly seen in patients with no other evidence of organic heart disease, although ventricular preexcitation is associated with a variety of congenital and acquired defects, including Ebstein's anomaly, mitral valve prolapse, and cardiomyopathies. Arrhythmias are seen more commonly in younger patients, but cardiac or pulmonary disease may induce these arrhythmias in susceptible individuals. Patients with a concealed accessory pathway may never have an arrhythmia until they are older and begin to develop PVCs or PACs that trigger an arrhythmia. The likelihood of arrhythmias may also be potentiated by sympathomimetic drug therapy used for various pulmonary diseases. In susceptible individuals, a variety of stimuli, such as anxiety, excess caffeine, alcohol, fatigue, and exercise can provoke these tachycardias. Similarly, any process that prolongs conduction in the AV node (e.g., ischemia) can result in "echo beats" and reentrant arrhythmias.

Natural History in the Various Settings

The natural history of PJT is not completely understood. Lundberg[6] and Giardina and colleagues[7] have reported the follow-up of children with PJT, both with and without evidence of antegrade ventricular preexcitation. A high percentage of neonates with WPW syndrome have spontaneous resolution of preexcitation and tachycardias during their first year of life. Some patients lose the capability for antegrade conduction through their accessory pathway but retain the capability for retrograde conduction and thereby the potential for development of AVRT. The capability for retrograde conduction may also be lost, however, as documented by the decreasing incidence of evidence of a concealed accessory pathway in progressively older groups of patients with PJT.[6,7]

The natural history of AVNR has also not been well documented. Wu and coworkers[8] found that 85% of adults with PJT had no evidence of an accessory pathway. In this series, the patients with AVNR were older than patients with AVRT (age 55 versus age 40) and had a higher incidence of underlying cardiac disease (50% versus 10%). This information suggests that there are two groups of patients with AVNR: (1) those with a congenital anomaly of the AV node, whose natural history is probably similar to that of patients with congenital accessory pathways; and (2) those with an acquired alteration of AV nodal conduction that is a part of a general cardiac problem. In the first group, tachycardias tend to resolve with age, whereas in the latter group, they appear with age.

General Methods of Treatment

NONPAROXYSMAL AV JUNCTIONAL TACHYCARDIAS

The treatment of nonparoxysmal AV junctional tachycardias (NPJT) is to remove the offending stimulus whenever possible. If the tachycardia is due to digi-

talis toxicity, the drug should be stopped. During the course of treating atrial fibrillation with digitalis, regularization of the rhythm with a rate above 60 beats per minute should suggest digitalis toxicity when both AV block and NPJT are present. If NPJT follows acute myocarditis, acute inferior myocardial infarction, or mitral valve replacement, there is no specific therapy. Fortunately, the rates are usually not that rapid and the tachycardias are well tolerated.

PAROXYSMAL AV JUNCTIONAL TACHYCARDIAS

Paroxysmal junctional tachycardias, whether AVNRs or AVRTs, are generally managed in the same way, except that the clinician must remember that under certain circumstances, digitalis and verapamil may speed accessory pathway conduction in AVRT (see later).

Acute Treatment. The acute management of PJTs is directed toward their termination. The strategy is to block conduction in one limb of the reentrant loop. In AVRT, the AV nodal limb of the tachycardia circuit is the usual focus of attack. In AVNR, the antegrade A (or "slow") pathway is most sensitive to intervention. Table 11–2 outlines the therapeutic approaches to these arrhythmias when they present acutely, beginning with a vagal maneuver and proceeding to drug therapy, cardioversion, or both, depending on clinical circumstances.

VAGAL MANEUVERS. The usual sequence is first to try a vagal maneuver such as carotid sinus massage. Chapter 4 outlines the proper administration of carotid massage and the effects of vagal maneuvers. The termination of PJT in response to a vagal maneuver is abrupt, despite the fact that the rate of the tachycardia may slow slightly before termination (see Fig. 11–11).

DRUG THERAPY. In hemodynamically stable patients, drug therapy is the second line of defense. My current preference is intravenous verapamil, because in selected patients, it has a high degree of safety and effectiveness (it successfully terminates PJT in 85% to 90% of patients). Verapamil causes slowing of AV nodal conduction with consequent slowing of the rate of the tachycardia that is either sustained or, more commonly, transient just before abrupt termination of PJT (Fig. 11–12). Verapamil is safe to use in PJT during sinus rhythm even in patients with known antegrade preexcitation, but it may result in cardiovascular collapse when given to such patients if they are in atrial fibrillation (see Chapter 10, page 229). Treatment with verapamil (as well as with β-blockers and procainamide) may result in hypotension, so that the blood pressure should be pharmacologically supported if the patient is initially mildly hypotensive (for example, blood pressure of 80 to 90 mmHg in a young person). Adenosine, a naturally occurring nucle-

**Table 11–2. METHODS FOR TERMINATING
PAROXYSMAL AV JUNCTIONAL TACHYCARDIAS**

Vagal Maneuvers	Valsalva maneuver, carotid massage, gagging, facial water immersion (diving reflex), ice water (cold pressor).
Pharmacologic Treatment	Verapamil: 5–10 mg IV over 2 min if BP stable; if no termination, repeat dose in 10 min.
	Adenosine: 6–12 mg IV as a rapid bolus.
	Digoxin: 0.5 mg IV followed by 0.25 mg IV in 30 min.
	Esmolol:* 500 μg/kg IV over 3–5 min followed by 50–100 μg/kg/min IV over 30 min; if no termination, increase by 50 μg/kg/min every 30 min until maximum of 300 μg/kg/min reached.
	Procainamide: 20–50 mg/min up to a loading dose of 12–17 mg/kg or a total dose of 1000 mg.
	Phenylephrine: 0.5–2.0 mg IV over 30 sec to increase BP to greater than 150 mmHg.
Nonpharmacologic Treatment	Atrial pacing, synchronized cardioversion.

BP = blood pressure; IV = intravenous.

*Because of the drug's rapid pharmacokinetics, the time to steady-state blood levels is rapidly achieved with a maintenance infusion, and the loading dose may be omitted.

oside, has been shown to have profound depressant effects on AV nodal conduction and was released for use in early 1990. It is given as a rapid intravenous bolus of 6 to 12 mg and is at least 90% effective in terminating PJTs. The side effects of flushing, chest pain, and dyspnea typically last less than 1 minute. Its brief half-life makes it safe to use even in patients with moderate hemodynamic compromise. It has also proved to be safe in patients with wide-QRS tachycardia. The drug has an important antiarrhythmic

role in PJT, as well as in the differential diagnosis of paroxysmal wide-QRS tachycardias, because of its potent depression of AV nodal conduction, its short half-life, and its excellent safety profile (see Chapter 15).

Patients with more profound hypotension require cardioversion as soon as possible. Those who have known antegrade conduction over an accessory pathway should not be given digitalis, as they may convert to atrial fibrillation with a very rapid ventricular response.

DIRECT-CURRENT CARDIOVERSION.
As previously noted, cardioversion of profoundly hypotensive patients should be effected as soon as possible, preferably with anesthesia if clinical circumstances permit. If a delay is unavoidable, the blood pressure should be increased with dopamine (2 to 5 μg/kg per minute) or norepinephrine (2 to 20 μg/mL), titrated to a systolic blood pressure above 90 mmHg, to maintain coronary and cerebral perfusion and to provide some time to analyze the problem. If titrated properly, these drugs

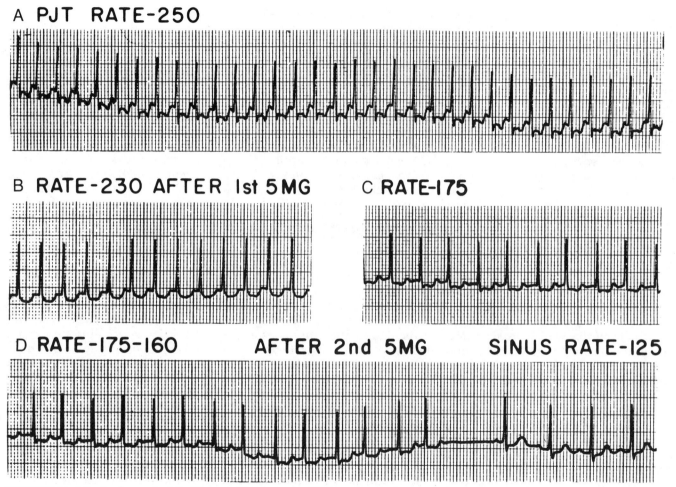

FIGURE 11–12. As shown in (*A*), (*B*), and (*C*), the rate of PJT gradually decreases from 250 to 175 beats per minute after a 5.0-mg intravenous infusion of verapamil. After a second 5.0-mg infusion of verapamil (*D*), transient alternating long and short cycle lengths are noted before the abrupt breaking of the tachycardia.

rarely aggravate the arrhythmia or cause other clinical problems.

Despite being alert and awake, these patients may be in profound shock. A check of the blood gases may reveal serious acidosis, hypoxia, or a base deficit reflecting poor perfusion. "Analysis paralysis" is a terrible disease affecting physicians who fail to notice that attached to every fascinating arrhythmia is a patient who may be deteriorating. A grave error is made when patients with rapid tachyarrhythmias are simply watched and not aggressively treated. Fortunately, most patients tolerate these arrhythmias with only mild degrees of hypotension.

Treatment of Recurrent Episodes of Paroxysmal Junctional Tachycardia.
Patients must be given a strategy for coping with these arrhythmias so that they feel neither frightened nor obligated to run to an emergency department with every episode of tachycardia. One method for management of intermittent PJT is to provide the patient with instructions (a "home recipe") for self-termination of the tachycardia (see example in the Appendix).

Most patients with occasional episodes of hemodynamically well-tolerated PJT do not need chronic prophylactic drug therapy, and a specific pharmacologic approach to treating each acute episode may be used. This approach consists of a single oral dose of either verapamil (120 mg) or a β-blocker such as propranolol (120 mg),

metoprolol (100 mg), or atenolol (100 mg) at the onset of the arrhythmia; the dose may be repeated in 1 hour if the arrhythmia has not converted. Alternatively, oral doses of digoxin (0.75 mg immediately followed by two to three doses of 0.25 mg at hourly intervals) may be used as acute home therapy in patients with no evidence of antegrade ventricular preexcitation. After a drug has been given, repetition of a vagal intervention such as the Valsalva maneuver frequently terminates the arrhythmia, even when the maneuver was unsuccessful initially.

Chronic Prophylaxis Against Recurrent PJT

DRUG THERAPY. Chronic therapy of paroxysmal AVNR and AVRT is indicated when PJT is frequent or when even infrequent episodes are associated with severe symptoms. Such prophylactic drug therapy is directed at either suppressing the premature beats that trigger the arrhythmia or altering conduction in some portion of the reentry circuit to prevent the arrhythmia from becoming sustained.

Just as with the acute treatment of PJT, drugs that primarily affect the AV node are helpful in preventing the arrhythmia. Digoxin is the cheapest, least toxic, and most convenient medication and can be used safely in patients without evidence of antegrade preexcitation. If the drug prolongs the refractory period of the AV node more than it slows conduction, it may

block conduction in this portion of the reentry circuit and prevent both AVNR and AVRT. The amount of digoxin needed to control PJT is usually larger than that given for treating heart failure; a dose of 0.375 or 0.5 mg daily is often necessary. The most common reason for digoxin to fail in this setting is inadequate dosing. In patients with manifest antegrade preexcitation, however, digitalis may speed conduction in the accessory pathway. Thus, even though the primary arrhythmia problem is orthodromic AVRT, these patients have an increased risk of atrial fibrillation, and digitalis is contraindicated unless EPS has been performed to determine the effects of the drug on the accessory pathway.

One of a variety of β-blockers, including propranolol, metoprolol, and atenolol, may be used to prevent episodes of either AVNR or AVRT. These agents may be used for each acute episode, as noted previously, or they may be given regularly to provide arrhythmia prophylaxis if the patient is having frequent episodes of tachycardia.

The class Ia drugs—quinidine, procainamide, and disopyramide—work primarily by preventing the premature beats that trigger the arrhythmias, but they also slow conduction in the accessory pathway and, to a lesser extent, in the retrograde pathway in the AV node. These drugs are potentially dangerous, however, and can cause torsades de pointes, a potentially lethal arrhythmia. They should be used only if no other therapy is tolerated, and even then they necessitate careful monitoring of the patient and attention to the QT interval.

The class Ic agents—flecainide and propafenone—are extremely effective in managing these arrhythmias. Only flecainide, however, has been approved for use with PJT, and then, only for a narrowly defined patient spectrum. Disadvantages of the class Ic agents include their expense, frequency of dosing, and potential for ventricular proarrhythmia (see Chapter 15). They all profoundly slow conduction in accessory pathways and may prove useful in patients with AVRT, particularly in those whose arrhythmia has failed to respond to more conventional therapy. They also slow AV nodal conduction and are effective in AVNR. Amiodarone is effective in treating PJT but is extremely toxic; patients who require this drug are likely candidates for nonpharmacologic management of their tachycardia.

NONPHARMACOLOGIC THERAPY. There are a number of nonpharmacologic approaches for the management of PJT. His bundle ablation by either catheter or surgical techniques cures the rapid ventricular rate in patients with AVNR and in some patients with AVRT. The approach is aggressive, however, and leaves the patient dependent on an artificial pacemaker. In addition, patients with AVRT who are treated by His bundle ablation may subsequently develop atrial fibrillation with a rapid ventricular response, owing to the intact accessory pathway.

The use of radio-frequency energy delivered by catheter techniques either to ablate accessory pathways (in patients with AVRT) or to modify AV nodal conduction characteristics (in patients with AVNR) is an extremely promising approach that can leave the patient with intact AV conduction and no recurrent tachycardia. Although still investigational, studies[9,10] have indicated a high rate of success in abolishing both types of AV junctional reentry tachycardias, with a low complication rate. Catheter ablation, antitachycardia pacing, and surgery are discussed in more detail in Chapter 17.

REFERENCES

1. Moe GK, Preston JB, and Burlington H: Physiologic evidence for dual A-V transmission system. Circ Res 4:357–375, 1956.
2. Bigger JT and Goldreyer BN: The mechanism of supraventricular tachycardia. Circulation 42:673–688, 1970.
3. Hoffman B and Cranefield PF: Electrophysiology of the Heart. McGraw-Hill, New York, 1960.
4. Horowitz LN: Electrophysiologic evaluation of patients with preexcitation syndromes. Cardiol Clin 4:447–457, 1986.
5. Lown B, Ganong WF, and Levine SA: The syndrome of short PR interval, normal QRS complex and paroxysmal rapid heart action. Circulation 5:693–706, 1952.
6. Lundberg A: Paroxysmal tachycardia in infancy: Follow-up study of 47 subjects ranging in age from 10 to 26 years. Pediatrics 51:26–35, 1973.
7. Giardina ACV, Ehlers KH, and Engle MA: Wolff-Parkinson-White syndrome in infants and children. Br Heart J 34:839–846, 1972.
8. Wu D, Denes P, Amat-y-Leon F, et al: Clinical, electrocardiographic and electrophysiologic observations in patients with paroxysmal supraventricular tachycardia. Am J Cardiol 41:1045–1051, 1978.
9. Jackman WM, Wang X, Friday KJ, et al: Catheter ablation of accessory atrioventricular pathways (Wolff-Parkinson-White syndrome) by radiofrequency current. N Engl J Med 324:1605–1611, 1991.
10. Calkins H, Sousa J, El-Atassi R, et al: Diagnosis and cure of the Wolff-Parkinson-White syndrome or paroxysmal supraventricular tachycardias during a single electrophysiologic test. N Engl J Med 324:1612–1618, 1991.

Ventricular Tachycardias

MARCEL GILBERT, MD,
GALEN S. WAGNER, MD, and
BARRY W. RAMO, MD

OUTLINE

In 1909, Sir Thomas Lewis published the first clinical report of ventricular tachycardia in a patient who had previously manifested ventricular premature beats,[1] and in 1922, Gallavardin noted that this arrhythmia could occur in presumably healthy young subjects with no objective manifestations of heart disease.[2] Ever since these early observations, this diverse group of arrhythmias has been the subject of intense scrutiny and controversy.

When the link between ventricular tachycardia and sudden death was noted, interest heightened even more, but it was not until the advent of coronary care units in the mid-1960s that a critical study of ventricular tachycardia in the setting of acute ischemia became possible. Lown and associates described a group of "warning arrhythmias" that were associated with the development of ventricular tachycardia and fibrillation.[3] Later, however, Lie and colleagues showed that ventricular tachycardia and fibrillation frequently occurred without such warning arrhythmias, and that warning arrhythmias could occur without progressing to ventricular tachycardia or fibrillation.[4] In other words, the development of ventricular fibrillation in the setting of acute myocardial infarction could not necessarily be predicted by some "baseline" rhythm status. Unfortunately, the relationship between ventricular premature beats and the development of ventricular tachycardia–fibrillation became inextricably linked, so that during the 1970s many patients without serious organic heart disease but with ostensibly serious ventricular arrhythmias were treated with what we have subsequently learned were dangerous antiarrhythmic drugs.

More recently, the development of techniques such as the intracavitary recording of electrical activity combined with ventricular stimulation and mapping has increased our understanding of ventricular arrhythmias and has opened the field to such new modes of treatment as implantable defibrillator-cardioverter devices, or surgical and catheter techniques for ablating abnormal arrhythmogenic substrates. Perhaps more important is our learning that the significance of ventricular arrhythmias depends on the specific clinical setting in which they occur. Those not associated with organic heart disease have a generally benign prognosis, whereas those associated with significant left ventricular dysfunction are associated with an increased risk of sudden death.

This chapter discusses the classification, mechanisms, diagnosis, and treatment of ventricular tachycardia. Because treatment depends on the specific clinical setting in which the arrhythmia occurs, the last section of this chapter discusses issues of treatment in those various settings.

CLASSIFICATION

Ventricular tachycardias arise below the branching of the His bundle. Because the intrinsic rate of a ventricular escape pacemaker is 30 to 40 beats per minute or less, any ventricular rhythm composed of three or more sequential beats (regardless of underlying mechanism) at a rate of 60 beats per minute or more is classified as ventricular tachycardia. Ventricular tachycardias are diverse in mechanism, configuration, duration, associated disease states, clinical significance, and a variety of other features. This diversity creates a fair amount of complexity when one attempts to classify the arrhythmia. Table 12–1 is an attempt to present this diversity as simply as possible.

Duration and Morphologic Features

One useful subclassification relates to the tachycardia's duration: *sustained* if the run is 30 seconds or longer, and *nonsustained* if the run includes three beats or more but is shorter than 30 seconds.

Ventricular tachycardia is also classified according to its morphologic constancy. Both the sustained and non-sustained varieties can be either monomorphic, with a single QRS configuration, or polymorphic, with either a fixed or a phasically variable QRS config-

Table 12–1. CLASSIFICATION OF VENTRICULAR TACHYCARDIA BY MECHANISM, DURATION, AND MORPHOLOGY

MECHANISM	DURATION	MORPHOLOGY
AUTOMATICITY	Nonsustained	Monomorphic
Enhanced	($\geq$3 beats and	
Abnormal	<30 seconds)	Polymorphic
Triggered		Torsades de pointes with long QT_c interval
REENTRY	Sustained	Torsades-like with normal QT_c interval
Focal	($\geq$30 seconds)	
Generalized		Bidirectional fixed variability

uration. An occasional patient may demonstrate two or more morphologically distinct QRS complexes at various times without changes in either the rate or endocardial origin as determined by catheter mapping of the ventricle. This variability, depending on the particular lead being monitored, may produce alternating upward and downward QRS complexes (so-called bidirectional ventricular tachycardia) or a more fixed variability.

Mechanism

Ventricular tachycardias may also be classified according to the underlying mechanism. Most are due to either increased pacemaker activity or reentry. Triggered activity has been suggested as the cause for ventricular tachycardia due to digitalis toxicity, drug-induced torsades de pointes, or exercise, but its exact role in these and other clinical ventricular arrhythmias is unknown.

MECHANISMS

Abnormalities of Impulse Formation (Enhanced Normal and Abnormal Automaticity)

One mechanism for ventricular tachycardia is enhanced normal automaticity, or the accelerated discharge of an ectopic focus with intrinsic phase-4 diastolic depolarization. Enhanced normal automaticity almost always occurs within the Purkinje system, where the cells normally have intrinsic pacemaker capability, and is due to the acceleration of the normal ionic mechanisms responsible for excitability.

Another mechanism is abnormal automaticity. Under normal circumstances, ventricular muscle fibers lack pacemaker properties. Accelerated pacemaker activity may develop, however, under abnormal circumstances such as acute ischemia or infarction, hypokalemia, hypomagnesemia, hypercalcemia, hypoxia, increased catecholamines, or digitalis intoxication. These stimuli accelerate phase-4 depolarization of these cells by abnormal ionic mechanisms. When their rate exceeds that of the sinus node, an accelerated ventricular rhythm also results (Fig. 12–1).

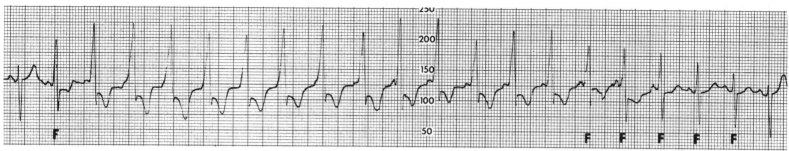

FIGURE 12–1. Pacemaker ventricular tachycardia. This electrocardiogram (ECG) begins with sinus tachycardia (rate: 111 beats per minute). The first beat is normally conducted, but the second is slightly premature with shortening of the PR interval, typical of atrioventricular (AV) dissociation. The second and third beats, with more evidence of AV dissociation, identify ventricular tachycardia with a peak rate of 125 beats per minute. The first premature beat, which is morphologically intermediate between sinus rhythm and the tachycardia, is a fusion beat (F) and also helps identify ventricular tachycardia. Toward the middle of the strip, the atrial rate speeds, because of a drop in output from the AV dissociation. A period of relative isorhythmicity between the atrial and ventricular rates creates a series of fusion beats followed by eventual complete sinus capture (last beat of the strip). The peak ventricular rate, the late coupling interval of the initiating beat, and the AV isorhythmicity are typical features of accelerated idioventricular rhythm (AIVR).

Such automatic ventricular tachycardias are commonly observed in the early period following an acute myocardial infarction and are due either to enhanced automaticity in Purkinje fibers or to abnormal automaticity in Purkinje fibers or in ischemic working myocardial cells. They seem to be particularly frequent in association with acute reperfusion following thrombolytic therapy, although by no means are they diagnostic of this event. They typically begin with a late coupling interval or a fusion beat, and therefore are more frequent during sleep, when the heart rate slows, or in response to the enhanced vagal tone associated with inferior myocardial infarction. They range in rate from 60 to 120 beats per minute and are nonparoxysmal, with a gradual onset and offset. They are usually regular, although exit block from the automatic focus may cause irregularity and the abrupt cessation that mimics a reentry ventricular arrhythmia. Because of their slow rates, there is often relative "isorhythmicity" with the atrial rate, resulting in atrioventricular (AV) dissociation rather than ventriculoatrial (VA) association (see Fig. 12–1). Suggested names for this arrhythmia have included *accelerated idioventricular rhythm (AIVR)* and *slow ventricular tachycardia*.

Abnormalities of Impulse Conduction (Reentry)

The usual mechanism for the more rapid ventricular tachycardias is reentry, wherein ventricular tissue is reexcited by the same impulse in a circuitous pattern (see Chapter 1, pages 15 to 18). Experimental models have demonstrated a complex interplay between a nonuniform state of refractoriness and slow, nonsynchronized conduction over abnormal regions of myocardial tissue, the "electroanatomic" substrate for the occurrence of reentry. Predisposing conditions include ischemia, fibrosis, and inflammation. Experimental infarct models have been used to illustrate this tachycardia that originates in the very ischemic regions adjacent to the infarct that also abuts "normal" tissue. The heterogeneity of this milieu creates marked differences in excitability, conduction velocity, and refractoriness in adjacent tissues. In such nonuniform states, with or without a sudden change in the basic rhythm, a single premature impulse can fail to propagate in one direction (unidirectional block) while propagating slowly through an alternate, neighboring pathway. If this wave front of depolarization continues to encounter excitable cells, sustained reentry ventricular tachycardia occurs (Fig. 12–2).

Most stable, chronic reentrant ventricular tachycardias are focal (microreentry), originating in heterogeneous ventricular muscle or in the junction between the endocardial Purkinje fibers and the ventricular muscle. The impulse cycles within this local area and then moves out as an advancing wave front over the remainder of the ventricles. The situation is analogous to the focal atrial or atrioventricular nodal reentry tachycardias, in which the electrical activity within the circuit is not visible on the surface electrocardiogram (ECG) and only the passively

responding atrial and ventricular depolarizations are seen. Ventricular microreentry occurs in an area so small that its electrical activity is not apparent on the surface ECG. One can only observe the sequential wide QRS complexes and T waves resulting from the alternating depolarization and repolarization of the passively responding parts of the ventricles, which are not included in the reentry circuit. In signal-averaged ECGs, this slow conduction through a scarred area of myocardium results in a late potential, occurring after the normal areas of the heart have depolarized (see Chapter 7, page 161).

In macroreentry, on the other hand, the circuit includes the mass of ventricular muscle, and the tachycardia is analogous to atrial flutter–fibrillation. The reentrant activity dominates the ECG, with no discrete QRS complexes or T waves apparent. "Ventricular flutter" has been also termed "ventricular tachycardia of the vulnerable period," and it occurs in the setting of acute myocardial infarction. It may be nonsustained, but if sustained and untreated, it rapidly progresses to ventricular fibrillation.

CLINICAL METHODS OF DIAGNOSIS

The differential diagnosis of a wide-QRS tachycardia includes ventricular tachy-

cardia and supraventricular tachycardia with aberration, as discussed in Chapter 8. Ventricular preexcitation due to an accessory pathway is often considered a third category, but it is really a form of aberration. The analysis of a wide-QRS tachycardia is a two-step process that includes differentiating ventricular tachycardia from supraventricular tachycardia with aberration and, if the tachycardia is ventricular, identifying the specific classification.

Aberrant conduction is present whenever a supraventricular impulse depolarizes the ventricles by an abnormal route, with a resulting change in QRS configuration. Two examples are a premature atrial complex (PAC) causing functional right bundle branch block (RBBB), and ventricular preexcitation with partial ventricular activation occurring through an accessory pathway. Abberration and criteria for its diagnosis are also discussed in Chapter 7 (pages 146 to 154), Chapter 8 (page 164), and Chapter 10 (pages 212 to 218). The following sections discuss those criteria that favor or identify a wide-QRS tachycardia as ventricular.

Clinical Criteria

Clues to the diagnosis of ventricular tachycardia from the patient's clinical history are presented in more detail in Chapter 2. When the tachycardia makes its initial appearance only after a myocardial infarction, ventricular tachycardia is

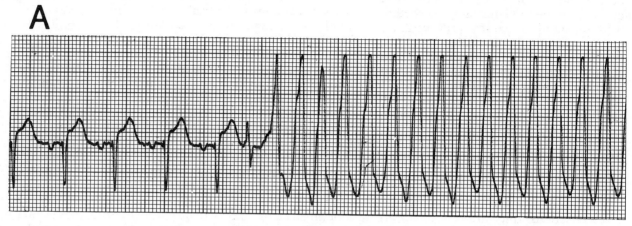

A

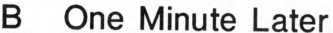

B One Minute Later

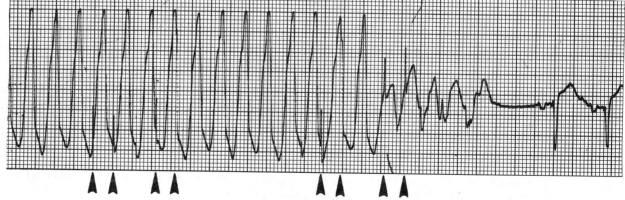

FIGURE 12–2. Reentry ventricular tachycardia. (*A*) Sinus tachycardia is interrupted by a premature ventricular complex (PVC) that, in turn, is followed by a rapid, wide-QRS tachycardia. The morphologic difference between the initiating beat, which is longer than 0.14 second in other leads, and the subsequent run is typical of reentry ventricular tachycardia. The regular variations in ST-T waves during the wide-QRS tachycardia may reflect ventriculoatrial (VA) conduction, another typical feature of ventricular tachycardia. (*B*) One minute later, the rhythm is terminated by ventricular pacing, which is yet another typical finding of this tachycardia. The arrowheads indicate pacing spikes.

likely. Conversely, a longstanding history of tachycardias or the presence of preexcitation on the ECG during sinus rhythm, or both, should suggest supraventricular tachycardia with aberration.[5] As discussed in Chapter 3, observation of arterial or venous pulses and cardiac auscultation may help in identifying signs of AV dissociation.

ECG Criteria

DYNAMIC CRITERIA

Dynamic criteria are highly predictive of ventricular tachycardia but are not particularly sensitive.

AV Dissociation. *Atrioventricular dissociation,* the phenomenon in which the atria and ventricles beat independently of each other with no electrical relationship, is one of the most reliable criteria for the diagnosis of ventricular tachycardia. In the presence of a wide-QRS tachycardia, therefore, AV dissociation establishes the origin as ventricular. Unfortunately, it is present in only about half of any series of patients with ventricular tachycardia, and it can be recognized from the surface ECG only about 25% of the time.[6]

Dissociated atrial activity is reflected by regular P waves "marching through" the QRS complexes and the ST-T waves (Fig. 12-3A). The presence of even a very subtle morphologic variation in the ST-T waves may be the only available clue to the presence of dissociated atrial activity. Distinct P waves may not be demonstrable, partic-

ularly if the heart rate is rapid. An inferiorly or anteriorly oriented lead is most likely to demonstrate atrial activity (Fig. 12-4B), although, when necessary, all leads should be carefully scrutinized (for example, Figure 12-3A, lead I). At times, either esophageal or intra-atrial recording is necessary to establish the AV relationship (see Chapter 5, pages 110 to 116).

Retrograde VA conduction is found in the other 50% of cases of ventricular tachycardia (see Fig. 12-3B); when it results in greater than a 1:1 VA ratio, the diagnosis of ventricular tachycardia is established (see Fig. 12-4B). An AV junctional tachycardia with preexistent or rate-related bundle branch block is also a remote possibility. When the atrial and ventricular rates are identical (Fig. 12-5A), the distinction between VA and AV conduction is not possible. The clinician must then try to distinguish ventricular tachycardia from supraventricular tachycardia with aberration by analyzing QRS morphologic characteristics, by dissociating atrial from ventricular activity with autonomic maneuvers (Fig. 12-5B), or by atrial pacing.

With atrial flutter, a regular, wide-QRS tachycardia may reflect either AV association with a constant degree of AV block and aberration, or the combination of atrial flutter and ventricular tachycardia (Fig. 12-6). Just as with sinus rhythm, an analysis of the relationship between atrial activity and ventricular activity is key to

the diagnosis. With atrial flutter, however, it is impossible to tell which flutter (or F) wave is conducting. The clinician must simply choose a fixed reference point for measurement, such as the first or second F wave in front of each QRS complex. With flutter and a regular, wide-QRS tachycardia, a constant F-QRS interval always indicates AV association and, therefore, a supraventricular rhythm with aberration, whereas a variable F-QRS interval indicates AV dissociation and, therefore, ventricular tachycardia.

Capture and Fusion Beats. *Capture* and *fusion beats,* defined as either normal or near-normal–appearing QRS complexes that are due to an atrial impulse "sneaking" through and depolarizing a part (fusion) or all (capture) of the ventricle, also indicate ventricular tachycardia (Fig. 12-7). Capture beats have a QRS morphology identical to the normal sinus QRS morphology. Fusion beats result from a collision between a conducted portion of the QRS complex and a ventricular beat. Both may result in a narrower QRS complex. These beats may be on time but are frequently a bit premature (Fig. 12-7A); capture beats are always premature. Fusion beats confirm that two foci are controlling the ventricles and (particularly when they are premature and narrow) that aberration cannot be the explanation for the wide-QRS complex tachycardia (Fig. 12-7B). Unfortunately, the ventricular rhythm's concealed retrograde conduction into the AV node usu-

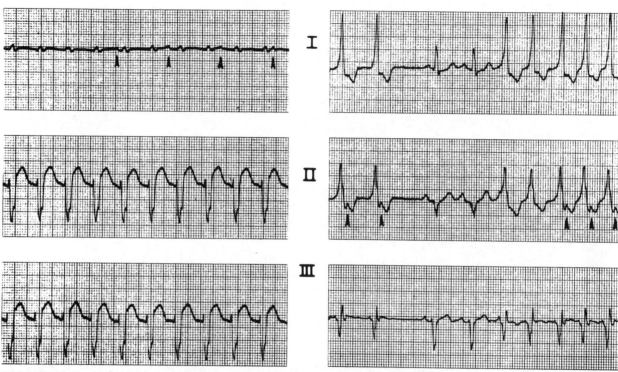

FIGURE 12–3. With a wide-QRS tachycardia, atrial activity must be identified in order to define the AV relationship. Often, the P waves are apparent in some leads but not in others, as in these examples of ventricular tachycardia with variable AV relationships. (*A*) Only lead I clearly shows the P waves (arrowheads). They identify an atrial rate that is slower than the ventricular rate, with variable PR intervals but constant RR and PP intervals, all typical features of AV dissociation. (*B*) The wide-QRS tachycardia, which terminates abruptly after two beats, is followed by two beats of sinus rhythm and then recurrent wide-QRS tachycardia. The P waves during the tachycardia are clearly apparent only in lead II (arrowheads), and they are associated with the preceding QRS complex but are independent of the sinus P waves, which is typical of VA conduction. When the tachycardia resumes, however, it does so with transient AV dissociation (note the on-time P wave in leads II and III, which merges with the first recurrent wide beat); this pattern is typical of ventricular tachycardia that eventually reestablishes VA conduction with retrograde P waves (last three arrowheads). Note also that the last complex of the initial run is a P wave, another finding suggesting ventricular tachycardia (or at least, a tachycardia that does not originate in the atria).

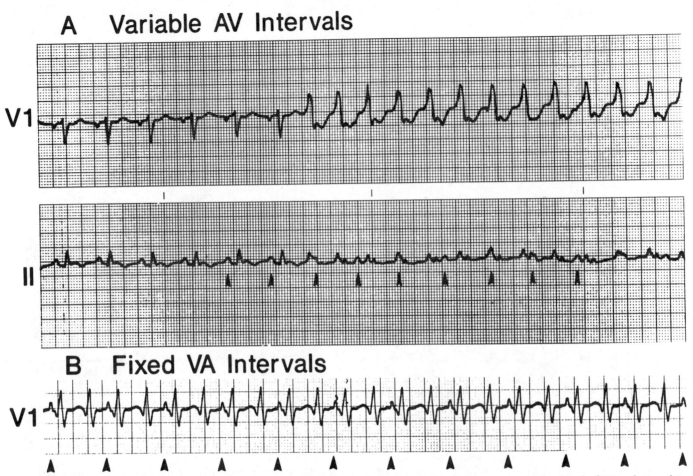

A Variable AV Intervals

V1

II

B Fixed VA Intervals

V1

FIGURE 12–4. Wide-QRS tachycardias in which either the lack of an AV relationship or a particular kind of VA relationship proves the diagnosis. (*A*) Lead V₁ falsely suggests P waves in the terminal part of most of the wide QRS complexes. Lead II, however, clearly shows P waves during the wide-QRS tachycardia. These P waves are "on time" in relation to the sinus P waves and bear no relationship to the wide QRS complexes, thus identifying AV dissociation due to ventricular tachycardia. (*B*) Atrial activity (arrowheads) is obvious and is fixed in relation to the QRS complexes but is one half of the ventricular rate. This pattern identifies 2:1 retrograde VA conduction and, therefore, ventricular tachycardia. (Compare this VA relationship with that of Fig. 12-5.)

FIGURE 12–5. These recordings of surface lead V_1 and an esophageal lead were obtained during a wide-QRS tachycardia before (*A*) and during (*B*) carotid sinus massage (CSM). Atrial activity cannot be accurately identified in the surface lead in either panel. In (*A*), the esophageal lead shows a 1:1 relationship between atrial (arrowheads) and ventricular activity but cannot differentiate ventricular tachycardia with retrograde VA conduction from an atrial tachycardia with aberration (albeit with a long PR interval). In (*B*), however, carotid sinus massage induces variable retrograde VA block (atrial electrogram indicated by arrowheads), establishing the diagnosis of ventricular tachycardia. The RP interval variability is typical of type I second-degree VA block. (Tracings provided by Seth Worley, MD.)

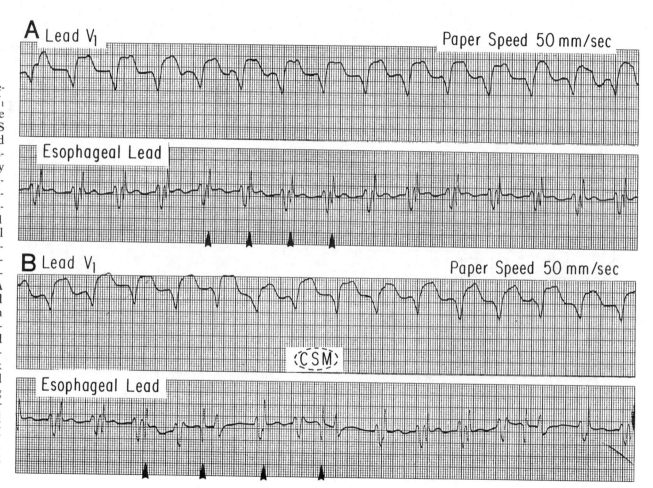

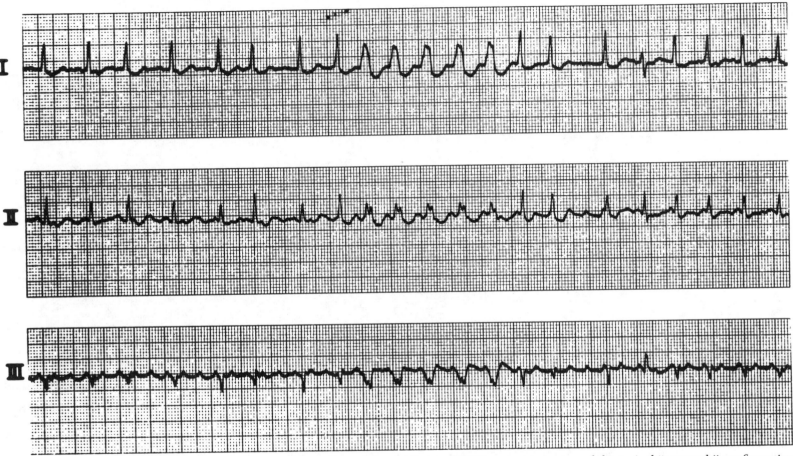

FIGURE 12–6. This patient, who was in atrial flutter (note the regular atrial rate of 300 beats per minute and the typical "sawtooth" configuration of atrial activity in lead III), developed a ventricular rhythm that was faster, more regular, and wider, raising the differential diagnosis of aberration versus ventricular tachycardia (midportion of the strip). Note the rate of this wide-QRS tachycardia (exactly half the atrial rate) and the absence of a pause following its termination, which are features typical of atrial flutter with 2:1 AV conduction and tachycardia-dependent left bundle branch block (LBBB) aberration.

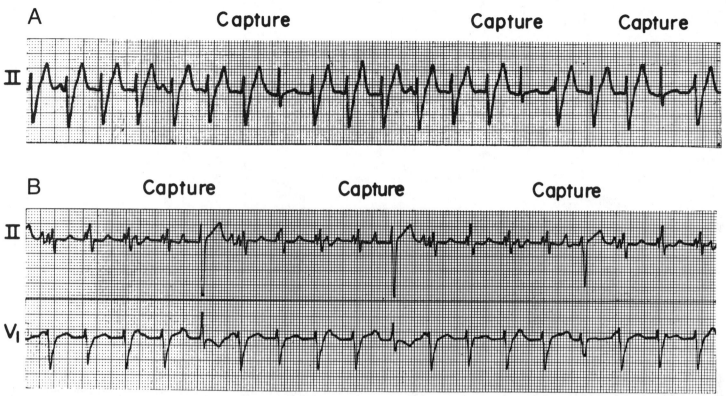

FIGURE 12–7. These ECGs were obtained in two different patients with wide-QRS tachycardias and intermittent narrow QRS complexes. In both examples, P waves that are independent of the wide-QRS beats are easily identified, indicating AV dissociation and, therefore, ventricular tachycardia. If no such identification of atrial activity were possible, however, one might be tempted to rely on the presence of intermittent QRS complexes that appear normal as indicative of atrial capture and, therefore, of ventricular tachycardia. In (A), this assumption would not be valid; the narrow complexes are on time, rather than premature, and can therefore be explained by intermittent normalization of aberrant conduction. (In this particular example, which has clear-cut evidence of AV dissociation and appropriately timed P waves, the narrow beats can be reliably identified as capture beats.) In (B), on the other hand, even if atrial activity were not identifiable, the assumption that the narrow complexes are capture beats would be valid, given that they are also premature and therefore cannot be explained by normalization of aberration. (The third narrow QRS complex is more nearly on time and is actually a fusion beat that is morphologically intermediate between that of the normally conducted QRS complex and the ventricular beat [best seen in lead V_1].)

Table 12–2. MECHANISMS FOR QRS NARROWING OR NORMALIZATION DURING WIDE-QRS TACHYCARDIA

CAUSE	MECHANISM
Fusion beat	1. Partial capture of the ventricle by a supraventricular beat during ventricular tachycardia.
	2. Simultaneous ventricular activation by the ventricular tachycardia focus and an ectopic focus arising from the opposite ventricle.
Capture beat	Completé capture of the ventricle by a normally conducted supraventricular beat during ventricular tachycardia.
Loss of aberration	1. Slowing of the tachycardia allows time for recovery of the affected bundle and normal conduction.
	2. Tachycardia-mediated autonomic and metabolic changes shorten the refractory period of the affected bundle and allow normal conduction.
	3. Loss of ventricular preexcitation occurs during sinus and other varieties of intra-atrial tachycardia.
	4. Rarely, the impulse encounters tissue during its supernormal phase of recovery, allowing conduction to proceed normally.

ally causes functional AV nodal block, particularly with rapid ventricular tachycardia. Capture and fusion beats, therefore, usually occur only with relatively slow ventricular tachycardia, where AV dissociation is also usually easier to demonstrate.

Narrowing of the QRS complexes during a wide-QRS tachycardia does not necessarily identify a ventricular origin unless they occur prematurely. Transient normalization of aberrant conduction during supraventricular tachycardia may also narrow the QRS complex by any one of several mechanisms listed in Table 12–2. Transient normalization of conduction that is not premature, therefore, may be seen in both supraventricular and ventricular tachycardias. Because definitive fusion or capture beats occur infrequently (in 10% or less of most series), they are a relatively insensitive diagnostic aid.

In summary, with a wide-QRS tachycardia, documentation that the atrial rate differs from the ventricular rate due to either AV dissociation or VA block is highly predictive of ventricular tachycardia. The clinician should use all available skills to determine the AV relationship, in conjunction with both the information from the physical examination and a careful analysis of the ECG. The presence of capture or fusion beats is a reflection of a varying AV relationship.

MORPHOLOGIC CRITERIA

Many criteria based on an analysis of QRS morphology have been proposed to help in distinguishing aberration from ventricular tachycardia.[6-10] Some criteria are met frequently and have high sensitivity but are not specific for a particular diagnosis. The few criteria that are highly specific tend to be infrequent and, therefore, insensitive. Combining certain morphologic features thus is necessary to enhance sensitivity while preserving specificity.

A 12-lead ECG should be obtained if possible; but frequently cannot be accomplished, particularly during nonsustained tachycardias. Leads V_1, V_2, and V_6 are helpful in evaluating for bundle branch block and QRS concordance; a combination of standard limb leads is used to determine the QRS axis. Various criteria purportedly indicating ventricular tachycardia or aberration are enumerated and discussed in the following sections.

QRS Configuration in Comparison with Sinus Rhythm. When the QRS complex of the tachycardia differs morphologically from that of sinus rhythm, the differential diagnosis between aberration and ventricular tachycardia is defined but not resolved. An exception to this rule occurs when the "normal" configuration is bundle branch block and that of the tachycardia differs morphologically; this markedly favors ventricular tachycardia.[10,11] This analysis depends, of course, on establishing the QRS configuration of sinus rhythm. A look in the trash may reveal discarded rhythm strips with both sinus rhythm (identifying the normal QRS configuration) and premature wide QRS complexes that are identical to those of the tachycardia. If these premature beats can be shown to be ventricular, then the tachycardia is also ventricular. If, on the other hand, they can be shown to be supraventricular with aberration, then the wide-QRS tachycardia is also supraventricular with aberration.

On the other hand, if the QRS configuration of the tachycardia is the same as in sinus rhythm, the tachycardia is supraventricular. It is, of course, necessary to establish the QRS configuration of sinus rhythm. The same techniques used during sinus rhythm to differentiate premature atrial complexes with aberration from ventricular ectopy can be applied to this problem (see Chapter 7, pages 146 to 154).

QRS Axis. Akhtar and colleagues have demonstrated that the QRS axis of ventricular tachycardia can be in any of the four axis-quadrants, although a normal axis is least likely.[12] Thus, whereas the axes of supraventricular tachycardias with aberration tend to lie between $-90°$ and $+180°$ (that is, in all except the right upper quadrant), there is considerable overlap with ventricular tachycardia. Patients with ventricular preexcitation demonstrate an axis that depends on the site of the accessory pathway, but the majority are also between $-90°$ and $+180°$ and overlap considerably with the axes of ventricular tachycardia. A tachycardia with extreme left axis deviation (more negative than $-90°$ and more positive than $+180°$—the "right upper quadrant") most likely is ventricular, except in children with com-plicated congenital heart disease producing severe right ventricular hypertrophy. Also, the combination of left bundle branch block (LBBB) and right axis deviation strongly favors ventricular tachycardia. With these latter two exceptions, however, the frontal plane axis is not very helpful in the differential diagnosis of wide-QRS tachycardias.

QRS Duration. The combination of a typical RBBB pattern and a QRS duration less than 140 milliseconds is characteristic of aberration. On the other hand, a QRS duration greater than 140 milliseconds with an RBBB morphology, or a QRS duration of 160 milliseconds or longer regardless of QRS morphologic features (in the absence of preexcitation or class Ia or class Ic drug therapy), favors ventricular tachycardia. QRS durations less than 160 milliseconds with an LBBB pattern can occur with aberration, and other QRS configurations less than 160 milliseconds can be seen with both aberration and ventricular tachycardia.

Bundle Branch Block Morphology: QRS Morphology in Leads V_1, V_2, and V_6. Earlier investigations suggested that RBBB with an upright QRS complex in lead V_1 is the most common variety of aberration. In reality, however, LBBB aberration is equally common and ventricular tachycardias frequently produce similar kinds of bundle branch block configurations, depending on the ventricle from which they arise. That is, a right ventricular tachycardia may produce a type of LBBB configuration. Nevertheless, a further evaluation of QRS morphology depending on whether the tachycardia demonstrates upright or negative forces in V_1 does have some utility. The following criteria, although by no means irrefutable, do provide the best "educated guess." In some cases (for example, the criteria outlined for a wide-QRS tachycardia with an LBBB pattern), the accuracy of the estimate may exceed 90%. Note that both V_1 and V_6 should be used to make the following evaluations. Left bundle branch block produces a negative deflection in V_1 and a positive deflection in V_6, whereas RBBB produces positive deflections in both leads.

Positive Deflection in V_1: RBBB.

Counting the number of peaks has some utility because a monophasic or biphasic QRS complex is more common in ventricular tachycardia and preexcitation than in RBBB aberrancy. This observation is not highly predictive of ventricular tachycardia, however, and it may be most helpful when combined with other clinical information such as the history, resting ECG morphology, and so forth. A triphasic QRS complex, though strongly touted as indicative of aberration, is not really a helpful discriminator unless the QRS duration is less than 0.14 second and the terminal R' wave is larger than the initial R wave.

NEGATIVE DEFLECTION IN V_1, V_2: LBBB.

Tachycardias with this morphology can be grouped in an LBBB subcategory. In the absence of preexcitation, certain features of the QRS complex in V_1, V_2, and V_6 have a high predictive accuracy for the presence of ventricular tachycardia, and the lack of these features has a high predictive accuracy for the absence of ventricular tachycardia.[10] In V_1 and V_2, these criteria include:

- An R wave duration greater than 30 milliseconds
- An interval greater than 60 milliseconds from the onset of the QRS complex to the nadir of the S wave
- Notching on the downslope of the S wave

In V_6, the criterion is a Q wave of any duration.

Each of these criteria alone has a low sensitivity for detecting ventricular tachycardia, but when ventricular tachycardia is diagnosed on the basis of a combination of criteria, the sensitivity surpasses 90%. It is important to evaluate both the V_1 and V_2 leads, recorded simultaneously, to be sure of the timing of the various QRS interval measurements (particularly the onset of the R wave).

QRS Concordance in Leads V_1 to V_6.

Concordance is present when all the QRS complexes are upright (positive concordance [Fig. 12–8]) or inverted (negative concordance) in leads V_1 to V_6. Concordance is found in only 10% to 20% of any given series of wide-QRS tachycardias, however. Positive concordance in the absence of ventricular preexcitation indicates ventricular tachycardia, but negative concordance is an unreliable criterion.

QRS Rate and Regularity.

The rates of supraventricular tachycardias with aberration or preexcitation overlap a great deal with those of ventricular tachycardia, although the supraventricular tachycardias with aberration due to ventricular preexcitation tend to be the fastest. A particular rate, therefore, is not a helpful differential point.

Similarly, irregularity can be misleading, particularly with nonsustained, wide-QRS tachycardias. When sustained, an irregularly irregular tachycardia strongly favors atrial fibrillation with either bundle branch block or ventricular activation via an anomalous pathway. Sustained ventricular tachycardia may be irregular, but the variation among RR intervals is typically less than 40 milliseconds.

Morphologically Distinct Ventricular Tachycardias.

Some varieties of ventricular tachycardia are so morphologically distinct that their ECG appearance is virtually diagnostic of a ventricular origin. Torsades de pointes is one example of such a tachycardia (Fig. 12–9). The ECG complexes seem to be physically expanding and contracting in amplitude as if they are "twisting" about a central reference point. True torsades de pointes occurs in association with a long-QT_c in-

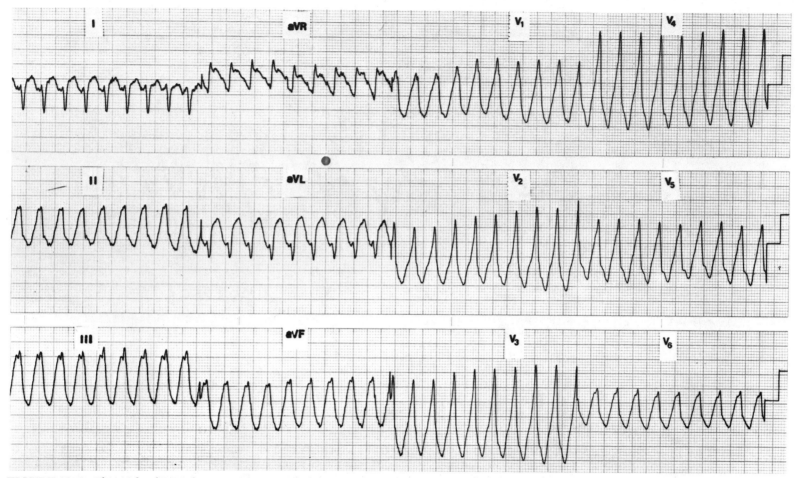

FIGURE 12–8. This 12-lead ECG shows a wide-QRS tachycardia with an axis that is rightward but not particularly helpful in discriminating between aberration and ventricular tachycardia. The positive concordance in the precordial leads, however, with no evidence of preexcitation, is highly suggestive of ventricular tachycardia.

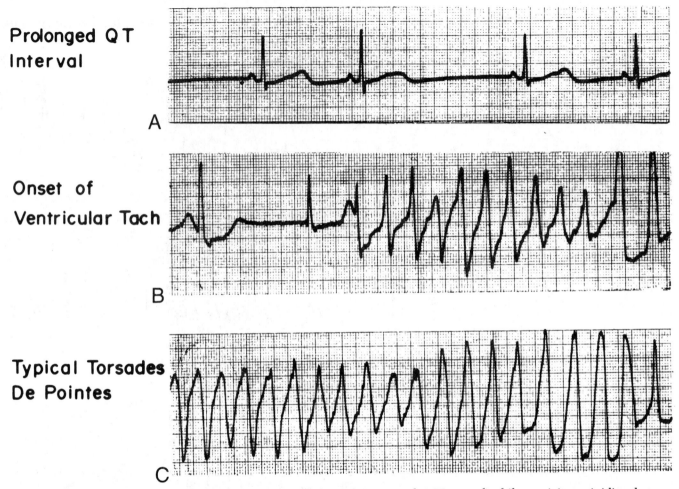

Prolonged Q T
Interval

A

Onset of
Ventricular Tach

B

Typical Torsades
De Pointes

C

FIGURE 12–9. (*A*) This patient developed a markedly prolonged QT interval (0.75 second) while receiving quinidine therapy. (*B*) A PVC occurs during the T wave and either initiates continuous ventricular reentry or is itself the result of a positive afterdepolarization wave that reaches threshold and is the first beat of a run of triggered ventricular activity. (*C*) The typical phasically alternating QRS pattern of torsades de pointes is apparent.

terval and has distinct implications as to mechanism and treatment. A similar-appearing "torsades-like" tachycardia can occur in association with a normal QT_c interval and should be distinguished from true torsades de pointes because of its different therapeutic response (e.g., it can respond to a class Ia drug). Some authors have suggested calling the latter *polymorphic ventricular tachycardia.*

Other varieties of ventricular tachycardia have configurations that are distinct from both torsades de pointes and monomorphic ventricular tachycardia. One variety is bidirectional ventricular tachycardia; in its most dramatic form, the morphology of the QRS complex in V_1 consistently indicates RBBB, but the frontal-plane QRS axis alternates between left and right axis deviation. The site and mechanism of this tachycardia remain controversial. A ventricular origin must be differentiated from a supraventricular tachycardia with aberration due to fixed RBBB in combination with alternating left anterior and posterior fascicular block. Bidirectional ventricular tachycardia commonly is the result of digitalis toxicity and advanced heart disease.

Another variety of morphologically distinct ventricular tachycardia demonstrates marked morphologic shifts from one QRS complex to another, such as from RBBB to LBBB. The shifts do not necessarily conform to any periodicity and may be due to variable pathways of exit from a given arrhythmogenic focus in the ventricle.

WIDE-QRS TACHYCARDIAS DURING ATRIAL FIBRILLATION

During atrial fibrillation, a wide-QRS tachycardia is most likely to be ventricular when:

1. There is fixed coupling of the initial wide beats to the previously conducted QRS complex.
2. There is a "compensatory" pause after the final wide-QRS beat.
3. The wide-QRS tachycardia is regular.
4. The wide-QRS tachycardia appears more frequently during periods when the narrow-QRS rhythm is relatively slow.
5. Isolated premature beats with a morphology identical to that of the wide-QRS tachycardia show fixed coupling to the previous narrow-QRS and are followed by relative pauses.
6. During periods of sinus rhythm, premature wide QRS complexes identical to those of the tachycardia can be shown to be ventricular by observing either AV dissociation or VA conduction.

These criteria are most helpful when multiple examples of the wide beats in question are available for review (see also Chapter 10).

INTERACTION WITH THE NERVOUS SYSTEM

Vagal maneuvers are typically applied to patients with tachyarrhythmias either to treat the patient or to help in diagnosis (see Chapter 4). Because parasympathetic innervation of the ventricle is minimal, however, vagal maneuvers rarely affect ventricular tachycardia.[13] During a wide-QRS tachycardia, therefore, if increased vagal tone causes ventricular slowing with or without normalization of the QRS complexes, ventricular tachycardia is excluded as a diagnosis for all practical purposes (Fig. 12–10; see Figs. 7–2, 7–4, and 7–5).

Vagal maneuvers and drugs affecting the AV node may alter VA conduction, if present, and lead to retrograde VA block. Dissociated or modified VA conduction may then be seen, establishing the diagnosis of ventricular tachycardia (see Fig. 12–5*B*). This finding is usually best demonstrated using ECG monitoring with special leads.

Sympathetic stimulation triggers certain types of ventricular tachycardia, particularly those produced by exercise (Fig. 12–11). Additionally, the increased sym-

A SLOW VENTRICULAR RATE   B NORMALIZE QRS COMPLEX

WIDE QRS TACH-150/MIN   CAROTID MASSAGE

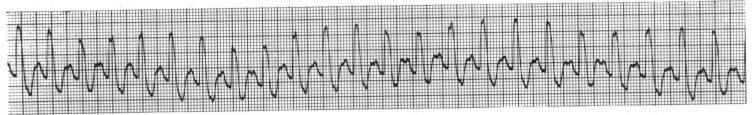

SINUS TACH-100/MIN   CAROTID MASSAGE   SINUS RHYTHM   90/MIN-NARROW QRS

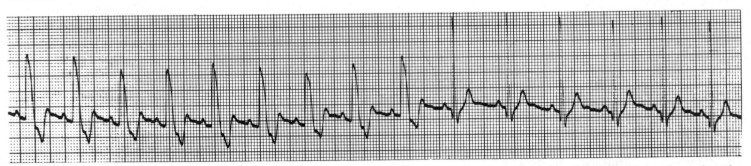

FIGURE 12–10. These two strips are sequential (but not continuous) from a patient who presented with a wide-QRS tachycardia. The notched T wave (*top*) is suggestive, but not diagnostic, of a contained P wave. Even if it were P-wave activity, however, it would not distinguish between AV and VA conduction, so the differential diagnosis would remain between aberration versus ventricular tachycardia. Carotid sinus massage (*bottom*), however, results in progressive slowing of the rate with an unchanged QRS configuration, permitting the diagnosis of sinus tachycardia with aberration. With further slowing of the rate to 90 beats per minute, the tachycardia-dependent aberration (in this case, LBBB) resolved, and a narrow QRS complex emerged.

During Exercise

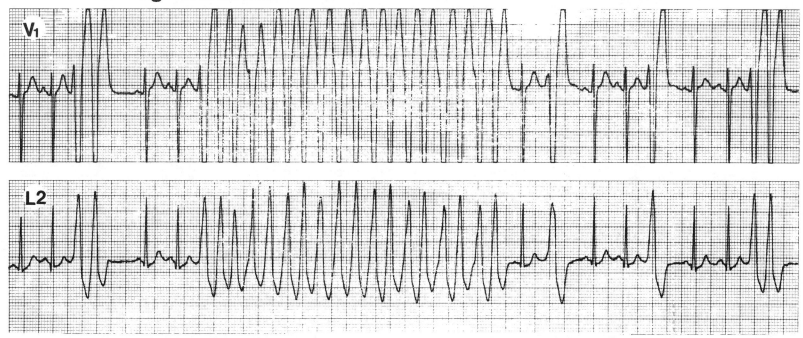

FIGURE 12–11. These simultaneous leads V_1 and II (L2) were recorded during exercise in a 33-year-old man with a history of exercise-induced syncope. They demonstrate a paroxysmal wide-QRS tachycardia that is identifiable morphologically as LBBB with right axis deviation. Intracardiac mapping studies have shown that this variety of morphologically distinct ventricular tachycardia originates from the right ventricular outflow tract.

pathetic tone associated with hypotension increases the rate of ventricular tachycardia.

USE OF INVASIVE ELECTROPHYSIOLOGY

Esophageal or Intra-Atrial Recording

Esophageal or right atrial intracavitary recordings are very useful when the atrial activity is not clearly defined on the surface ECG. Ventricular tachycardia can be diagnosed when either AV dissociation or VA association with less than 1:1 conduction is documented (Fig. 12–12). If there is either AV or VA association with a 1:1 ratio, neither esophageal nor intra-atrial recording alone resolves the differential diagnosis and a further intervention is necessary. For example, if atrial pacing at or above the tachycardia's rate either restores a normal QRS complex or induces AV dissociation, the diagnosis of ventricular tachycardia is confirmed. If the tachycardia terminates abruptly in response to atrial pacing, a supraventricular origin is most likely; if the tachycardia is abruptly terminated by ventricular pacing, on the other hand, a ventricular origin is most likely (Fig. 12–13; see Fig. 12–2). Ventricular pacing also can terminate paroxysmal junctional reentry tachycardia.

His Bundle Recording

Catheter recording of the His bundle electrogram can accurately and definitively differentiate between a ventricular versus a supraventricular origin for a wide-QRS tachycardia. In normal sinus rhythm, the H-V interval is 35 to 55 milliseconds. If the His bundle potential is related to and precedes the ventricular complex by 35 milliseconds or more, a supraventricular origin is confirmed. If the His bundle electrogram shows an H-V interval of less than 20 milliseconds, or if it is superimposed on or follows the ventricular complex (Fig. 12–14), the rhythm is ventricular and the His bundle deflection represents rapid retrograde activation from the ventricular focus. In about 80% of instances, however, the His bundle electrogram cannot be recorded during an episode of ventricular tachycardia either because of catheter malposition or because the His bundle electrogram is concealed within the QRS complex.

Electrophysiologic Stimulation

Electrophysiologic stimulation (EPS) often is of great clinical value in patients with hemodynamically or electrically significant ventricular arrhythmias or in patients with ventricular arrhythmias that are both hemodynamically and electrically significant. The methodologies are detailed in Chapter 6, and the following sections discuss applicability of electrophysiologic stimulation in various clinical situations.

CLINICAL FEATURES

Predisposing Clinical Settings and Natural History

Ventricular tachycardias occur in many different clinical situations and the prognosis and management, therefore, also vary greatly. In most instances, an accurate diagnosis of the underlying heart disease, if any, is equally as important as an accurate ECG diagnosis, underscoring the importance of the history, physical examination, and judicious use of ancillary diagnostic techniques.

ISCHEMIC HEART DISEASE

In patients with coronary artery disease, ventricular tachycardia can occur either in the presence or absence of ischemia. Prior to the development of myocardial infarction and scarring, ventricular tachycardia may appear during an episode of Prinzmetal angina or the earliest stage of acute myocardial infarction (that is, during acute, severe ischemia). After significant myocardial damage, however, the scarred left ventricle may become ar-

FIGURE 12–12. Leads I and III of the surface ECG are recorded simultaneously with an intra-atrial electrogram. The surface leads show a wide-QRS tachycardia (0.12 second); atrial activity cannot be defined. The intra-atrial tracing, however, clearly shows atrial electrograms (arrowheads), which occur at a constant interval relative to every other QRS complex. This atrial activity is most likely due to retrograde VA conduction with 2:1 VA block. Because it does show a gradual change in its timing, however (toward the end of the strip, the spike is slightly late and is superimposed on the R wave of the QRS complex instead of slightly preceding it), AV dissociation cannot be excluded. Nevertheless, either observation permits the diagnosis of ventricular tachycardia.

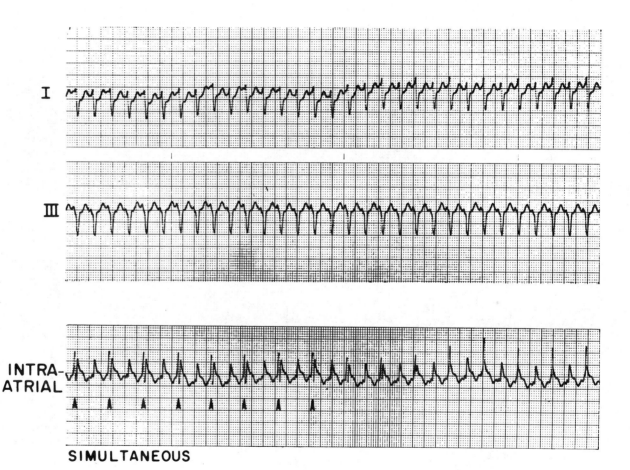

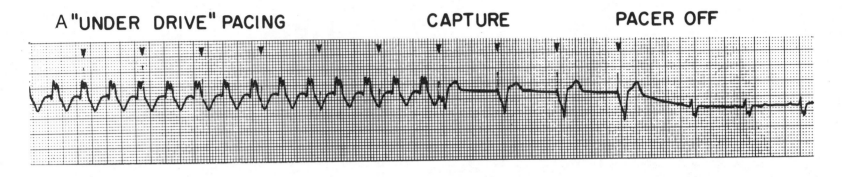

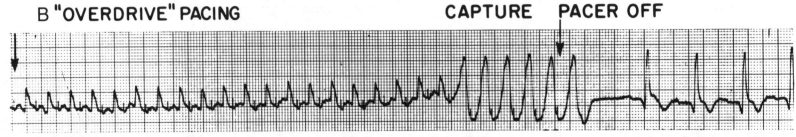

FIGURE 12–13. These tracings are from two different patients with wide-QRS tachycardias. They illustrate the utility of temporary transvenous pacing of the ventricle in differentiating ventricular from supraventricular tachycardia with aberration. (*A*) The pacemaker rate of 75 beats per minute is much slower than the rate of the tachycardia, which is 160 beats per minute. (The arrowheads indicate pacing spikes.) Eventually, however, the pacemaker effects ventricular capture and terminates the tachycardia. When the pacemaker is subsequently turned off, sinus rhythm emerges. (*B*) The pacemaker rate is faster than that of the native tachycardia. After a period of noncapture, it is eventually able to capture the ventricles and terminate the native tachycardia, replacing it with a paced rhythm at the slightly faster rate. When the pacer is subsequently turned off, normal sinus rhythm is the first rhythm to emerge. Both of these responses to ventricular pacing are typical of ventricular tachycardia. The arrow indicates the onset and termination of pacing.

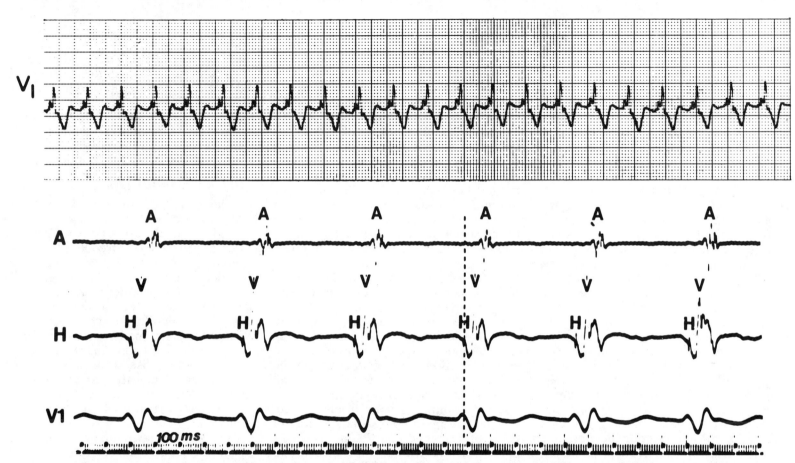

FIGURE 12–14. In this patient with a wide-QRS tachycardia, an analysis of lead V_1 does not permit differentiation of a ventricular versus a supraventricular origin. In the intracardiac recording, intra-atrial (A) and His bundle (H) electrograms are recorded simultaneously with lead V_1 at a more rapid paper speed. Atrial activity (A) occurs during the latter part of the QRS complex, with one P wave for each QRS complex. This pattern could reflect either VA conduction from ventricular tachycardia or an atrial tachycardia with an extremely long PR interval. The His bundle recording, however, resolves the question by showing that the His bundle spike occurs after the onset of the QRS complex (the dashed line denotes the timing of the His spike relative to the QRS complex in V_1). The diagnosis of ventricular tachycardia is therefore established. ms = milliseconds, V = ventricular depolarization.

rhythmogenic and a substrate for life-threatening ventricular tachycardias even in the absence of further ischemia. Intermittent, less severe ischemia does not appear to be a cause for premature ventricular complexes (PVCs) or ventricular tachycardia.

Sustained ventricular tachycardia during the acute phase of myocardial infarction is one manifestation of an unstable electrical state. Other manifestations include isolated unifocal or multifocal PVCs, ventricular couplets, nonsustained ventricular tachycardia, and ventricular flutter–fibrillation. These arrhythmias are relatively independent of the severity of muscle damage, so that the occurrence of ventricular tachycardia during the early stages of acute myocardial infarction is not of long-term prognostic significance.[14] Ventricular tachycardia after this initial phase (about 24 to 48 hours), however, usually characterizes more extensive myocardial damage and, consequently, carries a worse prognosis. Patients with large infarctions (for example, those with an anterior location and bundle branch block) have approximately a 33% risk of cardiac arrest due to ventricular fibrillation within the first 6 to 8 weeks following their infarction.[15] These arrhythmias may occur because of recurrent ischemia or infarction or may arise in an area of previously infarcted myocardium in the absence of any progression in underlying coronary artery disease.

Following either spontaneous or thrombolysis-induced reperfusion, ventricular tachycardia and fibrillation are possible but rarely observed clinically. Although such reperfusion is commonly associated with the slow form of ventricular tachycardia, AIVR, it does not have a high degree of predictive accuracy for reperfusion (see Fig. 12–1).[16] With AIVR, the modest heart rates (60 to 120 beats per minute) are usually not associated with hemodynamic impairment. Degeneration to ventricular fibrillation is rare and treatment is usually neither indicated nor necessary.

Ventricular tachycardia and fibrillation in patients with ischemic heart disease most often results from an underlying electrical abnormality produced by extensive ventricular scarring. This scarring may be associated with ventricular aneurysm formation, further potentiating the tendency to reentrant arrhythmias. Ambulatory ECG monitoring may detect frequent or complex or both variants of ventricular ectopy in approximately 50% of cases of sustained ventricular tachycardias associated with chronic myocardial scarring. The other half show no significant premonitory ventricular arrhythmias. Ventricular tachycardia is easily induced via EPS in over 90% of such patients (see Chapter 6, pages 135 to 139). Signal-averaged ECG techniques may reveal abnormal late potentials following the QRS complex, which are also a prom-

ising marker of the likelihood of significant ventricular arrhythmias, particularly when these are associated with left ventricular dysfunction. The absence of such late potentials similarly identifies patients at low risk for such arrhythmias, especially if ventricular function is normal or only mildly abnormal.[17]

DILATED CARDIOMYOPATHY

Dilated or congestive cardiomyopathies are associated with a very high incidence of sudden death, up to 15% to 30% per year. The presence of frequent PVCs and repetitive beating has been reported as an independent risk factor for sudden death in some series[18] but not in others.[19] Electrophysiologic study is more likely to yield a clinically significant arrhythmia when dilated cardiomyopathy is the result of severe, chronic valvular heart disease or coronary artery disease, as opposed to an "idiopathic" congestive cardiomyopathy, although the considerations regarding ventricular arrhythmias are essentially identical.

The role of antiarrhythmic therapy in altering the natural history of dilated cardiomyopathy is unknown. The only pharmacologic intervention that has been shown to alter the natural history of this disease is vasodilator therapy with either hydralazine and nitrates[20] or an angiotensin-converting enzyme inhibitor,[21] although the mechanism of this favorable effect remains speculative. Patients with nonsustained ventricular tachycardia, frequent PVCs, or significant ventricular dysfunction are at the highest risk for proarrhythmia from the class Ia and class Ic drugs, and asymptomatic PVCs and nonsustained ventricular tachycardia ordinarily should not be treated.

It is appropriate to consider treatment for patients with frequent PVCs, nonsustained ventricular tachycardia, or both, if they have symptoms of presyncope, syncope, or heart failure, and for those with sustained ventricular tachycardias, regardless of symptoms. As has been noted, however, these patients are at high risk for proarrhythmia and ambulatory monitoring has not been shown to be a successful tool for long-term prognostic stratification.[22] An NIH sponsored multicenter study (Multicenter Unsustained Tachycardia Trial or MUSTT), similar to the Cardiac Arrhythmia Suppression Trial (CAST), using EPS to guide drug therapy for ventricular tachycardia, is currently underway, but this study is subject to some of the same limitations and criticisms of the original CAST. It is quite likely that any relatively static, short-term measurement will have difficulty predicting favorable long-term success for a given drug regimen in patients who have changing anatomic and physiologic milieus over time.

Although ventricular tachycardia can be induced during electrophysiologic study (EPS) in only 50% of patients with nonischemic cardiomyopathy, EPS is still appropriate in patients who have experienced syncope or cardiac arrest. In choosing drugs to test during EPS, the clinician should remember that ventricular tachycardia is likely to be associated with poor ventricular function in this subgroup, and that the class Ia and class Ic antiarrhythmic drugs need to be carefully screened for their proarrhythmic effects. Disopyramide and flecainide are contraindicated because of their negative inotropic effects and tendency to worsen congestive heart failure. If EPS-guided therapy is ineffective, or if no clinical arrhythmia can be induced during EPS, patients with spontaneous ventricular fibrillation should be considered for an implantable cardioverter-defibrillator (ICD).

HYPERTROPHIC CARDIOMYOPATHY

In some patients with hypertrophic cardiomyopathy, ventricular tachycardia appears at a much earlier clinical stage than in patients with congestive cardiomyopathy. Ventricular tachycardia on ambulatory ECG monitoring appears to carry independent prognostic significance for sudden death.[23] Also at high risk for this complication are those with a positive family history of sudden death. Adrenergic-blocking drugs, disopyramide, and the calcium-channel–blocking drugs may be quite effective for patients with symptomatic arrhythmias. A single study has evaluated amiodarone, but its usefulness has

not been established.[24] A randomized, prospective trial of antiarrhythmic drug therapy in these patients has not been reported, so it is unproved whether such drugs can alter the natural history of this condition.

MITRAL VALVE PROLAPSE

Mitral valve prolapse has been reported to be associated with a variety of arrhythmias, even in the absence of significant mitral regurgitation or left ventricular dysfunction, or both. More rigid echocardiographic criteria for the diagnosis reduced its estimated frequency, but it is still the most commonly diagnosed valvular lesion. Its frequency in the general population complicates the analysis of a possible cause-effect relationship between it and arrhythmias. In addition, many reported series of patients with prolapse and arrhythmias are from tertiary care facilities, wherein patient selection biases are rarely controlled.

Prolapse is reportedly associated with PVCs; nonsustained ventricular tachycardia; and, rarely, sustained ventricular tachycardia (as well as a variety of supraventricular arrhythmias). For the most part, the ventricular arrhythmias occur in the absence of measurable left ventricular dysfunction.

Despite the frequency of the condition with and without, fewer than 100 cases of sudden death in association with mitral valve prolapse have been reported. Jeresaty's analysis of 35 cases of sudden death (including patients resuscitated from ventricular fibrillation) has identified certain risk factors. These include a history of presyncope or syncope; an apical late-systolic or holosystolic murmur; ST-T wave abnormalities in the inferior leads, precordial leads, or both; frequent PVCs; and pronounced prolapse with mild to moderate mitral regurgitation on left ventriculography.[25] The natural history of ventricular arrhythmias in patients with mitral prolapse without these risk factors is benign in the overwhelming majority of cases.

The treatment of patients with mitral valve prolapse and ventricular tachycardia is based on symptomatic status. In asymptomatic patients with normal ventricular function and nonsustained ventricular tachycardia, the benefit of therapy is questionable at best. If instituted (see next paragraph), it may make the clinician feel better but there is no proof of a favorable effect on the natural history. Indeed, the distinct risk of a proarrhythmia may produce exactly the opposite result.

In general, the treatment of nonsustained ventricular tachycardia in patients with mitral valve prolapse and no risk factors for sudden death should be reserved for those experiencing intolerable palpitations or other symptoms suggesting that their arrhythmia is hemodynamically or electrically significant. β-Blockers and calcium-channel blockers are relatively

safe choices and should be the only therapeutic agents considered at the moment. At the minimum, careful monitoring and follow-up regarding proarrhythmic drug effects are necessary. Drug therapy in patients with prolapse often leads to or compounds an underlying cardiac neurosis and seems to be associated with a high incidence of symptomatic side effects. Electrophysiologic studies in these patients are generally unrewarding and should be reserved for those with suspected hemodynamically or electrically significant arrhythmias.

LONG-QT$_c$ SYNDROMES (TORSADES DE POINTES)

Torsades de pointes occurs in two distinctive varieties of the long-QT$_c$ syndrome: pause-dependent and adrenergic-dependent. Patients with this syndrome may also develop nonsustained or sustained monomorphic ventricular tachycardia.

Pause-Dependent Long-QT$_c$ Syndrome. The pause-dependent variety is acquired and associated with any one or more of the following: (1) marked bradycardia, (2) electrolyte imbalance (usually hypokalemia or hypomagnesemia), or (3) drug therapy (particularly with the class Ia antiarrhythmic drugs, sotalol, phenothiazines, and tricyclic antidepressants), as well as a variety of other conditions including a liquid-protein weight reduction diet and coronary artery disease. *Pause-*

dependent relates to the mode of onset of the tachycardia, virtually always involving a PVC followed by a pause. The sinus beat following the PVC has a very long QT interval. A PVC falling on this long QT interval initiates the tachycardia of torsades de pointes (see Fig. 12–9B). Discontinuation of the offending drug, correction of the electrolyte-metabolic imbalance, increasing the heart rate, or some combination usually suppresses the ventricular tachycardia.

Adrenergic-Dependent Long-QT$_c$ Syndrome. The adrenergic-dependent long-QT$_c$ syndrome may be congenital (sometimes in association with deafness) or acquired (in association with severe illnesses such as subarachnoid hemorrhage). The prognosis is poor in the congenital varieties, with a death rate perhaps as high as 10% per year.[26] In the acquired varieties, however, the prognosis may be excellent when the causal agent can be identified and eliminated. β-Adrenergic–blocking drugs and diphenylhydantoin have been reported to be therapeutically useful. Patients with acquired long-QT$_c$ syndrome may be effectively managed with an atrial pacemaker or an ICD to prevent cardiac arrest.

POLYMORPHIC VENTRICULAR TACHYCARDIA WITH NORMAL-QT$_c$ SYNDROME

Some polymorphic ventricular tachycardias resemble torsades de pointes but occur in the absence of a long QT_c interval. Typical underlying clinical conditions include acute ischemic events, cardiomyopathy, and electrolyte abnormalities. This ventricular tachycardia can frequently be initiated during EPS by a PVC with a short coupling interval. It occurs with reasonable frequency as a *nonclinical arrhythmia* during EPS, in marked contrast to the torsades de pointes type of ventricular tachycardia, which occurs with a long QT_c interval and is rarely inducible at EPS. The normal-QT_c torsades-like ventricular tachycardia may also be associated with high-adrenergic tone. The ventricular arrhythmias associated with both long- and normal-QT_c syndromes may appear identical on ECG. A distinction requires careful measurement of the QT interval and attention to other parameters such as concomitant therapy with drugs likely to be a cause.

IATROGENIC VENTRICULAR TACHYCARDIAS OTHER THAN TORSADES DE POINTES

Extensive clinical experience and ambulatory monitoring have shown that all antiarrhythmic drugs are capable of producing significant ventricular arrhythmias.[27] These arrhythmias may be of the torsades de pointes variety (particularly with class Ia drugs), but also may be either nonsustained or sustained monomorphic ventricular tachycardia (particularly with class Ic drugs).[28,29] All of these arrhyth-

mias may degenerate into ventricular fibrillation. The proarrhythmic effects from the class Ia drugs are most likely to occur with quinidine and sotalol in association with hypokalemia or hypomagnesemia and prior QT_c prolongation. The class Ic drugs are most likely to have proarrhythmic effects at higher dosages, in patients with poor left ventricular function, in the elderly, or in patients with preexistent sustained ventricular tachycardia (see also Chapter 15, pages 353 to 354, 370 to 372, and 375).

VENTRICULAR TACHYCARDIA IN PATIENTS WITH OTHERWISE NORMAL HEARTS

Several varieties of ventricular tachycardia occur in patients with no evidence of underlying cardiovascular disease. Two are morphologically distinct. One is ventricular tachycardia with LBBB and right axis deviation. This morphology itself is predictive of a ventricular origin. This arrhythmia generally occurs as salvos of monomorphic, nonsustained ventricular tachycardia (which, on occasion, can be sustained) and has been termed *repetitive monomorphic ventricular tachycardia*. It can often be precipitated by exercise or rapid pacing; triggered automaticity has been suggested as a mechanism. Endocardial mapping studies have suggested a site of origination in the right ventricular outflow tract. It tends to respond well to β-adrenergic–blocking

drugs, as well as to calcium-channel blockers and ablation.

The second variety of morphologically distinct ventricular tachycardia shows a pattern of RBBB and left axis deviation (Fig. 12–15). This morphology does not reliably predict ventricular tachycardia (it would have to be differentiated from supraventricular tachycardia with right bundle branch–left anterior hemiblock aberration), but ventricular tachycardia with this morphology has several interesting characteristics. It can be induced by rapid atrial pacing as well as by programmed ventricular electrical stimulation. Reentry is the most likely mechanism, and patients have responded well to either β-adrenergic– or calcium-channel–blocking agents. In addition, it tends to occur in younger patients, is well tolerated, and carries a good prognosis.

Nonsustained ventricular tachycardia with a variety of other QRS morphologies may occur in patients with no evidence of organic heart disease. These patients are often asymptomatic, and because the natural history is benign, such patients are not candidates for either EPS or empiric antiarrhythmic drug treatment. In patients whose symptoms necessitate therapy, class Ib and class Ic drugs are typically well tolerated. The class Ic drugs are usually more effective and do not have prohibitively high proarrhythmic risks in patients with no structural heart disease.

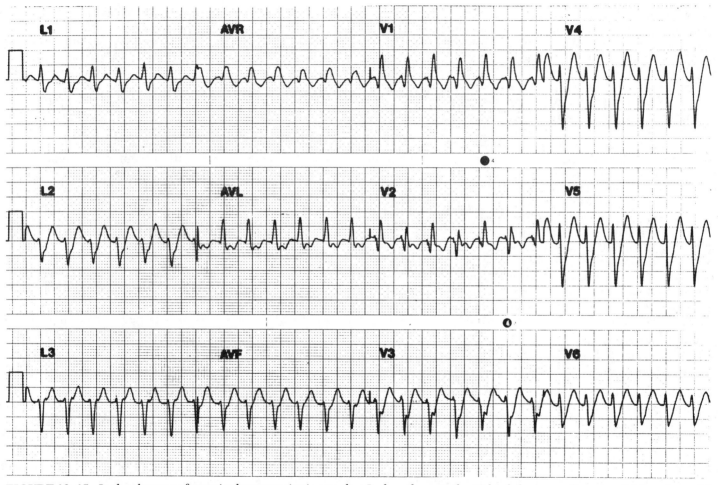

FIGURE 12–15. In the absence of ventricular preexcitation or class Ic drug therapy, the 12-lead electrocardiogram of this patient with a wide-QRS tachycardia provides one key observation that permits identification of a ventricular origin: The QRS duration is 0.16 second or longer (note particularly lead V₆). The tachycardia also displays the distinct pattern of right bundle branch block (RBBB) with left axis deviation.

Methods of Treatment

CARDIOVASCULAR COLLAPSE AND ARREST

When cardiovascular collapse or complete arrest occurs during ECG monitoring, the most common rhythm is ventricular flutter–fibrillation (Fig. 12–16). Out-of-hospital cardiac arrest usually is ultimately due to ventricular fibrillation, but in many cases is preceded by ventricular tachycardia. Q-wave myocardial infarction becomes evident in only about one third of such patients, although over 90% have significant coronary artery disease. The prognosis for patients who are resuscitated following sudden death in the presence of acute myocardial infarction is no different from that for similar patients who do not have a cardiac arrest. Patients who do not develop evidence of myocardial infarction, however, are at high risk for recurrent sudden death, and EPS is indicated to plan optimal therapy. If ventricular fibrillation or ventricular tachycardia is induced during EPS, a drug trial with repeated EPS is indicated until the arrhythmia is no longer inducible. The empiric use of amiodarone has been favored by some, but the recurrence rate of ventricular tachycardia or fibrillation is still significant. Implantable cardioverters-defibrillators should be considered for patients whose arrhythmia cannot be suppressed by drugs, or for those in whom no arrhythmia can be induced with EPS. ICDs are also being used more frequently because of the unpredictable and toxic long-term side effects of many of the antiarrhythmic drugs.

If a defibrillator is immediately available, the treatment of ventricular tachycardia with cardiovascular collapse and ventricular fibrillation is immediate countershock with 200 joules. If unsuccessful in restoring an effective rhythm, a second shock at 200 to 300 joules should be applied, followed quickly (as necessary) by a third shock of 360 joules. If these measures are unsuccessful, or if no defibrillator is immediately available, basic and advanced cardiac life support must be instituted immediately.

NONSUSTAINED VENTRICULAR TACHYCARDIA

The significance of nonsustained ventricular tachycardia (NSVT) must be determined rapidly prior to initiating drug therapy by addressing the following questions:

1. Is the arrhythmia hemodynamically significant?
   a. Is it associated with impaired cardiac output causing hypotension or shock?
   b. Is it occurring in a patient with ischemic heart disease in whom a significant increase in myocardial oxygen consumption could lead to angina, an acute myocardial infarction, or increased size of a recent infarction?
2. Is the arrhythmia electrically significant? That is, does it have the potential for producing ventricular fibrillation?

For NSVT, the answers to these questions are usually critically dependent on additional clinical factors such as the status of left ventricular function and presence or absence of concomitant cardiac disease. Nonsustained ventricular tachycardia may be one of the most threatening and emergent ventricular arrhythmias in certain clinical situations because of its potential for hemodynamic and electrical significance. For example, during the early phases of acute myocardial infarction and in other situations where cardiac status is unstable (e.g., electrolyte abnormalities, severe heart failure, and altered respiratory function leading to hypoxia and acidosis), it may be the harbinger of sustained ventricular tachycardia–fibrillation. It is often encountered following defibrillation in response to cardiac arrest, when it may portend a recurrence of ventricular fibrillation. The diagnosis of this arrhythmia is generally simple unless the patient is in atrial fibrillation, wherein runs of wide QRS complexes due to aberration are a frequent confounding variable. Nonsustained ventricular tachycardia may be monomorphic or polymorphic. Even though the episodes may persist for only a few seconds, they can some-

A   WIDE QRS TACH   PVCS   VENT FLUTTER

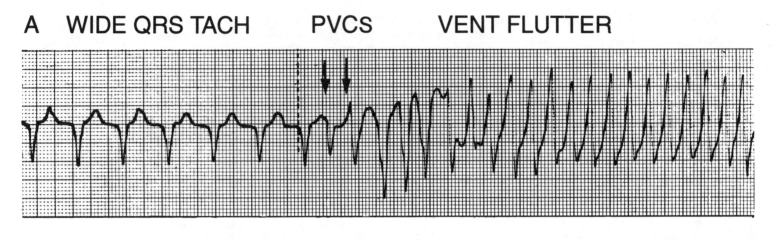

B   AFTER 1 MINUTE   VENT FIBRILLATION

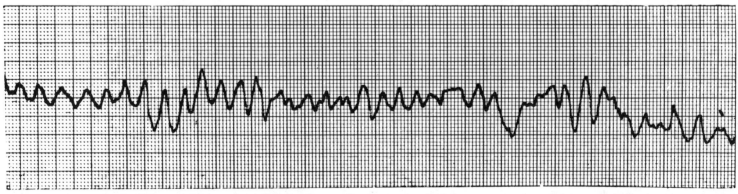

FIGURE 12–16. These tracings illustrate the progression from a more stable, relatively slow ventricular tachycardia (116 beats per minute) to ventricular fibrillation. During the ventricular tachycardia, PVCs occur and initiate a different type of ventricular reentry at a much more rapid rate (ventricular flutter at 300 beats per minute). No intervention occurred in this patient, and the ventricular flutter rapidly degenerated to the more disorganized pattern of ventricular fibrillation.

times cause hypotension and loss of consciousness.

Contributing factors such as hypoxia and hypokalemia should be corrected, but their presence is often difficult to document rapidly. These patients are often hypotensive and therefore the use of all antiarrhythmic drugs is limited. The hypotension should be corrected immediately by elevating the legs and, if necessary, employing an appropriate adrenergic agent. Clinicians often are reluctant to correct hypotension with drugs in this situation, believing that the arrhythmia alone is responsible and that the blood pressure will return to normal with its correction. Hypotension, however, tends to confound the problem and may even potentiate the arrhythmia. On occasion, the arrhythmia may be unresponsive to drug therapy while the patient is hypotensive but become much less frequent or treatable once hypotension is corrected.

Cardioversion is not useful in this setting, because patients are repetitively and spontaneously converting on their own. In the setting of myocardial infarction, lidocaine is the drug of choice; a standard loading regimen of a 75-mg bolus, followed by three additional boluses of 50 mg every 5 minutes, along with the simultaneous initiation of a continuous infusion at 2 to 4 mg per minute is one common standard. For patients with significant heart failure or hepatic insufficiency, the initial 75-mg bolus should be followed by only one additional 50-mg

bolus, and the infusion rate should be decreased to 1 mg per minute. Intravenous procainamide, bretylium, and, if the hemodynamics are acceptable, a β-blocker are therapeutic alternatives.

It may not be possible to stop all of the episodes of NSVT with clinically tolerable drug dosages; then the clinical goal would be prevention of sustained ventricular tachycardia or ventricular fibrillation. On occasion, however, when progression to more significant arrhythmias occurs despite adequate drug therapy, ventricular pacing can be used to speed the ventricular rate and suppress the ventricular tachycardia.

SUSTAINED VENTRICULAR TACHYCARDIA

In patients with sustained ventricular tachycardia, therapy has two objectives: (1) termination of the arrhythmia, and (2) prevention of its recurrence (and thereby the risk of ventricular fibrillation). Management of patients with terminated sustained ventricular tachycardia, therefore, is the same as that previously indicated for those resuscitated from cardiac arrest. In this section, we consider how to achieve the previous two objectives in various clinical situations.

With an Unstable Patient. When sustained ventricular tachycardia is associated with hemodynamic instability, the first goal is to terminate the arrhythmia quickly and safely. Diagnostic measures that unduly delay treatment are not justi-

fied. A grave error is made when patients with rapid tachyarrhythmias are simply watched or exposed to complex diagnostic procedures and not aggressively treated. If hemodynamic impairment is severe, the tachycardia should be immediately terminated by synchronized cardioversion. In alert patients, this procedure should be accomplished under appropriate anesthesia or sedation if possible, but in the hemodynamically deteriorating patient, there may not be time to initiate either of these measures. If there is to be a delay, hypotensive patients should have their blood pressure increased with dopamine or norepinephrine to maintain coronary and cerebral perfusion. Often a patient exhibits profound shock despite being alert and awake; a check of arterial blood gases reveals severe metabolic acidosis reflecting poor perfusion. If discrete QRS complexes are present, a synchronized shock should be employed to avoid inducing ventricular fibrillation, although at times even this may not be feasible. If the patient's hemodynamic stability permits, a 1-mg/kg bolus of lidocaine should be administered while the defibrillator is being prepared for the procedure. With ventricular flutter, synchronization of the DC shock should not be attempted because no discrete "vulnerable period" exists.

With a Stable Patient. When a wide-QRS tachycardia is sustained and hemodynamically well tolerated, the patient should be clinically evaluated for findings

**Table 12–3. DRUG THERAPY OF STABLE
VENTRICULAR TACHYCARDIA**

DRUG	DOSAGE	COMPLICATIONS
Lidocaine*	75 mg IV q 5 min × 3 doses or 1 mg/kg IV bolus with 0.5 mg/kg q 8 min until VT resolves or total of 3.0 mg/kg given†	Paresthesias, somnolence, coma, seizures
Procainamide‡	20 mg/min to total 1 or NSR	Hypotension
Bretylium§	5–10 mg IV over 2 min	Hypotension, induction of ventricular fibrillation

IV = intravenous; NSR = normal sinus rhythm; VT = ventricular tachycardia.

*These regimens differ from that used for ventricular arrhythmia prophylaxis during acute myocardial infarction.

†This regimen is recommended by the American Heart Association.

‡Procainamide can be used sequentially if initial lidocaine therapy is unsuccessful.

§Bretylium should be used only if ventricular tachycardia is recurrent following cardioversion.

typical of ventricular tachycardia. A 12-lead standard ECG also should be obtained to aid in differentiating aberration from ventricular tachycardia, and to serve as a template of the patient's spontaneously occurring tachycardia for comparison with arrhythmias induced by EPS, should laboratory study become necessary.

Hemodynamic stability allows more latitude for drug therapy before moving to cardioversion. Considerations in the selection of antiarrhythmic agents include ease of administration, low incidence of hemodynamic and electrophysiologic complications, and promptness of onset of action. Table 12–3 outlines pharmacologic regimens to convert sustained ventricular tachycardia. Lidocaine is usually recommended but is effective for termination of ventricular tachycardia in only about 10% of patients, even with more aggressive regimens. Importantly, however, its use does not preclude subsequent treatment with other agents. The next drug of choice, procainamide, can terminate ventricular tachycardia in 20% to 30% of patients and decreases the rate of the tachycardia in others. Bretylium may terminate ventricular tachycardia but may also produce ventricular fibrillation because it initially causes an acute release of catecholamines.

If pharmacologic agents fail, the tachycardia should be terminated electrically using either synchronized cardioversion or, particularly with hemodynamically stable sustained ventricular tachycardia, ventricular pacing (see Chapter 17, pages 416 to 418).

CONSIDERATION OF PROARRHYTHMIA

Ventricular tachycardia is but one of a variety of proarrhythmias that may be induced by antiarrhythmic drugs (see Chapter 15, pages 353 to 354). Proarrhythmia should be suspected when an existing ventricular tachycardia or other arrhythmia is aggravated (becoming more frequent, faster, or more sustained) or when a new arrhythmia appears; in both cases, the patient's underlying clinical status is not changed, and there is no other evidence of drug toxicity. Random variability in an arrhythmia's frequency is a common confounding variable, however.

The first line of treatment is to stop the drug (or drugs) precipitating the arrhythmia. Class Ic drugs, in particular, may precipitate an incessant ventricular tachycardia which requires a prolonged resuscitation attempt, presumably related to the time necessary to clear the drug from the patient's system.

Indeed, in the CAST study, this may have been the mechanism for the doubling of the mortality rate in the encainide- and flecainide-treated patients as compared with those receiving placebo.[22] It is remarkable that this enhanced mortality occurred in patients whose NSVT had been shown by ambulatory monitoring to be suppressed by a given drug. Furthermore, this proarrhythmic death rate was relatively linear and cumulative over the period of follow-up, an observation underscoring the difficulty of predicting the timing and occurrence of ventricular proarrhythmia.

Torsades de pointes is the most easily recognized proarrhythmic event. It represents a special type of NSVT that is particularly prone to produce ventricular fibrillation. This arrhythmia most commonly arises in patients receiving class Ia drugs (quinidine, disopyramide, or procainamide) but is also associated with hypokalemia, hypomagnesemia, phenothiazines, tricyclic antidepressants, and, more rarely, other antiarrhythmic drugs. Torsades de pointes does not respond to any of the usual antiarrhythmic drugs. In particular, the class Ia drugs, even if they are not responsible for this arrhythmia in the first place, do not stop it and, of course, can make it worse. Acceleration of the sinus rate shortens the QT interval and often results in the cessation and prevention of recurrent torsades de pointes. Increased sinus rates can be progressively and transiently induced by isoproterenol, but atrial or ventricular pacing, or both, at rates of 80 to 120 beats per minute is the treatment of choice (Table 12–4). Therapy can be discontinued when the precipitating drug has been cleared by the body or the electrolyte-metabolic imbalance has been corrected, or when both treatment goals have been achieved.

PREVENTIVE THERAPY

When adequate information regarding the cause of a given arrhythmia is available, prophylactic therapy against recurrence should be instituted that is as specific as possible for that arrhythmia. For instance, the use of β-adrenergic–receptor blocking agents is preferable in patients with ventricular tachycardia associated with exercise or emotion (catecholamine induced). β-adrenergic–receptor blocking agents are also indicated post myocardial infarction independent of ventricular rhythm status. With acute ischemic heart disease, intravenous lidocaine is the drug of choice, with procainamide a reasonable alternative. Bretylium

Table 12–4. TREATMENT OF TORSADES DE POINTES

1. Stop offending drug
2. Replace potassium and magnesium as necessary:
   KCl at rates up to 40 mEq/h* IV
   MgSO₄ 2 g IV over 20 min, then 2 mg/min infusion
3. Increase the ventricular rate:
   Ventricular or atrial pacing (80–120 beats/min)
   Drug therapy:
   Atropine 0.5 mg IV q 5 min to a total dose of 2.0 mg
   Isoproterenol 2–20 μg/min IV:
   Titrated to effective suppression of torsades

IV = intravenous; KCl = potassium chloride; MgSO₄ = magnesium sulfate.

*This dosage is recommended to treat life-threatening arrhythmia in the setting of hypokalemia. In other situations, 10 mEq per hour is the recommended maximal rate.

can be an effective adjunct to electrical cardioversion or ventricular pacing. High doses of procainamide have proved useful in patients with chronic ischemic heart disease who present with ventricular tachycardia. Hypokalemia should be considered if diuretic therapy, vomiting, diarrhea, alcoholism, or trauma (including surgery) are present.

It is mandatory to prevent sustained ventricular tachycardia even if the patient is asymptomatic, because it carries a risk of ventricular fibrillation. A systematic approach should be used, beginning with a baseline evaluation of left ventricular function by either invasive or noninvasive techniques, for reference and for guidance in drug selection.

Ambulatory ECG Monitoring and EPS. The two most widely studied methods for arrhythmia evaluation in this situation are ambulatory ECG monitoring and programmed electrophysiologic stimulation during EPS, but the efficacy of both remains hotly debated. The former has been suggested for the ambulatory patient to document spontaneously occurring arrhythmias and to evaluate therapeutic efficacy; the latter has been used to test drug regimens acutely. From CAST, we have learned that although a given drug can suppress spontaneous ventricular arrhythmias, this suppression does not predict freedom from subsequent sudden death. Ambulatory ECG monitoring according to the ESVEM study[30] is as valuable as programmed electrophysiological stimulation to predict drug efficacy in patients with ventricular tachycardia.

Table 12–5 presents a tentative approach to using these two methods in various clinical situations. When there has

Table 12–5. AMBULATORY ECG MONITORING VERSUS ELECTROPHYSIOLOGIC STUDY IN THE EVALUATION AND MANAGEMENT OF VENTRICULAR TACHYCARDIA

PATIENT SUBGROUPS	AMBULATORY ECG MONITORING*	ELECTROPHYSIOLOGIC STUDY
High risk for VT-VF	For risk stratification; frequent or complex ventricular arrhythmia to be considered in context of other variables such as ventricular function and signal-averaged ECG	Controversial No definitive recommendation pending ongoing studies
Documented NSVT; low risk for VT-VF	No data that evaluation or therapy should be guided by monitoring Used for correlation between arrhythmia and symptoms	Not likely to yield useful information
Documented sustained VT	Recommended	Recommended
Resuscitated from VT-VF or sudden death	Only if EPS is negative†‡	Recommended

NSVT = nonsustained ventricular tachycardia; VT-VF = ventricular tachycardia–ventricular fibrillation.

*Ambulatory ECG monitoring can be combined with telemetry depending on clinical circumstances.

†Ambulatory ECG monitoring is often used to evaluate proarrhythmia following electrophysiologic study.

‡These patients may be candidates for implantable cardioverter-defibrillator.

been no previously documented life-threatening ventricular tachycardia (sustained ventricular tachycardia or ventricular fibrillation), a therapeutic decision for further evaluation can usually be reached by information from ambulatory ECG monitoring. Patients with frequent serious ventricular arrhythmias, poor left ventricular function, and a positive signal-averaged ECG, are at high risk for sudden death. Unfortunately, ideal treatment has yet to be defined. These patients should be considered for ongoing prospective research studies (e.g., MUSTT, see 287). If no significant arrhythmias are documented on baseline ambulatory ECG monitoring, the potential for serious sustained ventricular arrhythmias is low, and neither treatment nor programmed stimulation is indicated.

With sustained ventricular tachycardia, both EPS and ambulatory ECG monitoring can be used. However with ventricular fibrillation the EPS is the evaluative choice. After the initiation of EPS-guided drug therapy, ambulatory monitoring can be used to evaluate for ventricular proarrhythmia.

Treadmill Exercise Testing and the Signal-Averaged Electrocardiogram.
Treadmill exercise testing has not proved sufficiently sensitive in the majority of patients in various clinical settings, although in some patients it may reveal clinically significant arrhythmias that are not detected by other methods.

Evaluation of the signal-averaged ECG, looking for "splintering" or late potentials in the terminal portion of the QRS complex, is currently a very promising technique to aid in the clinical evaluation of patients with known or suspected ventricular arrhythmias. Patients with ischemic heart disease who demonstrate a negative signal-averaged ECG, particularly if they have normal or minimally abnormal ventricular function, appear to have a low risk for significant ventricular arrhythmias. Further studies of large numbers of patients using all of these techniques, however, are required to determine the sensitivity, specificity, and predictive accuracy of each in the evaluation and management of ventricular tachycardia–fibrillation.

Selection of Drugs and Nonpharmacologic Therapy.
Selecting the treatment for each patient is often done by empiric trial and error. It is prudent to test a drug (or drugs) systematically and base decisions on the principle of cause-oriented management. It is not clinically practical, however, to test all of the drugs one after another in sequence in each individual patient, because of the prohibitive costs of extended hospitalization as well as the cost and risk of repetitive laboratory procedures. A new practical approach, based on the ESVEM study, is to use sotalol as the preferred drug unless there are serious side effects or contraindications.[31] If this agent fails to reduce the

arrhythmia (either spontaneous or elicited by programmed stimulation), one of five subsequent approaches may be initiated:

1. Using a second-generation (class Ic) agent alone
2. Using a combination of a class Ib agent with either a class Ia or class Ic drug or sotalol
3. Initiating amiodarone therapy[32]
4. Catheter or surgical ablation of the arrhythmogenic focus or foci[33-36]
5. Implanting an antitachycardia pacemaker[37] or the ICD, or both devices[38] (see Chapter 17, pages 419 to 422).

If drug therapy is selected, it is important to determine whether the response is beneficial or deleterious. A relatively high incidence of proarrhythmia with all of the *antiarrhythmic* drugs has been well documented.[28,29] The goal of testing is to identify an agent capable of either reducing the level of ambulatory arrhythmias below a threshold level,[39] or preventing ventricular arrhythmias induced by programmed stimulation in the laboratory. It is important to monitor blood levels of the various pharmacologic agents to maximize efficacy and minimize the likelihood of side effects. The dosage of a drug may be increased until either a therapeutic response, intolerable side effects, or the upper level of the recommended therapeutic window is reached.

LIMITATIONS OF EVALUATION TECHNIQUES

Though clinically valuable, the results of ambulatory ECG monitoring may vary from day to day in the same patient, and even more from one week or month to the next. Interim changes in underlying clinical status are another potential confounding variable. Therefore, at least 48 hours of baseline ambulatory monitoring should be performed before initiation of antiarrhythmic therapy, and repeat monitoring should be performed with the onset of new symptoms or other clinical events. Another limitation of ambulatory monitoring is that it has shown a sensitivity of only about 50% for detecting significant arrhythmias in patients who have had life-threatening arrhythmias documented by other means. In such patients, therefore, the absence of either numerous or complex ventricular arrhythmias on ambulatory monitoring should not be considered as evidence of low risk for recurrence of the serious ventricular arrhythmias.

In many clinical settings, the sensitivity of the programmed stimulation technique is also quite low. A higher sensitivity can be gained only by introducing a more aggressive stimulation protocol, which then may sacrifice specificity by producing clinically irrelevant nonsustained or sustained polymorphic ventricular tachycardia.

Because of these limitations, we hope that newly emerging techniques such as the assessment of spontaneous heart-rate variability, ECG signal-averaging, and the AICD will add significantly to the diagnostic and therapeutic options available for the care of patients at risk for ventricular tachycardia–fibrillation.

REFERENCES

1. Lewis T: Paroxysmal tachycardia, the result of ectopic impulse formation. Heart 1:262–282, 1909–1910.
2. Gallavardin L: Extra-systolie ventriculaire: a paroxysmes tachycardiques prolonges. Arch Mal Coeur Vaiss 15:298–306, 1922.
3. Lown B, Fakhro AM, Hood WB, and Thorn GW: The coronary care unit: New perspectives and directions. JAMA 199:188–198, 1967.
4. Lie KI, Wellens HJ, van Capelle FJ, and Durrer D: Lidocaine in the prevention of primary ventricular fibrillation. A double blind randomized study of 212 consecutive patients. N Engl J Med 291:1324–1326, 1974.
5. Tchou P, Young P, Mahmud R, Denker S, Jazayeri J, and Akhtar M: Useful clinical criteria for the diagnosis of ventricular tachycardia. Am J Med 84:53–56, 1988.
6. Akhtar M, Shenasa M, Jazayeri M, Caceres J, and Tchou P: Wide QRS complex tachycardia: Reappraisal of a common clinical problem. Ann Intern Med 109:905–912, 1988.
7. Marriott JHL: Differential diagnosis of supraventricular tachycardia and ventricular tachycardia. Geriatrics 25:91–101, 1970.
8. Wellens HJJ, Bar FWHM, and Lie KI: The value of the electrocardiogram in the differential diagnosis of a tachycardia with a widened QRS complex. Am J Med 64:27–33, 1978.
9. Kindwall KE, Brown J, and Josephson ME: Electrocardiographic criteria for ventricular tachycardia in wide complex left bundle branch morphology tachycardia. Am J Cardiol 51:1279–1283, 1988.
10. Dongas J, Lehmann M, Mahmud R, Denker S, Soni J, and Akhtar M: Value of preexisting bundle branch block in the electrocardiographic differentiation of supraventricular from ventricular origin of wide QRS tachycardia. Am J Cardiol 55:717–721, 1985.
11. Kremers M, Black W, Wells P, and Solodyna M: Effect of preexisting bundle branch block on the electrocardiographic diagnosis of ventricular tachycardia. Am J Cardiol 62:1208–1212, 1988.
12. Ahktar M, Shenasa M, Tchou P, and Jazayeri M: Role of electrophysiologic studies in supraventricular tachycardia. In Brugada P and Wellens HJJ (eds): Cardiac Arrhythmias: Where to Go from Here? Futura Publishing, New York, 1987, pp 233–242.

13. Waxman MB and Wald RW: Termination of ventricular tachycardia by an increase in cardiac vagal drive. Circulation 56:385–391, 1977.

14. Cobb LA, Baum RS, Alvarez H, and Schaffer WA: Resuscitation from out-of-hospital ventricular fibrillation: Four years follow-up. Circulation 52(Suppl III):223–228, 1975.

15. Lie KI, Liem KL, Schuilenberg RM, David GK, and Durrer D: Early identification of patients developing late in-hospital ventricular fibrillation after discharge from the coronary care unit. A 5½-year retrospective and prospective study of 1897 patients. Am J Cardiol 41:674–677, 1978.

16. Goldberg S, Greenspon AJ, Urban PL, Muza B, Berger B, Walinsky P, and Maroko PR: Reperfusion arrhythmia: A marker of restoration of antegrade flow during intracoronary thrombolysis for acute myocardial infarction. Am Heart J 105:26–32, 1983.

17. Kuchar DL, Thorburn CW, and Sammel NL: Late potentials detected after myocardial infarction: Natural history and prognostic significance. Circulation 74:1280–1289, 1986.

18. Unverferth DV, Magorien RD, Moeschberger ML, Baker PB, Fetters JK, and Leier CV: Factors influencing the one-year mortality of dilated cardiomyopathy. Am J Cardiol 54:147–152, 1984.

19. Huang SK, Messer JV, and Denes P: Significance of ventricular tachycardia in idiopathic dilated cardiomyopathy: Observations in 35 patients. Am J Cardiol 51:507–512, 1983.

20. Cohn JN, Archibald DG, Ziesche S, Franciosa JA, Harston WE, Tristani FE, Dunkman WB, Jacobs W, Francis GS, Flohr KH, Goldman S, Cobb FR, Shah PM, Saunders R, Fletcher RD, Loeb HS, Hughes VC, and Baker B: Effect of vasodilator therapy on mortality in chronic congestive heart failure: Results of a Veterans Administration cooperative study. N Engl J Med 314:1547–1552, 1986.

21. The CONSENSUS Trial Study Group: Effects of enalapril on mortality in severe congestive heart failure: Results of the Cooperative North Scandinavian Enalapril Survival Study (CONSENSUS). N Engl J Med 316:1429–1435, 1987.

22. Cardiac Arrhythmia Suppression Trial Investigators: Mortality and morbidity in patients receiving encainide, flecainide or placebo. N Engl J Med 324:781–788, 1991.

23. McKenna WJ, England D, Doi YL, Deanfield JE, Oakley C, and Goodwin JR: Arrhythmias in hypertrophic cardiomyopathy. I. Influence on prognosis. Br Heart J 46:168–172, 1981.

24. McKenna WJ, Oakley CM, Krikler DM, and Goodwin JF: Improved survival with amiodarone in patients with hypertrophic cardiomyopathy and ventricular tachycardia. Br Heart J 53:412–416, 1985.

25. Jeresaty RM: Mitral Valve Prolapse. Raven Press, New York, 1979, p 219.

26. Schwartz PJ: The long QT syndrome. In Wellens HJJ and Kulbertus HE (eds): Sudden Death. Martinus Nijhoff, The Hague, 1980, p 355.

27. Velebit V, Podrid P, Lown B, Cohen BH, and Graboys TB: Aggravation and provocation of ventricular arrhythmias by antiarrhythmic drugs. Circulation 65:886–894, 1982.

28. Morganroth J: Risk factors for the development of proarrhythmic events. Am J Cardiol 59:32E–37E, 1987.

29. Zipes D: Proarrhythmic effects of antiarrhythmic drugs. Am J Cardiol 59:26E–30E, 1987.

30. Mason JW: For the electrophysiologic study versus electrocardiographic monitoring investigators: A comparison of electrophysiologic testing with Holter monitoring to predict antiarrhythmic-drug efficacy for ventricular tachyarrhythmias.

31. Mason JW: A comparison of seven antiarrhythmic drugs in patients with ventricular tachyarrhythmias. N Engl J Med 329:452, 1993.

32. Herre JM, Sauve MJ, Malone P, et al: Long term results of amiodarone therapy in patients with recurrent sustained ventricular tachycardia or ventricular fibrillation. J Am Coll Cardiol 13:442–449, 1989.

33. Morady F, Scheinman MM, DiCarlo LA Jr, et al: Catheter ablation of ventricular tachycardia with intracardiac

shocks: Results in 33 patients. Circulation 75:1037–1049, 1987.

34. Cox JL: Patient selection criteria and results of surgery for refractory ischemic ventricular tachycardia. Circulation 79 (Suppl I):163–177, 1989.

35. Page PL, Cardinal R, Shenasa M, Kaltenbrunner W, Cassette R, and Nadeau R: Surgical treatment of ventricular tachycardia: Regional cryoablation guided by computerized epicardial and endocardial mapping. Circulation 80 (Suppl I):124–134, 1989.

36. Mickleborough LL, Usui A, Downar E, Harris L, Parson I, and Gray G: Transatrial balloon technique for activation mapping during operation for recurrent ventricular tachycardia. J Thorac Cardiovasc Surg 99:227–233, 1990.

37. Kelly PA, Cannom DS, Garan H, et al: The automatic implantable cardioverter-defibrillator: Efficacy, complications and survival in patients with malignant ventricular arrhythmias. J Am Coll Cardiol 11:1278–1286, 1988.

38. Winkle RA, Mead RH, Ruder MA, et al: Long term outcome with the automatic implantable cardioverter-defibrillator. J Am Coll Cardiol 13:1353–1361, 1989.

THE IMPORTANT ARRHYTHMIA PROBLEMS: BRADYCARDIAS

CHAPTER 13

Bradycardias Due to Pacemaker Failure

GALEN S. WAGNER, MD

OUTLINE

Even total failure of sinus node function need not be accompanied by significant clinical symptoms. Although the heart rate might be slowed and the "atrial kick" or transport function lost, neither syncope nor presyncope should occur, because pacemakers located elsewhere in the atria or lower in the atrioventricular (AV) junction or Purkinje tissues ordinarily escape and maintain a cardiac rhythm. Sinus node dysfunction, therefore, would be expected to produce clinical symptoms only with simultaneous dysfunction of all other escape pacing sites. Because these sites are so numerous, it is rare that all fail simultaneously, producing symptomatic bradyarrhythmias.

Global pacemaker dysfunction, however, can occur owing to a variety of intrinsic or exogenous factors, or some combination of both factors. When pacemaker failure is observed, the clinician should attempt to determine which of these mechanisms (or perhaps a combination of them) appears to be at work. This chapter discusses a systematic approach to the understanding and treatment of failures of pacemaker function. Although it deals mostly with the sinus node as a prototypic example of pacemaker tissue, the concepts hold true for pacemakers from all areas of the heart.

CLASSIFICATION

By Electrophysiologic Mechanisms

Pacemaker failures can be classified by electrophysiologic mechanisms into three broad groups, including those caused by (1) inhibition of impulse formation following premature activation and resetting of the pacemaker *(over-drive suppression)*,[1] (2) primary failure of impulse formation *(arrest* of the pacemaker), and (3) blocking conduction of the impulse or depolarizing wave front from the pacemaker site to the surrounding myocardium *(exit block)*.

By Contributing Pathophysiologic Factors

Pacemaker failure can also be classified according to the pathophysiologic processes responsible for producing or accentuating any one or a combination of these electrophysiologic mechanisms. These processes include (1) intrinsic disease in or around the pacemaker site or in both locations, (2) autonomic dysfunction from enhanced parasympathetic stimulation or sympathetic withdrawal, and (3) dysfunction due to drug effects or, more rarely, electrolyte imbalance. These three different groups have corresponding differences in therapeutic implications and prognosis.

MECHANISMS

Electrophysiologic Mechanisms

Although these three basic electrophysiologic mechanisms are well-documented processes, arrest and exit block are more difficult to diagnose and their relative individual importance as causes of pacemaker failure is debated. For example, whether permanent "arrest" of the myriad pacemaker cells from a primary pacing site such as the sinus node ever occurs short of its virtual destruction is conjectural. Accordingly, the concept that exit block accounts for most examples of prolonged failures of pacemaker activity has been proposed; for all practical purposes, however, no significant clinical advantage accrues from aggressively pursuing the differential diagnosis of these two mechanisms.

Any of the three basic electrophysiologic mechanisms can be precipitated or exacerbated, or both, by any one or more of the previously cited pathophysiologic factors.

INHIBITION OF IMPULSE FORMATION FOLLOWING PREMATURE ACTIVATION (OVERDRIVE SUPPRESSION)

Overdrive suppression is a normal electrophysiologic event that becomes pathologic or clinically significant by the degree of escape pacemaker suppression. Overdrive suppression can follow premature activation of pacemaking tissue by either isolated early beats or a series of early beats such as occur with tachycardias. With premature activation, the cell becomes hyperpolarized due to increased intracellular potassium content. In its least complicated form, the cell simply takes longer to spontaneously depolarize to the threshold potential. Another important factor can be a change in the rate of diastolic depolarization following premature activation, a process that is very sensitive to autonomic balance and circulating catecholamines. In some instances, a more positive threshold potential may be an additional factor.[1]

Clinically, overdrive suppression techniques have been used to assess the function of intrinsic cardiac pacemakers such as the sinus node. (See Use of Invasive Electrophysiology later in this chapter.) Normal overdrive suppression of the sinus node lasts for only a second or two. With enhanced sympathetic tone, the degree of overdrive suppression of the sinus

node is frequently minimal and inapparent on the rhythm strip. With enhanced parasympathetic tone, on the other hand, the rate of phase-4 diastolic depolarization may be markedly slowed, and both factors (more negative membrane potential and rate of change in diastolic membrane potential) lead to a prolonged pause. Similarly, drug effects and intrinsic disease may both contribute to the degree of hyperpolarization and slow the rate of spontaneous diastolic depolarization following premature activation. In general, the lower the escape pacing site is located in the hierarchy of pacemaking tissues, the longer the duration of overdrive suppression. Sinus node cells, for example, are highest in the hierarchy and are least susceptible, but under certain circumstances, even single premature atrial beats can produce pathologic overdrive suppression of the sinus node (Fig. 13-1A).

On other occasions, the premature atrial beats may occur repetitively, contributing to a sustained slowing of the effective heart rate, as illustrated in Figure 13-1B. This patient had developed marked fatigue and limited exercise tolerance in the setting of a persistently slow pulse rate. Blocked premature atrial complexes (PACs), rather than sinus node dysfunction, were found to be causing the bradycardia. Treatment with a class I drug resulted in sinus rhythm, an increase in ef-

fective heart rate, and an improvement in clinical symptoms.

Because lower pacemakers in the His-Purkinje region are most susceptible to overdrive suppression, the development of sudden AV block may be associated with long periods of asystole (one mechanism for the classic syncope of heart block). Even in patients with heart block and a stable escape ventricular rhythm, the development of premature ventricular contractions can be associated with prolonged pauses and syncope. Similarly, when temporary pacing is used for maintenance of a ventricular rhythm in patients with AV block, overdrive suppression may be enhanced, with prolonged periods of asystole in the event of failure of the temporary pacing system.

In some patients, significant overdrive suppression only occurs following termination (by whatever mechanism) of an ectopic or reentrant tachycardia. A period of asystole follows the termination, interrupted only when the first cell with pacemaking capability is able to resume its function (Fig. 13-2). A more rapid or longer-lasting ectopic or reentrant tachycardia generally results in greater overdrive suppression. Associated sinus node disease can contribute to prolonged periods of asystole following the termination of an atrial tachycardia; in addition, such patients frequently have spontaneous episodes of sinus bradycardia and sinus ar-

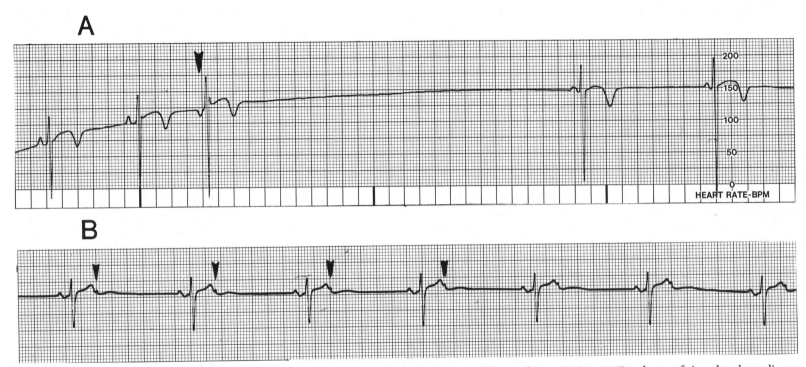

FIGURE 13–1. Sinus pauses: Resetting and overdrive suppression due to premature atrial complexes (PACs). (*A*) Two beats of sinus bradycardia are followed by a single conducted PAC (arrowhead). This sequence initiates a prolonged sinus pause of 4.84 seconds, which is terminated by a probable sinus escape beat with subsequent sinus bradycardia at an even slower rate. This pause and subsequent sinus slowing reflect abnormal overdrive suppression of both the sinus pacemaker and all escape pacemakers. (*B*) This electrocardiogram (ECG) of a 78-year-old man shows sinus rhythm with blocked PACs (arrowheads) in a bigeminal pattern that simulates sinus bradycardia (an effective heart rate of 41 beats per minute). Apparent sinus node dysfunction is not present; the problem is enhanced impulse formation.

Lead II

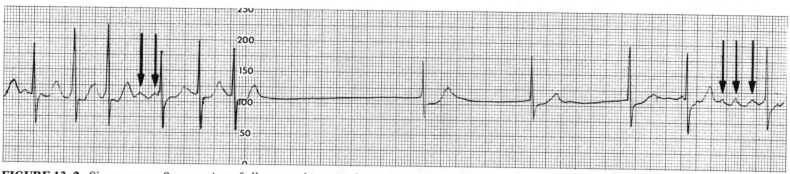

FIGURE 13–2. Sinus pauses: Suppression of all pacemaking sites by a reentrant supraventricular tachycardia. Atrial fibrillation (arrows) terminates abruptly and is followed by a 2.5-second pause. Suppression of all potential atrial, junctional, and ventricular escape pacemakers during the tachycardia continues after its cessation, until an escape junctional rhythm eventually emerges. At the end of the recording, atrial fibrillation recurs.

rest that also may be symptomatic. Most antiarrhythmic drugs used to treat tachycardias worsen the degree of posttachycardia overdrive suppression and can contribute to the development or worsening of symptoms such as presyncope or syncope. For example, the initiation of class I antiarrhythmic drug therapy in patients with paroxysmal atrial fibrillation may lead to prolonged periods of posttachycardia asystole.

Lown[2] noted that patients with either longstanding atrial fibrillation or a slow ventricular response are not suitable candidates for cardioversion. Patients with prolonged atrial fibrillation have a high incidence of postcardioversion sinus node instability and a high likelihood of reversion to atrial fibrillation. Those with slow ventricular responses frequently have associated AV conduction disease and may have remarkable suppression of all pacemaker activity when cardioverted. These likelihoods have led to the recommendation that such patients be electrically cardioverted only if sinus rhythm is deemed absolutely necessary. Also, electrical cardioversion itself directly causes the release of acetylcholine from cholinergic nerve endings and may further worsen overdrive suppression. The bradyarrhythmias induced by electrical shock may be prevented or treated by the administration of appropriate adrenergic or anticholinergic medication.

FAILURE OF IMPULSE FORMATION (ARREST)

Failure of the sinus node pacemaker to depolarize (a synonym is *sinus arrest*) may rarely reflect intrinsic disease of the pacemaking cells (for example, complete replacement of the sinus node with fibrous tissue, or some intrinsic abnormality of the action potential). Most commonly, it is due to a more transient, reversible depression of function from parasympa-

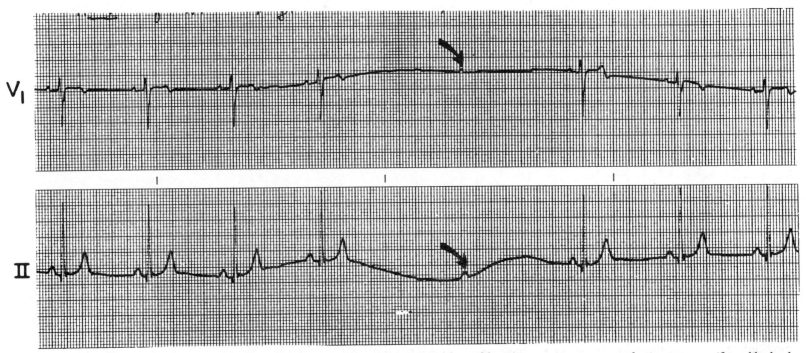

FIGURE 13–3. In this simultaneous recording of leads V_1 and II, vomiting caused a sudden increase in parasympathetic tone, manifested by both slowing of the sinus rate and atrioventricular (AV) block (note nonconducted P wave [arrows]). The increase in parasympathetic tone also suppressed junctional escape pacemakers; the pause of 3.44 seconds was interrupted only by the return of sinus rhythm.

thetic stimulation (Fig. 13–3) or drug effects. Not uncommonly, factors may combine, as when a patient with borderline adequacy of sinus node function becomes symptomatic when the heart rate is slowed even more by β-blocker therapy.

FAILURE OF IMPULSE CONDUCTION (EXIT BLOCK)

Electrical conduction from pacemaker cells to surrounding muscle typically proceeds through adjacent cells with pace-

making capability, which have low-amplitude action potentials and a slow rate of rise of phase 0 (see Chapter 1, pages 4 and 8). Conduction through such cells to the surrounding myocardium is therefore slowed and, at times, may even be totally blocked. As mentioned, drugs or parasympathetic stimulation, either alone or in combination with intrinsic disease of the pacemaker site, can contribute to the likelihood and severity of exit block. Conduction from a pacemaker site may be slowed (first-degree exit block), complete (third-degree exit block), or intermittent (second-degree exit block).

Pathophysiologic Factors in Pacemaker Failure

INTRINSIC DISEASE

The sinus node and other pacemaking tissues are subject to the same pathologic processes that affect other tissues of the heart, including inflammation, hemorrhage, ischemia, infarction, and fibrosis. In the elderly, such processes are the most common cause of clinically significant bradycardias, particularly when accompanied by superimposed problems due to autonomic dysfunction or drug effects. In some instances, the structural changes are part of a more generalized process such as atherosclerosis or myocarditis. In others, the changes are idiopathic.

The function of the sinus node can be remarkably well preserved despite extensive destruction, particularly in the absence of superimposed stresses such as drugs. In other patients, however, perinodal pathology may be dominant and presumably contributes to sinus exit block. Not uncommonly, when treatment with a new drug seems to produce clinically important pacemaker dysfunction for the first time, a review of previous (or subsequent) drug-free electrocardiograms (ECGs) shows evidence of preexistent and undetected intrinsic sinus node disease. That is, a combination of factors was necessary to produce clinical symptoms.

AUTONOMIC IMBALANCE

The rate of pacemaker impulse formation is normally determined by the sympathetic-parasympathetic balance. Intense parasympathetic stimulation can result in a sudden marked slowing or even cessation of all pacemaking activity within the heart. Perhaps the most common cause of such global pacemaker depression is the common faint or vasovagal reaction. Furthermore, excess parasympathetic tone is frequently accompanied by AV nodal block, so that any sinus or atrial escape beats that do occur may not be capable of capturing the ventricles (see Fig. 2–8). Indeed, the most common rhythm observed during vagally induced syncope is marked sinus bradycardia combined with the absence of an escape response from lower pacemakers, with or without accompanying AV nodal block (see Fig. 13–3).

Either parasympathetic excess or sympathetic deficiency can contribute to pacemaker dysfunction. For example, α-methyldopa, a centrally acting anti–α-adrenergic agent, commonly causes pathologic bradycardias by decreasing sympathetic tone in the sinus node and elsewhere.

DRUG EFFECTS AND ELECTROLYTE IMBALANCE

Drugs, particularly the β-blockers, calcium antagonists, and the class Ia and class Ic agents, also commonly result in global pacemaker depression, although clinically significant slowing usually occurs only when they are superimposed on one or both of the other processes. Digitalis enhances phase-4 diastolic depolarization (particularly of normally latent atrial, junctional, and ventricular pacemakers), but it also has significant parasympathomimetic effects. These effects, when superimposed on intrinsic disease, occasionally can cause significant slowing or exit block from pacemaker sites.

Digitalis and quinidine are the quintessential drugs cited in the older literature as causing inappropriate sinus bradycardia or sinus exit block. Frequently sinus exit block accompanies digitalis-induced type I, second-degree AV block. With the more careful use of digitalis and the availability of an increasing array of alternatives to quinidine, however, clinicians today see fewer bradyarrhythmias due to these drugs. Nevertheless, the newer antiarrhythmic drugs mentioned above also are capable of producing clinically significant depressions of sinus node and lower-pacemaker function and have more than filled the void.

Disorders of potassium and calcium balance also may contribute to problems of pacemaker function. Hyperkalemia usually just lowers the amplitude of the P waves, but on occasion they may disappear, raising the possibility of sinus arrest versus sinus exit block. Rarely, patients with hyperkalemia may show evidence of continued sinus function with conduction of the impulse through the atrium but without atrial activation. That is, there is no P wave, but the atrial rhythm remains responsive to factors that normally influence the sinus node—the so-called sinoventricular rhythm. All of these changes are usually dramatically reversible on correction of the hyperkalemia. On rare occasions, hypercalcemia due to iatrogenic or disease-related causes (particularly with concomitant digitalis therapy) has pathologically slowed the sinus node and caused exit block as well.

CLINICAL METHODS OF DIAGNOSIS

Definitions

A pathologic abnormality of pacemaker function is defined by the observation of either an inappropriately low resting heart rate or a heart rate (low or otherwise) that does not increase appropriately with stress or activity. Whether the heart rate is "inappropriate" requires clinical correlation; for example, long-distance runners frequently demonstrate resting heart rates that might prompt the insertion of a pacemaker in symptomatic patients. A significant problem with impulse formation may also be defined when normal sinus rhythm is interrupted by a sudden pause of 3 or more seconds.

Terms such as *sick sinus syndrome* have been used to describe all varieties of bradycardia wherein P waves either occur at inappropriately slow rates or are absent. Prolonged pauses or remarkably slow heart rates, however, require failure of pacemaker activity from all potential escape pacing sites rather than from the sinus node alone, and are more likely due to parasympathetic or drug excess than to any intrinsic "sickness" within the sinus node or other potential pacing sites.[3] Although the term sick sinus syndrome is therefore misleading, it is firmly embedded in the literature. In this text, we keep its usage to a minimum. Similarly, the term *bradycardia-tachycardia syndrome* is also commonly used but merely describes the observation that the patient has both a bradycardia and a tachycardia. The term is not helpful for classifying or understanding the two coexisting arrhythmias.

ECG Documentation

A significant bradycardia due to failure of impulse formation requires ECG documentation to differentiate the other causes of pathologically slow heart rates, such as AV block or bigeminal rhythms wherein the coupled atrial or ventricular premature beats are not apparent (e.g., the occult PACs in Figure 13–1*B*). Ambulatory ECG monitoring is a widely available technology that may both diagnose the bradycardia and document a convincing relation between the recorded bradyarrhythmia and the patient's symptoms. Sometimes, however, sinus bradycardias or pauses of striking degree occur without a convincing relationship to the patient's symptoms. The picture is further complicated by the occurrence of comparable bradyarrhythmias in asymptomatic "control" populations. For example, patients may have sinus pauses of up to 3 seconds or longer with no symptoms. Even marked *sinus arrhythmia* with periods of sinus bradycardia alternating with sinus tachycardia in phase with the respiratory cycle is frequently asymptomatic (Fig. 13–4). It is important to recognize that in the absence of any symptomatic correlates, these particular bradycardias are benign.

During marked sinus bradycardia, the mechanisms producing a bigeminal pulse may be different from those of classic ventricular bigeminy. With very slow sinus rates, both premature junctional and ven-

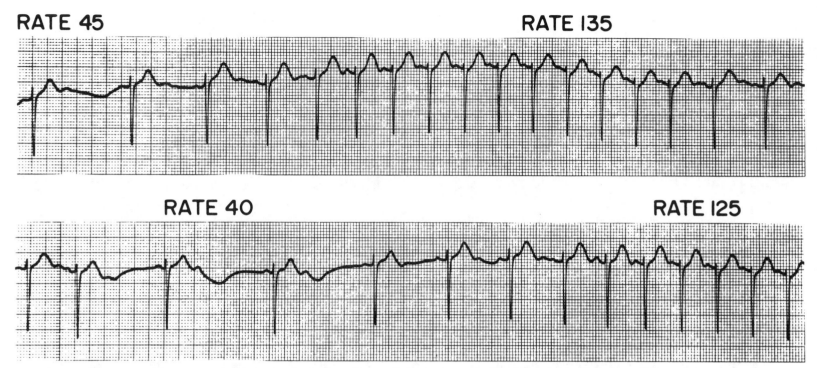

FIGURE 13–4. Successive PP intervals in sinus arrhythmia may vary from a minimum of 0.12 second to the extremes shown here. Note the phasic speeding and slowing of the sinus pacemaker, in this case synchronous with the respiratory cycle.

tricular beats are more likely to be interpolated between two successive sinus beats, producing a couplet cadence rather than bigeminy (Fig. 13–5). When a bigeminal cadence does occur, one common cause is *escape-capture bigeminy*. The slow rhythm allows junctional or ventricular escape beats to occur, which may then conduct retrograde and capture the atrium. The atrial beat in turn may conduct antegrade to the ventricle, producing a coupled sequence with the first beat of the couplet due to the escape beat and the second due to the atrial capture beat (Fig. 13–6A). This phenomenon is often seen with artificial ventricular pacemakers. Alternatively, sinus slowing may be associated with AV dissociation and independent atrial activity. Whenever this activity occurs far enough away from the preceding QRS complex, it conducts and

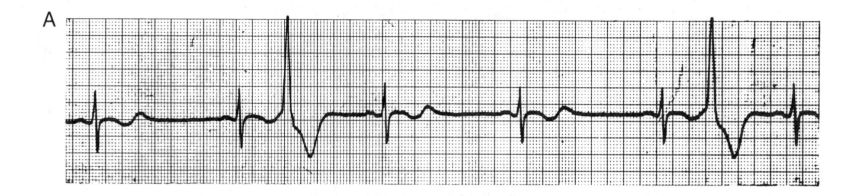

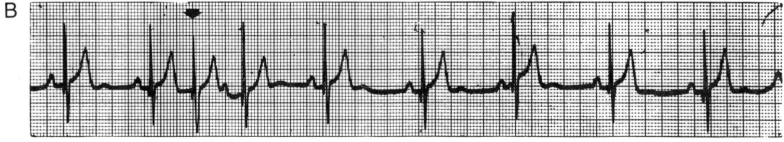

FIGURE 13–5. When the intrinsic rate is slow, either ventricular (*A*) or junctional (*B*) premature beats are much more likely to be "interpolated," because the bradycardia allows ample time for the AV node to recover and for the next on-time P wave to conduct. As shown in (*A*), even with late premature ventricular complexes (PVCs), extreme sinus bradycardia allows complete recovery of the AV node; the subsequent P waves conduct normally. With a relatively late premature junctional complex (PJC), indicated by the arrowhead in (*B*), even less extreme sinus bradycardia still allows AV nodal recovery and conduction of the following on-time P wave, albeit with a longer PR interval. The latter is due to "concealed" retrograde conduction from the PJC, which increases AV nodal refractoriness and delays antegrade conduction of the next normal beat.

A

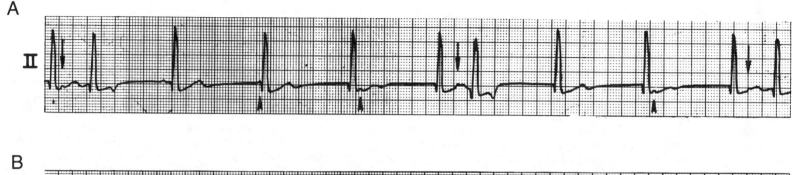

B

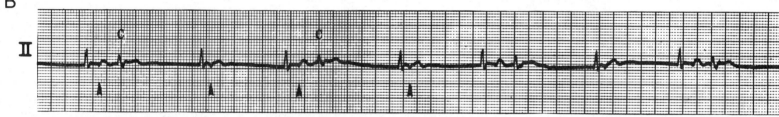

FIGURE 13–6. Two mechanisms for escape-capture bigeminy are illustrated. (*A*) The occurrence of AV dissociation is due to sinus slowing with a junctional escape pacemaker. Whenever P waves follow the QRS complex by sufficient intervals (arrows), producing a bigeminal sequence, AV conduction occurs. Other P waves that follow the QRS complex by slightly earlier intervals, or that occur just before or during the QRS complex, are blocked (arrowheads). (*B*) Slowing of the sinus rate permits a junctional escape rhythm at 50 beats per minute with subsequent retrograde ventriculoatrial (VA) conduction. These retrograde (inverted) P waves (arrowheads) follow each escape junctional beat with a type I conduction pattern. The longer RP intervals are associated with ventricular capture beats (C) that conduct aberrantly and reset the junctional pacemaker. The resetting-induced pause allows the next RP interval to shorten, and there is no associated "echo" beat of ventricular capture. While this ECG illustrates the basic principles behind one mechanism of escape-capture bigeminy, the overall pattern in this particular case produces an "escape-capture trigeminy" sequence.

contributes to an occasional coupled sequence (Fig. 13–6*B*).

Pauses During Sinus Rhythm and Following Tachycardia

With pauses during sinus rhythm, the diagnosis hinges mainly on determining whether a blocked PAC (the most common cause) is the culprit (see Fig. 13–1*B*). If no blocked PAC is apparent, further evaluation requires, at a minimum, reviewing additional ECG leads and, on occasion, even proceeding to esophageal or intra-atrial recordings, depending on the clinical circumstances. When blocked PACs have been excluded as a cause, the diagnosis by default becomes sinus arrest or sinus exit block.

Because the time of discharge of the sinus pacemaker cells cannot be determined on the surface ECG, the conduction time to the atrium cannot be measured and first-degree sinus exit block (or sinoatrial [SA] block) can never be reliably identified. With third-degree sinus exit block, the atrial rhythm is typically captured by whatever lower pacemaker is dominant, and a slower ectopic atrial or junctional rhythm is most often noted. Third-degree sinus exit block, therefore, also can never be diagnosed reliably.

Second-degree sinus exit block produces intermittent pauses in atrial activity which may be either regular or irregular. When these pauses are regular, reflecting easily recognized, reproducible patterns (such as pauses that are exact multiples of the basic PP interval), a diagnosis of sinus exit block from the surface ECG may be possible (Fig. 13–7). Rarely (most often with digitalis toxicity), type I sinus node exit block (or Wenckebach SA block) may occur with patterns analogous to type I second-degree AV block. Wenckebach SA block is diagnosed when progressive shortening of the PP interval is followed by a pause that is less than twice the shortest PP interval. Commonly, however, the basic sinus rate is not regular, either due to the effects of respiratory reflexes (respiratory-phasic sinus arrhythmia), or for no apparent reason. This variability complicates the analysis of the PP intervals in proximity to pauses, because the diagnosis of sinus exit block depends on the ability to compare a basic PP interval during sinus rhythm to the pause, or depends on the occurrence of a series of beats with progressively shortening PP intervals. When there is no reproducible PP pattern for comparison, the diagnosis of second-degree sinus exit block cannot be made.

Thus, further differentiation between sinus arrest and SA block is frequently not possible. In addition, although exit block and arrest are important mechanistic concepts in understanding failures of pacemaker function, there are no data showing that it is clinically important to make such a distinction. For all practical purposes, therefore, pauses not due to PACs can be considered to be due to either sinus exit block or sinus arrest, and little time should be expended in this portion of the analysis. It is more important to determine the etiology of the bradyarrhythmia—intrinsic disease, autonomic imbalance, drug-electrolyte effects, or some combination.

Since a pathologic bradycardia may occur only after the cessation of rapid tachycardias, it is important to observe the pattern of resumption of pacemaker activity following a tachycardia's termination (see Fig. 13–2). Normally, the sinus pause should be less than 3 seconds, followed by gradual speeding of the pacing rate to the baseline level. A pause of 3 or more seconds in this setting may indicate pacemaker dysfunction. If an ECG of the termination of the patient's spontaneously occurring tachycardia is not available, the sinus node recovery time (SNRT) can be determined by inducing and terminating the tachycardia during electrophysiologic testing (see the next section in this chapter and Chapter 6, pages 130 to 131).

The Importance of the Clinical Setting

The clinical setting of the bradycardia (discussed further later in this chapter) is frequently key to the diagnosis. For example, bradycardias due to vasovagal effects occur during venipuncture; blood donation; or in warm, crowded environments. Just as in the evaluation of AV

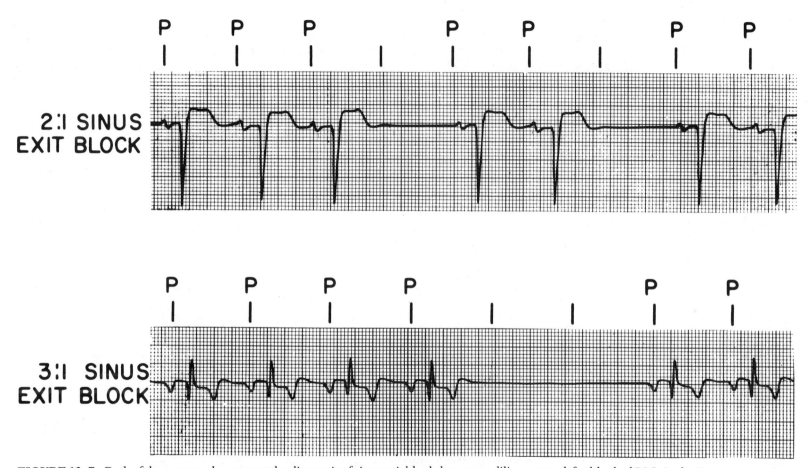

FIGURE 13–7. Both of these examples suggest the diagnosis of sinus exit block, because a diligent search for blocked PACs in the T waves preceding the pauses is negative, and the PP intervals encompassing the pauses are a multiple of the baseline PP interval. In the top panel, the duration of the atrial pauses is twice the baseline PP interval. In the bottom panel, the atrial pause is three times the baseline PP interval.

block, a detailed, accurate drug history is absolutely vital. For example, any patient developing pathologic sinus bradycardia or pauses while taking digitalis should be carefully evaluated for digitalis toxicity. Particular note should also be made of the use of any β-blockers or calcium blockers, centrally acting antiadrenergic blood pressure medications (e.g., rauwolfia alkaloids, α-methyldopa), and virtually all of the antiarrhythmic medications (see Chapter 15).

INTERACTION WITH THE AUTONOMIC NERVOUS SYSTEM

Autonomic balance is influenced by a variety of stimuli, and autonomic stress testing may be useful in the differential diagnosis of bradycardias due to failure of impulse formation. A dysfunctional sinus node due to intrinsic disease, for example, may fail to increase its rate in response to postural changes, exercise, or atropine, whereas sinus bradycardia due to parasympathetic excess would be expected to correct with exercise or atropine. A pathologic bradycardia may occur only with vagal stimulation. The various maneuvers described in Chapter 4, (pages 23 to 76), which stimulate the parasympathetic nervous system, may elicit failure of impulse formation or conduction and precipitate the patient's symptoms. It may also be helpful to monitor the ECG during activities that can enhance parasympathetic tone, such as swallowing, micturition, defecation, or head turning, to see whether there is any inhibition of pacemaker activity. Finally, monitoring the rhythm and blood pressure while the patient is tilted on a tilt table, with or without isoproterenol provocation, may provide valuable insight into the cause of syncope from vagally mediated bradycardias due to stimulation of intracardiac receptors.[4]

USE OF INVASIVE ELECTROPHYSIOLOGY

Various intracardiac stimulation techniques, sometimes in combination with drug response protocols, have been developed and evaluated for clinical utility in diagnosing sinus node function in particular, or in testing patients with unexplained syncope in general. The potential for overdrive suppression by electrical pacer-induced tachycardias or even single premature beats can be determined during electrophysiologic study (EPS). Following termination of either a train of stimuli or a single stimulus, the duration of overdrive suppression of the sinus node (the SNRT) is routinely recorded in an attempt to assess sinus node function[5] (see Chapter 6, pages 130 to 131). On occasion, striking postpacing overdrive suppression provides convincing evidence of a cause-effect relationship between the bradycardia and the patient's symptoms. A normal result, however, does not exclude parasympathetically induced sinus arrest as a cause for the patient's symptoms, because most such episodes appear to be related to paroxysms of enhanced vagal tone. In other words, a pacing test of sinus node function at a given time may not reflect how the sinus node performs under other conditions of autonomic balance at other times. There also may be problems in determining whether the paced stimuli conduct into the sinus node and capture the pacemaker. For a variety of reasons, therefore, these techniques are generally not able to differentiate problems of intrinsic pacemaker dysfunction from problems due to enhanced parasympathetic activity.[6]

In any clinical series of patients with enigmatic syncope subjected to EPS and tilt, bradyarrhythmias due to sinus node dysfunction are an infrequent cause. Ventricular and supraventricular tachycardias and *neurocardiogenic syncope* are much more common causes.[7] The role of EPS in evaluating sinus node function is detailed in Chapter 6.

CLINICAL FEATURES
Predisposing Clinical Settings

A great variety of settings predispose to the occurrence of a vasovagal reaction or a "faint." Among these are sudden fright, noxious stimuli such as pain or the sight of blood, and being enclosed in a warm, crowded environment. In addition, a vasovagal reaction may occur any time approximately 20% of the circulating blood volume is removed from the effective circulation, as in acute blood loss or venous pooling. Vasovagal reaction can occur after standing motionless for long periods and is the mechanism for soldiers fainting while standing at attention. Hypersensitivity of the carotid sinus, in combination with physiologic functions such as swallowing, micturition, and so forth, also causes vagally mediated bradycardias.

Profound myocardial ischemia (as during Prinzmetal angina or acute myocardial infarction) is a common setting for a bradycardia due to pacemaker dysfunction. In this setting, the problem usually reflects enhanced parasympathetic stimulation and responsiveness, rather than ischemia of the cells with pacing capability. It is more common with right coronary occlusion, probably because of the greater accumulation of postganglionic parasympathetic fibers in the posterior aspect of the myocardium.[8,9] Medications used for pain relief, particularly potent venous vasodilators such as nitroglycerin, may initiate the bradycardia. Intense parasympathetic stimulation may also cause vasodilation, worsening the hypotension and the clinical symptoms.

Failure of pacemaker activity due to intrinsic disease is more common with advancing age; in addition to ischemia, hemorrhage, infarction, and fibrosis, it may be caused by inflammatory or degenerative conditions such as sarcoidosis, acute rheumatic fever, collagen vascular diseases, and myocarditis.[10,11] The ECGs in Figure 13–8 were obtained in a 37-year-old man who presented for evaluation of syncope and was found to have suppression of sinus node impulse formation as well as impaired AV conduction. There was no evidence of other heart disease and he was treated with a permanent pacemaker. One year later, sinus rhythm with normal AV conduction had returned, raising the possibility that a transient disease process such as a myocarditis predominantly affecting the specialized tissues in the sinus node and AV junction was responsible for both his bradyarrhythmias and tachyarrhythmias.

Drugs that decrease sympathetic input to the heart (β-adrenergic blockers, rauwolfia alkaloids, α-methyldopa) or that block electrophysiologically important channels (calcium-channel blockers, class Ia and class Ic antiarrhythmic drugs, and amiodarone) can seriously potentiate pacemaker dysfunction (see Chapter 15). Such drugs should be considered the culprit in any patient with pathologic bradycardias or pauses until proven otherwise.

Natural History in the Various Settings

When the bradycardia is due to intrinsic disease of cells with pacemaking capability, the problem tends to progress. Fortunately, however, such progression may be slow, particularly in the elderly. Although artificial pacing may ameliorate symptoms due to the bradycardia, there are no data that pacing increases longevity in patients with intrinsic sinus node disease.

Pacemaker dysfunction due to parasympathetic excess occurring in the setting of acute myocardial ischemia or infarction tends to be transient and to appear only during the very early stages. The natural history of fainting in the supine position is not known, since drug therapy and assistance with leg raising are also available in most instances where the patient is being monitored. In one small series, however, three of the four patients observed had no spontaneous return of pacing activity and expired.[12]

When problems with pacemaker failure are due to drug therapy or hyperkalemia, the problem is reversible with appropriate recognition and treatment, and the natural history is usually that of the underlying condition. When the cause is missed, however, resulting arrhythmias can produce significant morbidity and even death.

Methods of Treatment

Vasovagal episodes usually occur in the upright position and resolve when venous return to the heart is increased, as when a recumbent position is attained (either voluntarily or involuntarily). A faint occur-

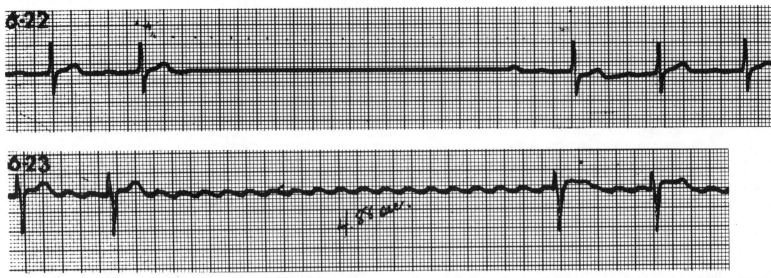

FIGURE 13–8. (*Top*) Sinus rhythm with first-degree AV block is interrupted by a 4.68-second pause that is due to sinus arrest (no blocked PAC was found on intra-atrial monitoring). An escape P wave occurs but does not conduct, and the pause is finally terminated by a junctional escape beat and then resumption of sinus rhythm with first-degree AV block. (*Bottom*) One day later, atrial flutter with sudden complete (or at least high-degree) AV block and a pause of 4.88 seconds occurs. These two tracings indicate problems with both impulse formation and impulse conduction, a combination that is common in patients with sinus node dysfunction.

ring while the patient is already recumbent may be resolved by elevating the legs or using Military Anti-Shock Trousers (MAST), which compress the legs and lower abdomen and move venous blood centrally.[13] Indeed, paramedics in field situations should put MAST trousers in place before administering vasoactive agents such as nitroglycerin for patients with symptoms of acute coronary insufficiency. Since the effect of nitrates may be enhanced by other agents such as lidocaine or morphine, sequential medications should be given at intervals of no less than 5 minutes. Subsequent episodes of severe bradycardia can be prevented by administering intravenous fluids, because volume expansion inhibits the redevelopment of the vasovagal episode.

If, in the acute situation, enhanced parasympathetic activity causes recurrent symptomatic bradycardias that are unresponsive to leg raising or intravascular volume expansion or both, management with intravenous atropine is indicated. Even when successful acutely, however, chronic parasympatholytic therapy with oral agents is rarely successful, and permanent pacing may be required. One should first use a temporary pacemaker, however, to test whether pacing prevents the development of symptoms, because the peripheral vascular vasodepressor aspects of vasovagal episodes persist during pacing. If these are dominant, they may continue to cause hypotension and syncope despite prevention of the bradycardia.

When the specific cause of a vasovagal response has been identified, future episodes may be prevented if that stimulus is avoided. For example, a hypersensitive carotid sinus should no longer produce profound bradycardia if the patient refrains from wearing tight collars and exercises care during shaving or head turning.

When bradyarrhythmias result from drug therapy, switching to a different drug with less impact on impulse formation or conduction may solve the problem. On occasion, however, pacemaker therapy may be necessary to allow the continued use of drugs considered essential, such as β-blockers for angina, or antiarrhythmic drugs for the tachycardia component of a bradycardia-tachycardia syndrome.

If the bradyarrhythmia is due to intrinsic pacemaker dysfunction, atrial pacing alone is usually contraindicated because of the high probability of accompanying problems with conduction through the AV junction (see Fig. 13–8). Atrioventricular sequential pacing (in selected patients) or ventricular demand pacing is the treatment of choice. More informa-tion on the use of pacing in patients with symptomatic bradycardias appears in Chapters 14 and 16.

REFERENCES

1. Vassalle M: Electrogenic suppression of automaticity in sheep and dog Purkinje fibers. Circ Res 27:361–377, 1970.
2. Lown B: Electrical reversion of cardiac arrhythmias. Br Heart J 29:469–488, 1967.
3. Thormann J, Schwarz F, Ensslen R, and Sesto M: Vagal tone, significance of electrophysiologic findings and clinical course in symptomatic sinus node dysfunction. Am Heart J 95:725–731, 1978.
4. Almquist A, Goldenberg IF, Milstein S, et al: Provocation of bradycardia and hypotension by isoproterenol and upright posture in patients with unexplained syncope. N Engl J Med 320:346–351, 1989.
5. Mandel W, Hayakawa H, Danzig RF, and Marcus HS: Evaluation of sino-atrial node function in man by over-drive suppression. Circulation 44:59–66, 1971.
6. Strauss HC, Prystowksy EN, and Scheinman MM: Sino-atrial and atrial electrogenesis. Prog Cardiovasc Dis 19:385–404, 1977.
7. Sra JS, Anderson AJ, Sheikh SH, et al: Unexplained syncope evaluated by electrophysiologic studies and head-up tilt testing. Ann Intern Med 114:1013–1019, 1991.
8. Rokseth R and Hatle L: Sinus arrest in acute myocardial infarction. Br Heart J 33:639–642, 1971.
9. Adgey AAJ, Geddes JS, Mulholland HC, Keegan DAJ, and Pantridge JF: Incidence, significance and management of early bradyarrhythmia complicating acute myocardial infarction. Lancet 2:1097–1101, 1968.
10. Lev M: Aging changes in the human sinoatrial node. J Gerontol 9:1–9, 1954.
11. Thery C, Gosselin B, Lekieffre J, and Warembourg H: Pathology of sino-atrial node. Correlations with electrocardiographic findings in 111 patients. Am Heart J 93:735–740, 1977.
12. Warren JV and Lewis RP: Beneficial effects of atropine in the pre-hospital phase of coronary care. Am J Cardiol 37:68–72, 1976.
13. Zydlaw SM Jr: A suit for all seasons. Emergency Product News, August 1977:35.

CHAPTER 14

Bradycardias Due to Failure of Atrioventricular Conduction

Robert A. Waugh, MD, and
Michael Rotman, MD

OUTLINE

CLASSIFICATION
  Degrees of AV Block
  Sites of AV Block

MECHANISMS
  First-Degree AV Block
  Higher Degrees of AV Block

CLINICAL METHODS OF DIAGNOSIS
  Degree of AV Block
  Site of AV Block

INTERACTION WITH THE
  AUTONOMIC NERVOUS SYSTEM

USE OF INVASIVE
  ELECTROPHYSIOLOGY

CLINICAL FEATURES
  Predisposing Clinical Settings
  Natural History in the Various
    Settings
  Methods of Treatment

The atrioventricular (AV) junction is the area of the heart that electrically connects the atria to the ventricles. Anatomically, its principal components are the AV node, the His bundle, and the proximal portions of the bundle branch system. Functionally, besides the important task of conducting the electrical impulse, the AV junction serves two additional key roles: varying the speed of AV conduction, and escape pacing when either AV conduction or higher pacemakers fail.

The AV node resides in the floor of the right atrium below and slightly cephalad to the membranous portion of the interventricular septum. It is continuous with the His bundle, which penetrates the right fibrous trigone and then courses along the inferior edge of the membranous portion of the interventricular septum. At the apex of the muscular interventricular septum, the His bundle branches into the right and left bundles. The right bundle extends as a discrete fascicle to the apex of the right ventricle; the left bundle branches into two broad subdivisions— the anterior and posterior fascicles. The His bundle and bundle branches, collectively, are referred to as the *His-Purkinje system.*

Rarely, a strand of atrial tissue may connect the atria and ventricles at a site remote from the AV node and His-Purkinje system. Such extra connections are called *Kent fibers* or *bundles;* they constitute bypass tracts or accessory pathways which provide an additional route for electrical connectivity between atria and ventricles. When such pathways support antegrade conduction, ventricular preexcitation occurs (for example, the Wolff-Parkinson-White syndrome). They may also support bidirectional conduction or only retrograde ventriculoatrial (VA) conduction and produce atrial preexcitation. Such pathways may also be considered to be part of the AV junction (see Chapter 11, pages 240 to 249, for a more detailed discussion of ventricular preexcitation).

The AV node and His bundle are the gate through which supraventricular impulses must pass before activating the ventricle. They are electrically insulated from surrounding tissue and, as such, are well-documented loci for disturbances in AV conduction. The more proximal portions of the three major divisions (or fascicles) of the bundle branch conduction system are also electrically insulated from adjacent tissue until they "insert" (i.e., connect electrically) into ventricular muscle, and can also be considered as part of the AV junction. Like the AV node and His bundle, they are part of the "gate" in AV conduction and can also participate in failures of AV conduction.

The AV junction can also vary the speed of AV conduction. This important function resides almost entirely within the AV node and allows the appropriate timing of atrial systole relative to ventricular systole under widely varying conditions, ranging from the sinus bradycardia of sleep to the sinus tachycardia of maximum exercise. This ability is tightly linked to AV node autonomic balance. Understanding the physiology of this modulation is important in understanding the behavior of AV nodal block and in using the autonomic nervous system as an aid in the diagnosis of AV block locations (see Chapter 1, pages 11 and 14 to 15, and Chapter 4, pages 82 to 88).

A third important function of the AV junction is escape pacing—initiating an electrical impulse when no conducted impulse occurs because of either AV block or failure of atrial escape pacing. Purkinje cells located in the AV node–His junction and His bundle and throughout the bundle branches are capable of spontaneous phase-4 diastolic depolarization and can function as escape pacing sites. The intrinsic rate and reliability of these escape pacing sites becomes progressively less the more distal their location is in the conduction system. In addition, the more distal escape pacing sites are less responsive to physiologic demands for rate increases. These characteristics of escape pacemakers (intrinsic rate, reliability, and physiologic responsiveness) explain the relationship between prognosis and the site of AV conduction failure.

This chapter discusses failures of AV conduction located primarily in the AV node, His bundle, and bundle branch system, and stresses the important electro-

Table 14–1. CHARACTERISTICS OF AV BLOCK ACCORDING TO ANATOMIC SITE

| SITE OF BLOCK | DEGREE OF AV BLOCK | | | | SITE OF ESCAPE PACER | QRS WIDTH OF ESCAPE PACER | ETIOLOGIES |
| | FIRST | SECOND | | THIRD | | | |
		TYPE I	TYPE II				
AV node	Yes	Yes	No	Yes	Distal AV node–His bundle	Narrow*	Enhanced parasympathetic tone; digitalis; β-blockers; calcium blockers; inferior infarction
His bundle	No†	No	Yes	Yes	Distal His bundle, proximal bundle branches	Usually narrow*	Congenital disruption (e.g., corrected transposition); idiopathic fibrosis; erosion by adjacent calcification
Bundle branches	Yes	No	Yes	Yes	Distal bundle branches	Wide	*Idiopathic fibrosis; erosion by adjacent calcification; anterior infarction; inflammation (e.g., Chagas' disease)

AV = atrioventricular.

*In AV nodal block, the escape pacemaker displays a narrow-QRS width unless aberration occurs.

†For all practical purposes, conduction time through the His bundle is usually too short to contribute significantly to prolongation of the PR interval.

physiologic features that facilitate recognition of the site of AV block. It also explains the marked differences in the clinical behavior of AV block from different sites, and the therapeutic implications of these differences. Table 14–1 summarizes these important features of AV block according to site.

CLASSIFICATION
Degrees of AV Block

Atrioventricular block may be classified by amount (or degree) into three straight-forward subgroups, first-, second-, and third-degree (see Fig. 1–7). Corresponding definitions are also simple. In first-degree AV block, all impulses conduct from the atrium to the ventricles, but they do so more slowly than normal. Second-degree AV block is the most colorful subgroup. Although simply defined as the failure of conduction of some impulses, the category encompasses a broad spectrum of AV conduction ratios, as well as two electrocardiographically distinct subcategories, type I and type II, to be discussed later. With third-degree AV block, no AV conduction is present.

Sites of AV Block

Atrioventricular conduction failure may also be classified according to its anatomic site into nodal and infranodal subgroups, each with distinctly different connotations in terms of etiology, natural history, and treatment. In many instances, a reliable clinical judgment as to site, while circumstantial, may be made by assessing a variety of readily available clues (see pages 324 to 336), but in other instances, invasive electrophysiologic study (EPS) may be necessary (see pages 336 to 338 and Chapter 6).

Second-degree AV block may be further subgrouped (or "subtyped") into type I and type II. This "typing" is an electrocardiogram (ECG) definition hinging on whether the PR interval changes (type I) or remains constant (type II) with variations in the related RP intervals (see Chapter 1, pages 11 to 15 and Fig. 1–8). When so defined, the "type" of AV block bears a close relationship to site: type I predominantly involves the AV node, and type II, the His–bundle-branch system. Consequently, the types are also closely related to both prognosis and therapy. In reality, the lessons learned about the behavior of AV conduction as related to type of block can be extrapolated to both first- and third-degree AV block in terms of predicting the site of involvement and, therefore, prognosis; in this regard, type can be considered as independent of the degree of AV block.[1,2]

MECHANISMS

The important electrophysiologic differences in the behavior of cells from the AV node versus those from the His–bundle-branch system are detailed in Chapter 1 (pages 4 to 6). Included in that discussion are the topics of how these differences explain the dissimilar behavior of the various parts of the AV conduction system, and how these behavioral differences are important in the clinical diagnosis and management of AV block.

First-Degree AV Block

First-degree AV block differs from the other degrees in that intra-atrial conduction time contributes to the interval, in addition to the conduction time through the AV junction (that is, the AV node and His-Purkinje system). A prolonged conduction time in any one area may be the primary cause of a prolonged PR interval, or, rarely, conduction times at the upper limits of normal in each area may summate to produce an overall prolongation of the PR interval. Intra-atrial block is most often related either to physical discontinuities (such as ostium primum atrial septal defects) or to atrial enlargement with a consequent increase in the duration of the P wave. Clinically it has never been shown to produce higher degrees of AV block.

Delayed conduction in the AV node is the most common cause of first-degree AV block and is even more likely if the PR interval is markedly prolonged (greater than 0.30 second). Infranodal first-degree AV block is rarely due to His bundle delay; more commonly, it reflects preexistent disease in two of the three major fascicles, with prolonged conduction in the remaining fascicle. This cause of AV block is associated with a wide QRS complex.

Higher Degrees of AV Block

Advanced degrees of AV block may occur because of conduction failure anywhere in the AV junction. The mechanisms responsible for second- and third-degree AV block are identical to those causing first-degree AV block, except that intra-atrial block is not a contributing factor. They vary from congenital or acquired physical discontinuities in the pathway (including alterations in geometry that contribute to decremental conduction) to physiologic variations in the electrical function of the conducting tissues in the pathway. Both anatomic and physiologic dysfunction may be superimposed on an underlying disorder of the action potential, such as incomplete repolarization (i.e., diminution in resting membrane potential), a diminution in maximum volume ($\dot{V}_{max}$) of phase 0, and alterations in the relative and absolute refractory periods.

When the site of the block is the AV node, usually the prognosis is not much different from that of first-degree AV block; such block most often is the result of an increase in drug effect, parasympathetic tone, or ischemia. It is usually reversible, although rarely it may be permanent, as when infarction destroys the AV node, creating anatomic discontinuity.

Infranodal block is rarely due to reversible impairment of physiologic function, such as the transient AV block that follows localized hyperkalemia caused by septal infarction, when the conduction system is not physically destroyed. Most often, fixed, anatomic disease accounts for AV block, such as the anatomic discontinuity between the AV node and the His bundle typical of congenital complete heart block. Progression of AV block is usually associated with further, often irreversible, destruction of the conduction system, related again to fixed anatomic disease (for example, erosion of the His bundle from calcification of an adjacent aortic valve or aortic or mitral annulus). Idiopathic degeneration or fibrosis of the Purkinje fibers of the conduction system itself (Lenegre's disease) is a slowly progressive condition that accounts for the majority of fascicular and AV blocks in the aged United States population.[3] In South America, Chagas' disease accounts for the majority of fascicular block. Regardless of the cause, progression of infranodal AV block beyond first-degree carries with it a quantum leap in significance and mandates for action.

A relatively discrete single "lesion" in the AV node or His bundle may cause AV conduction failure. For conduction failure to occur in the bundle branches, however, it requires much more extensive involvement of the involved fascicle proximal to its site of insertion into ventricular muscle, *along with* simultaneous or, more likely, preexistent conduction failure in the remaining fascicles.

CLINICAL METHODS OF DIAGNOSIS

The patient history (Chapter 2) and physical examination (Chapter 3) provide important clues to the presence, degree, site, and etiology of failures of AV conduction. A wide variety of pharmacologic agents can perturb AV conduction, and a detailed drug history is extremely important in the evaluation of patients with failures of AV conduction. Once AV block is suspected, the clinician should proceed expeditiously to ECG, to determine the degree and probable site of AV block. An excellent-quality ECG rhythm strip with clear P waves is invaluable for measuring the various intervals (PP, RR, PR, RP, and QRS) that allow accurate characterization of AV block. A good set of calipers greatly aids in this endeavor. Ambulatory ECG monitoring also can be an invaluable aid in the diagnosis of AV conduction disturbances, as it allows the relationship between the patient's daily activities, symptoms, and rhythm status to be evaluated and used to plan appropriate therapy. A monitoring period of at least 24 hours, including both daytime activities and periods of sleep, ensures a more accurate assessment of the effects of variable autonomic balance on AV conduction.[4]

Degree of AV Block

FIRST-DEGREE AV BLOCK

The degree of AV block is an ECG definition hinging on the PR interval and whether all, some, or none of the P waves are electrically related (associated) to the QRS complex. With first-degree AV block, the PR interval is more than 0.20 second, and all P waves are associated (Fig. 14–1A). In the highly conditioned athlete, the PR interval may be a bit longer than normal, and some have suggested allowing a PR interval of 0.21 to 0.22 second to be within the range of normal in the setting of sinus bradycardia. The PP intervals may be regular or vary. With a regular rate, the PR interval is constant, but the PR interval may shorten following the pause after a premature beat, for example, with an AV nodal site of block (Fig. 14–1B). The upper range for a PR interval that can still be believed to have conducted is controversial, but PR intervals above 0.5 second that show evidence of AV association are unusual.

SECOND-DEGREE AV BLOCK AND TYPING

Over a given period of observation, second-degree AV block may be sustained, demonstrating a repetitive pattern of dropped P waves or, on the other hand, it may appear suddenly, with one or a series of dropped P waves. In the former situation, either the PR interval is fixed, with the regularity of the RR intervals determined solely by the regularity of the AV conduction ratios (Fig. 14–2A), or the PR interval varies, with resulting variability in the RR interval due to this PR variability or that of the AV conduction ratios, or due to variability in both (Fig. 14–2B).

Variability in the PR interval leading up to the dropped beat is the hallmark of type I, second-degree AV block; a closer in-

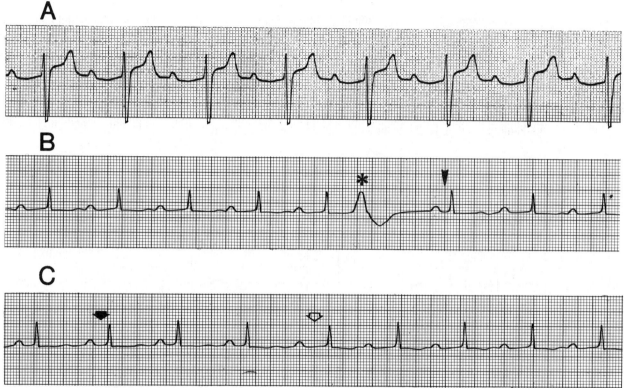

FIGURE 14–1. First-degree atrioventricular (AV) block. (*A*) This constant PR interval of 0.44 second defines first-degree AV block. (Longer rhythm strips confirmed AV association.) (*B*) Sinus rhythm with first-degree AV block is interrupted by a premature ventricular complex (PVC), indicated by an asterisk. The first PR interval following the pause (arrowhead) is shortened because the AV node is allowed to "rest and recover." Subsequent PR intervals increased. Such type I periodicity (reciprocal RP-PR variability), even without progression to second-degree AV block, identifies the AV nodal origin of the first-degree AV block. (*C*) In the same patient, spontaneous PR interval variability (solid arrow versus open arrow) also occurred repeatedly, with no corresponding change in heart rate or in underlying rhythm, and with no progression to second-degree AV block. The variability was most marked during sleep, suggesting a centrally mediated enhancement of parasympathetic tone and illustrating the dynamic nature of autonomic control of AV nodal conduction.

A

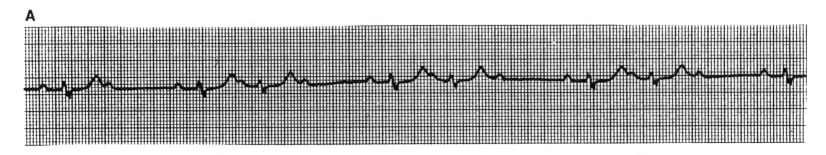

B

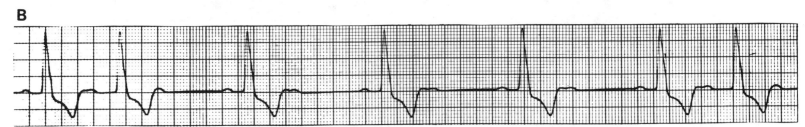

FIGURE 14–2. (*A*) and (*B*) are from two different patients with bundle branch block in association with second-degree AV block. In (*A*), note the constant PR intervals both before and after the blocked P waves, as well as the wide QRS pattern of the conducted beats (a right bundle branch block [RBBB] was present). This pattern represents type II block that is due to conduction failure in the Purkinje system of the left bundle branches. In (*B*), left bundle branch block (LBBB) occurs in association with second-degree AV block. The variation in the PR intervals of the conducted beats, however, defines type I block and, therefore, an AV nodal site of the block.

spection will show a reciprocal RP-PR interval pattern. Thus, when the prior RP interval lengthens (measured from the prior conducted R wave to the next conducted P wave), the subsequent PR interval shortens and vice versa. For all practical purposes, this type I pattern of conduction identifies an AV nodal site of block. The shortening of the PR with lengthening of the prior RP reflects the improvement in AV node conduction that occurs with "rest and recovery" (see Fig. 14–2*B*). When reciprocal variability in the RP-PR intervals is absent, type II AV block is present (see Fig. 14–2*A*).

Note that AV block can only be typed when the RP interval varies. Thus, when the AV conduction ratio is fixed (e.g., 2:1,

3:1, 4:1, and so forth), additional observations are necessary. For example, an intervention that changes autonomic balance, such as exercise or atropine, may change the AV conduction ratios. The resulting variability in the RP interval may allow typing of the block (Fig. 14–3).

THIRD-DEGREE AV BLOCK

Third-degree AV block is present when P waves occur that are more than 0.20 second in front of the QRS complex, and also follow the T wave of the prior QRS complex in association with a variable PR interval and a regular RR interval. In other words, the varying PR and regular RR intervals define AV dissociation, whereas the P waves that should have conducted, but did not, define AV block (Fig. 14–4).

PITFALLS IN ASSESSING DEGREE OF AV BLOCK

Determining the degree of AV block is usually simple and straightforward, given adequate ECG information. On some occasions, however, third-degree AV block may masquerade as apparent second-degree AV block. In any single, brief rhythm strip, for example, there may be a fortuitously constant PR interval that falsely suggests AV conduction (Fig. 14–5A). Frequently these difficulties are related to inadequate periods of observation, because the change in timing between the P waves and QRS complexes may be too subtle to detect in a short rhythm strip. A maneuver

that changes autonomic tone, or simply observing the rhythm for a longer period of time, may reveal that what was apparently second-degree AV block is really third-degree AV block (Fig. 14–5B).

On other occasions, no P waves are seen that allow a judgment of whether conduction would have occurred. With isorhythmic AV dissociation, for example, the P wave and QRS complexes occur at a similar rate, and the P waves typically never "march out" far enough from the QRS complex to allow a judgment of their capability for conducting. Once again, longer observation or an intervention to change the P-QRS relationship may be necessary to evaluate AV conduction (Fig. 14–6).

When second-degree AV block is present with a fixed AV ratio (e.g. 2:1, 3:2, 4:1, and so forth), some P waves may be concealed in the preceding ST-T waves. This is particularly likely with sinus tachycardia or marked ST-T wave distortion, such as may be seen with acute myocardial infarction. Observation of multiple surface leads, esophageal or intra-atrial leads with or without a vagal intervention may be necessary to identify the atrial rate and regularity and to facilitate identification of the correct sequence of AV relationships.

At times, it is not possible to determine whether third-degree AV block exists, because of circumstances independent of the ECG information available for review.

For example, when complete AV dissociation occurs with an accelerated junctional or ventricular rhythm, it is possible that some of the atrial beats might have conducted if the rapid ventricular rate (with its retrograde concealed conduction into the AV junction) were not present. It is best to designate such rhythms as complete AV dissociation and then to describe the cause of the accelerated ventricular rate (e.g., accelerated junctional rhythm, ventricular tachycardia, and so forth). Of course, the "slower" the ventricular rate in this setting, the more likely is the presence of underlying significant conduction disease in the AV junction. Conversely, the faster the ventricular rate, the more likely the AV dissociation solely reflects interference from concealed retrograde conduction into the AV junction.

Site of AV Block

Whenever any degree of AV block is diagnosed, the next task is to try to determine its site. The two most helpful clues in predicting site are the type of AV block and the width of the QRS complex during escape as well as during periods of AV capture. A third clue is provided by the QRS morphology.

SIGNIFICANCE OF TYPE OF AV BLOCK

A type I conduction pattern (that is, a reciprocal RP-PR relationship), particularly with a narrow QRS complex, almost al-

A MCL₁ - Initial Tracing

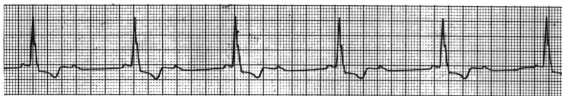

MCL₁ - Subsequent Tracing

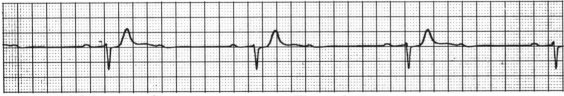

B MCL₁ - Initial Tracing

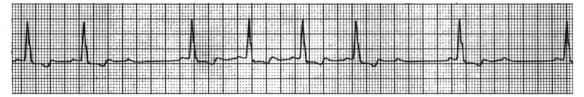

MCL₁ - Subsequent Tracing

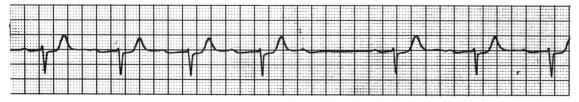

FIGURE 14–3. The initial tracings in (*A*) and (*B*) both show sinus rhythm with 2:1 second-degree AV block. The fixed AV conduction ratio prevents "typing" of these blocks (i.e., the constant RP intervals produce constant PR intervals regardless of the site of block). In the subsequent tracings obtained later the same day, the AV conduction ratios have changed. In (*A*), despite the RP variability, the PR interval remains constant, identifying type II, second-degree AV block. In (*B*), the PR intervals varied reciprocally in response to RP-interval variation, identifying type I, second-degree AV block. On the left is a classic "Wenckebach sequence" (5:4 AV conduction ratio).

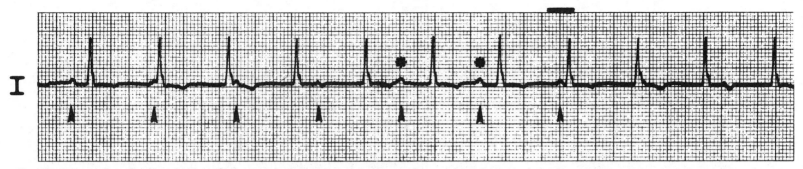

FIGURE 14–4. The arrowheads identify the regularly occurring P waves. The regular RR intervals and varying PR intervals define AV dissociation. Note that even those P waves that occur after the T waves of the preceding beat and more than 0.2 second before the next beat (asterisks) fail to conduct, defining third-degree AV block. The accelerated ventricular rate (80 beats per minute) may be contributing to the degree of AV block through concealed retrograde conduction into the AV junction. I = lead I.

ways identifies an AV nodal site of block. Rarely, a type I conduction pattern due to block in the His bundle–Purkinje system may be demonstrable on a routine 25-mm-per-second rhythm strip, but this is usually the stuff of which case reports are made. More typically, the demonstration of type I conduction in the His-Purkinje system requires an electrophysiologic laboratory with rapid recording speeds, and so forth.

A type II pattern, on the other hand, almost always identifies an infranodal site of AV block. Intra-His block is unusual enough that, for all practical purposes, the block may be assumed to reside in the bundle branch system, particularly when the type II pattern occurs with a wide QRS complex. When simple observations of the surface ECG and the clinical setting fail to identify the site of AV block, however, recourse to EPS with timing of the His bundle depolarization may be indicated, depending on the potential clinical implications (see pages 336 to 338, and Chapter 6, pages 131 to 133).

SIGNIFICANCE OF QRS WIDTH

Another observation from the surface ECG that is independent of the type or degree of AV block but that is useful in identifying its site is QRS duration (see Fig. 1–15). When the QRS is "narrow" (less than 0.12 second), a supraventricular site (AV node or, much less frequently, His bundle) is certain. When the QRS complex is "wide" (more than 0.12 second), however, the site of the AV block may be infranodal, or, if preexistent bundle branch block is present, it may be in the AV node; recourse to other clues then becomes necessary.

SIGNIFICANCE OF QRS MORPHOLOGY: HEMIBLOCKS

Disturbances of conduction within the bundle branches (fascicles) produce variable QRS abnormalities indicative of intraventricular conduction delay. Thus the recognition of the variable patterns of fascicular block may provide important clues in predicting the site of AV conduction failure. Neither complete left nor right bundle branch block (RBBB) usu-

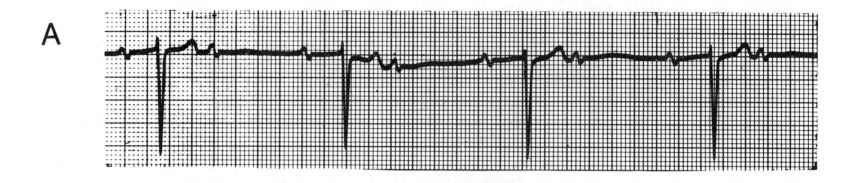

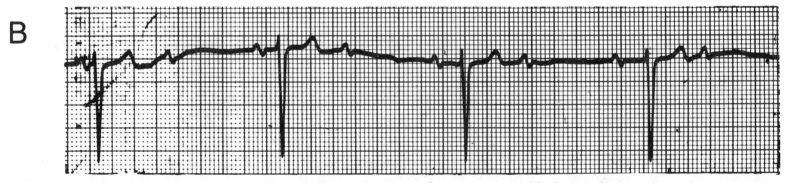

FIGURE 14–5. (*A*) The relatively constant PR interval preceding each QRS complex suggests 2:1 AV block. (*B*) A short time later, obvious variation in the PR intervals, with regular RR intervals, defines AV dissociation. The numerous P waves that should have conducted, but did not, define third-degree AV block.

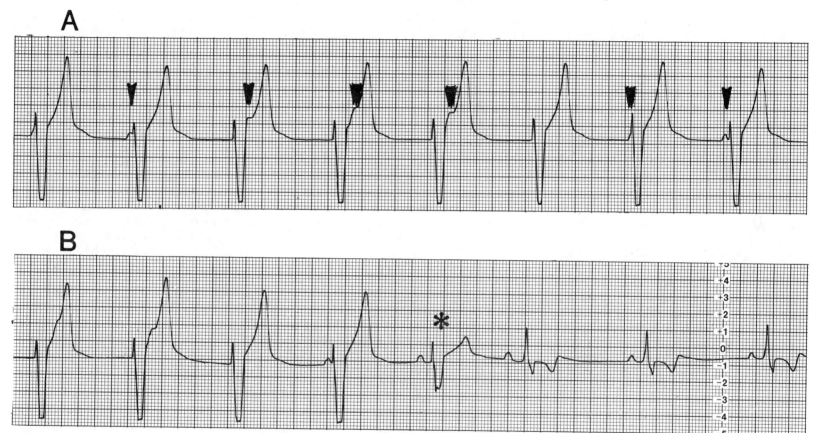

FIGURE 14–6. (*A*) This tracing illustrates the difficulty in determining the presence of AV block when isorhythmic AV dissociation is present. Although there is no evidence of AV conduction, neither are there any P waves (arrowheads) that occur after a T wave or more than 0.20 second before a QRS complex. The status of AV conduction, therefore, cannot be assessed. (*B*) After the patient performs three sit-ups in bed, the sinus rate speeds and, with atrial capture, shows that AV conduction is intact. Note that the first capture beat (asterisk) is a fusion beat between the idioventricular escape rhythm and the normally conducted beat. Despite subsequent slowing of the sinus rate, sinus rhythm persists because of overdrive suppression of the idioventricular pacemaker.

ally results in significant mean-frontal-plane QRS axis deviation, so that the axis with these blocks usually remains between −30° and +90°.

Focal delays in either the anterior or posterior fascicle of the left bundle branch, left or right ventricular hypertrophy, and inferior or high lateral myocardial infarction, however, all result in axis deviations. Axis deviations due to infarction can be differentiated from those due to the other conditions because the Q wave (that is, an initial force) rather than the S wave is abnormally directed. The primary differential diagnosis, therefore, for significant left axis deviation is left anterior fascicular block (LAFB) versus left ventricular hypertrophy, and, for right axis deviation, left posterior fascicular block (LPFB) versus right ventricular hypertrophy.[5] Left ventricular hypertrophy rarely produces an axis more negative than −45°, so that requirement of an axis of −60° or more for identification of LAFB is more predictive. Right ventricular hypertrophy and LPFB, however, can both produce similar extremes of right axis deviation. Left posterior fascicular block (or hemiblock) should be considered if the axis is more positive than +120°, but the possibility of right ventricular hypertrophy still exists. It should be noted that with an axis more negative than −60° or more positive than +120°, the QRS complex is more positive than negative in lead aVR. This lead, therefore,

should be observed first for the diagnosis of either LAFB or LPFB. Because aVR is perpendicular to lead III, one may then observe whether the QRS complex is predominantly positive or negative in lead III to determine whether the axis, and therefore the diagnosis, is LAFB (negative QRS complex in lead III) or LPFB (positive QRS complex in lead III).

Lesser degrees of axis deviation may be produced by either type of fascicular block, but can be considered diagnostic of this condition only when they occur abruptly in the absence of a clinical situation that could have produced either sudden left or right ventricular pressure overload, such as acute systemic hypertension or cor pulmonale. In both varieties of isolated unifascicular block, the QRS duration is usually only slightly prolonged. Ventricular hypertrophy, on the other hand, frequently produces QRS prolongation that may, with severe hypertrophy, exceed 0.12 second. In Figure 14–7, the typical appearances of both LAFB and LPFB are demonstrated as alternating patterns of rate-related aberrant conduction following premature atrial complexes.

SIGNIFICANCE OF QRS MORPHOLOGY: BUNDLE BRANCH BLOCKS

The key lead for differentiating complete left versus right bundle branch block is lead V_1, because it is located perpendicular to the interventricular septum

(Fig. 14–8). Left bundle branch block (LBBB) produces late activation of the posteriorly located left ventricle, with forces at the end of the QRS complex that are directed away from lead V_1—a notched S wave. Right bundle branch block produces late activation of the anteriorly located right ventricle, resulting in a late positive deflection in lead V_1 or an R′ wave. Because the left ventricle is thicker than the right ventricle, complete LBBB usually results in a QRS complex of at least 0.14 second. Complete RBBB, on the other hand, usually results in less prolongation of the QRS complex (greater than 0.12 second but less than 0.14 second). At times, LBBB and RBBB may alternate in a single rhythm strip. In Figure 14–9, for example, the underlying conduction disturbance was RBBB, but LBBB followed premature ventricular complexes (PVCs). No obvious change in the PR interval accompanies these changes and this variability between RBBB and LBBB can be explained by either a post-PVC improvement in conduction (that is, following the pause, conduction improved in the right bundle but slowed conduction was unmasked in the left bundle), or a deterioration in conduction (following the pause, conduction slowed in the left bundle, forcing the right bundle to become competent). Both explanations imply that complete bundle branch block on the scalar ECG may be due to slowed conduction in that bundle

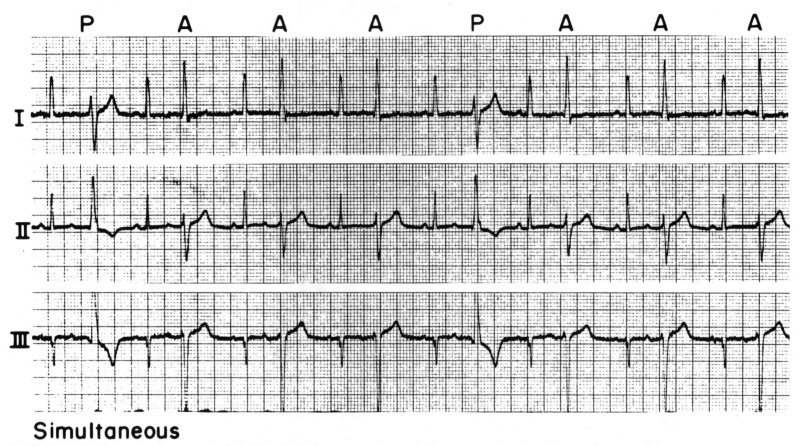

Simultaneous

FIGURE 14–7. These simultaneous leads I, II, and III show premature atrial beats occurring in a bigeminal pattern. The normal sinus impulses conduct with no axis deviation, but each premature beat conducts aberrantly through the ventricles. The first and fifth premature beats conduct with extreme right axis deviation, indicating left posterior fascicular block (P), whereas the remaining beats conduct with extreme left axis deviation, indicating left anterior fascicular block (A).

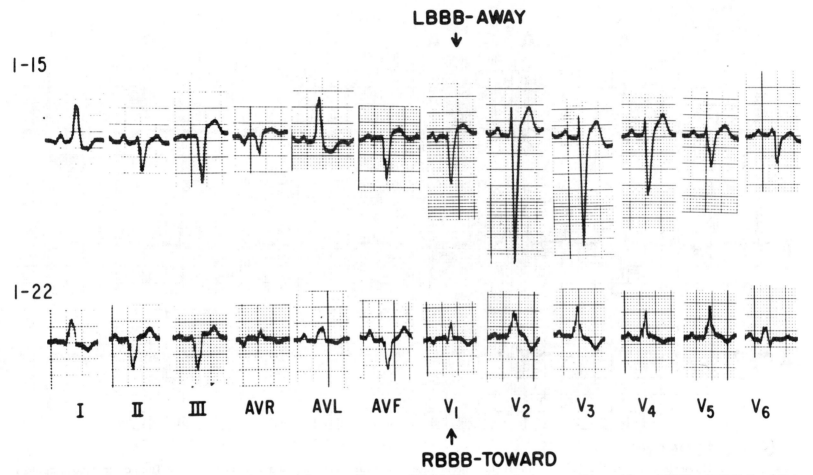

FIGURE 14–8. During the week between these two electrocardiograms (ECGs), the conduction pattern changed from LBBB to RBBB. Lead V₁ is the key for identifying the involved bundle. In the top row, late forces are directed toward the posterior or left ventricle and away from the anterior precordium, producing a wide, slurred S wave in lead V₁ and indicating LBBB. In the bottom row, late activation occurs in the anterior right ventricle, producing terminal anterior forces (i.e., an R′ wave) in lead V₁ and indicating RBBB.

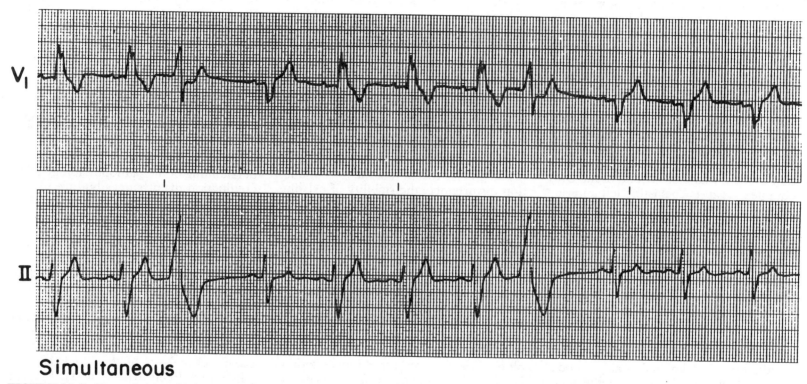

Simultaneous

FIGURE 14–9. Normal sinus rhythm with a wide QRS response is interrupted by two premature ventricular beats (the third and eighth QRS complexes). Marked axis deviation is present for all conducted beats (note the negative QRS in lead II), but the intraventricular conduction pattern changes markedly after each PVC (lead V_1). Initially, RBBB is present, but, after each PVC, it changes to LBBB. This pattern is transient for one beat after the first PVC, but after the second PVC, it persists to the end of the strip and may reflect either an improvement or a deterioration in intraventricular conduction (see text).

branch rather than due to complete block. Clinically, however, it is best to assume complete block, with its implied instability and unreliability of AV conduction and the potential for an unstable rhythm, because simultaneous failure of conduction in both bundle branches would produce third-degree AV block with a unpredictable escape rhythm.

Right bundle branch block may be accompanied by block in one of the two fascicles of the left bundle. Complete RBBB accompanied by extreme left axis deviation of the initial 0.08 second of the QRS complex suggests coexisting left anterior fascicular block. Complete RBBB with right axis deviation of the initial 0.08 second of the QRS complex suggests accompanying LPFB (Fig. 14–10).

The ECG findings other than the bradyarrhythmia itself can give clinical clues to the underlying cause and site of the conduction disturbance and thereby guide clinical decisions. With an accompanying acute inferior myocardial infarction, any degree of AV block with no associated bundle branch delay makes an AV nodal site of block very likely. A stable junctional escape pacemaker with a reasonable rate and eventual reversibility to normal or near-normal electrical conduction almost always occurs. With an accompanying acute anterior (and rarely inferior) myocardial infarction, on the other hand, any degree of AV block with an accompanying bundle branch delay makes a distal site of block most likely. In this setting, the risk is high of a sudden increase in the degree of AV block; slow, unstable escape rhythms; and permanence of the conduction disturbance.[6]

INTERACTION WITH THE AUTONOMIC NERVOUS SYSTEM

The precise location of the AV conduction disturbance, the stability of existing conduction, and the capability of escape pacing sites distal to the site of block may be further evaluated by methods that change autonomic tone, including vagotonic maneuvers, parenteral atropine or β-adrenergic–agonist drugs, and exercise.[7] The ability of the AV node to vary its conduction time and hence the manifest surface ECG marker of this conduction time, the PR interval, provides an important clue to the diagnosis of the site of block. Because this variability is modulated by the autonomic nervous system, modifying autonomic balance is a readily available clinical tool to help in investigating any given situation involving AV block. Vagal blockade, increased sympathetic tone, or both, usually improve AV nodal conduction, producing less block and shortening the PR interval. The reverse occurs with enhanced vagal tone or reduced sympathetic tone. Neither the His bundle nor its branches participate significantly in this variability in conduction time with changes in autonomic balance.

USE OF INVASIVE ELECTROPHYSIOLOGY

Invasive EPSs have enhanced our understanding of the pathophysiology of AV conduction disturbances but are usually not necessary either to diagnose the site of AV block or to plan effective therapy. The site of AV block can be deduced with reasonable accuracy by combining information from the clinical setting with the routine ECG rhythm strip. This is especially true in patients with a narrow QRS complex and in those with recurring symptoms (heart failure, presyncope, syncope) and documented ECG evidence of AV block. In patients with a narrow QRS complex, the site of the block is overwhelmingly likely to be AV nodal. In other patients, the site is irrelevant because in these patients, urgent pacemaker therapy is indicated.

His bundle studies can be used to determine the site of the conduction disturbance in the intermittently symptomatic or even the asymptomatic patient who has

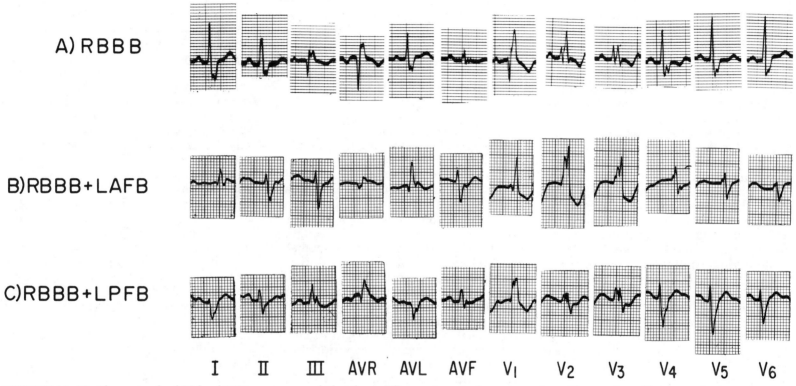

FIGURE 14–10. These standard 12-lead ECGs were recorded at three different times in the same patient. Observation of lead V_1 indicates that right bundle branch block (RBBB) is present on all three occasions. (*A*) The frontal-plane QRS axis is indeterminate. (*B*) Three years later, the axis has shifted markedly leftward, with terminal QRS forces directed away from inferior leads II, III, and aVF, a pattern typical of left anterior fascicular block (LAFB). (*C*) Two days later, the axis has shifted markedly rightward, with the terminal QRS forces directed away from leftward leads I and aVL, a pattern typical of left posterior fascicular block (LPFB).

any degree of AV block, an adequate ventricular rate, and a wide QRS complex.[8] These studies are also helpful in evaluating the causative role of a medication such as digitalis, which produces block in only one area (the AV node).

Electrophysiologic study in asymptomatic patients with varied combinations of fascicular conduction delays have not been useful in defining a subgroup at sufficiently high risk for subsequent high-degree AV block. Although marked prolongation of the His-to-ventricle conduction time can identify a subgroup at increased risk of progressing to higher degrees of AV block, the time course of progression is greatly variable, and the overall risk is not sufficiently high to justify prophylactic pacing of the entire subgroup.[9,10] The patient with intermittent neurologic symptoms suggestive of globally decreased cerebral perfusion, who also shows ECG evidence of involvement of either two or three fascicles (and in whom the clinical evaluation has revealed no other cause of the symptoms) presents a difficult therapeutic problem. The decision to implant a permanent pacemaker may be made with greater confidence when an invasive EPS demonstrates either significant prolongation of the His-to-ventricle interval (greater than 70 milliseconds), or second-degree AV block below the His bundle with incremental atrial pacing.[8] Unfortunately, the former observation provides only circumstantial evidence for a bradycardia as the cause of syncope, and the latter rarely occurs.

CLINICAL FEATURES

Predisposing Clinical Settings

Atrioventricular conduction disturbances can occur with or without underlying heart disease or clinical symptoms. For example, the increased vagal tone of a conditioned athlete with a normal heart can lead to either first-degree or second-degree type I AV block at rest or during sleep, and yet, when exercise inhibits vagal tone and increases sympathetic tone, all AV block disappears and world-class athletic performance may occur.

On the other hand, the entire etiologic spectrum of cardiac disease can be related to disturbances of AV conduction. Congenital heart block due to discontinuity of the AV junction at varied levels can occur as an isolated defect or in association with other cardiovascular malformations, such as congenitally corrected transposition of the great vessels. Left anterior fascicular block occurs in association with ostium primum atrial septal defects, and RBBB is seen with a variety of congenital malformations affecting the right ventricle.[11]

Coronary artery disease, in the acute stage of myocardial infarction, can effect reversible or irreversible changes in the AV conduction system. Atrioventricular nodal block may occur during Prinzmetal angina, when the AV node's blood supply is jeopardized. Myocardial infarction is the only manifestation of coronary artery disease that has been documented to cause bundle branch block, however. Furthermore, bundle branch blocks are usually associated with large myocardial infarctions, because the bundles lie deep within the superior aspect of the interventricular septum. Thus, in patients with bundle branch block but no other evidence of myocardial infarction, a cause other than ischemic heart disease must be assumed.

Acute rheumatic fever causes AV nodal conduction disturbances, presumably due to nodal inflammation. Fibrosis and calcification of the *left side of the cardiac skeleton* in proximity to the AV junction (Lev disease[12]) may lead to intraventricular conduction disturbances (most often RBBB and LAFB) as well as to AV conduction disturbances. In patients with AV block and a narrow QRS complex who are over 70 years of age, injury of the penetrating portion of the His bundle due to Lev disease is a common finding. Similarly, calcific aortic valve stenosis may extend from the bases of the aortic cusps, erode the conduction system, and disrupt either the His bundle or the bundle branches, leading to AV block. Cardiomyopathies from any cause can produce AV block in any part of the AV conduction system. Other conditions affecting AV conduction include the collagen vascular diseases (scleroderma, rheumatoid arthritis, and systemic lupus erythematosus) as well as sarcoidosis, amyloidosis, infectious endocarditis, and iatrogenic injury during cardiac catheterization or surgery.

Numerous drugs have been associated with AV conduction disturbances. At the AV nodal level, digitalis, β-blockers, and calcium blockers (principally verapamil and, to a lesser extent, diltiazem) frequently prolong the PR interval. When these drugs are given in nontoxic doses and in the absence of preexistent slowing of AV nodal conduction, the PR prolongation is rarely clinically significant. With intrinsic disease or superimposed vagal tone, or both, however, impressive bradycardias may result. Digitalis toxicity may affect both the conduction and pacing functions of the AV junction, with varying degrees of AV nodal block or acceleration of His bundle pacing rates, or both consequences. At the His-Purkinje level, many antiarrhythmic drugs can slow conduction and cause intraventricular and AV conduction delays.

When associated congenital, myocardial, coronary, and valvular heart diseases, as well as calcification of the cardiac skeleton, have been excluded (particularly when the AV block occurs in association with bundle branch block), Lenegre's disease is the most likely cause.[3]

Natural History in the Various Settings

The natural history of an AV conduction disturbance, in general, depends on the clinical setting in which it occurs, as this usually determines the site of AV block and, therefore, the prognosis. Judging the prognosis by the degree of AV block can be notoriously misleading. Second-degree AV block can vary from the benign situation of sinus rhythm at 80 beats per minute with a Wenckebach sequence, in which for every 11 atrial beats, 10 are conducted (11:10 AV conduction), to sinus rhythm at 80 beats per minute, in which only every fourth beat is conducted (4:1 AV conduction). With the former rhythm, a well-preserved ventricular rate persists, but the latter rhythm results in a severe bradyarrhythmia if there is concomitant failure of escape junctional and ventricular pacemakers.

The significance of AV block with acute myocardial infarction varies depending on both its anatomic site and the extent of infarction. With no concomitant cardiac failure, the natural history varies depending on the site of AV block. With congestive heart failure, however, the prognosis and natural history are more influenced by the severity of cardiac dysfunction.[13] Atrioventricular nodal block usually develops within 1 to 3 days of the onset of infarction, progresses gradually, and is rarely persistent. It typically resolves within days (infrequently lasting as long as 10 to 14 days) and usually does not influence the mortality rate.[14] Even in the thrombolytic era, it appears that the prognosis of patients with advanced AV block and acute inferior myocardial infarction is still very much related to the degree of ventricular dysfunction rather than the AV block.[15] Conduction disturbances in the bundle branches also appear early in the course of infarction, but they have a very different natural history and prognosis. Fascicular blocks typically occur first, and subsequent AV block occurs suddenly, often with abrupt progression from normal AV conduction to third-degree AV block. Furthermore, the escape rhythms are typically slow (less than 40 beats per minute) and unstable, with frequent asystole and syncope.

Bundle branch block with intact AV conduction occurring in the setting of acute infarction has a variable prognosis and natural history, depending on which (and how many) fascicles are involved acutely, and on the presence or absence of (1) first-degree AV block, (2) old fascicular block, and (3) severe cardiac failure. In the absence of severe cardiac failure, patients with acute myocardial infarction and bundle branch block can be divided into subgroups at low, medium, and high risk of developing sudden, high-grade AV block. The risk is greatest (31% to 38%) in patients with newly developed bilateral bundle branch block (RBBB and left anterior hemiblock, RBBB and LPFB, or RBBB alternating with LBBB). Medium risk (19% to 20%) is present in patients with first-degree AV block and either new bundle branch block (left or right) or old bilateral bundle branch block. The lowest risk (9% to 13%) occurs in patients who have only one or none of the three variables (first-degree AV block, new bundle branch block, or old bilateral bundle branch block).[16]

The natural history of patients who survive acute infarction complicated by bundle branch block varies depending on the presence or absence of the progression to high-degree AV block in the hospital. At highest risk for sudden death are those who develop transient high-degree AV block with their bilateral bundle branch block.[17] Infarction rarely directly destroys either the AV node or the bundle branches, so that conduction disturbances (particularly nodal disturbances due to enhanced parasympathetic tone) are typically transient during the acute stages. Atrioventricular nodal block is also not associated with later recurrences

of AV block; fascicular involvement, however, is more often associated with later recurrences.[17] This difference probably results from the intramyocardial location of the bundles; as the surrounding infarcted myocardium heals, the bundles may be damaged by fibrosis and scarring.

The natural history of drug-induced AV conduction disturbances depends on the severity of the underlying heart disease as well as on the recognition and withdrawal of the causative agent.

The natural history of patients with chronic first- and second-degree AV nodal block has been documented to be excellent over a long period of follow-up.[18] A good prognosis is also seen with isolated congenital heart block. When associated with other congenital abnormalities, the outcome depends on the severity of the other defects. Even when associated with congenitally corrected transposition with no associated cardiac shunts and normal pulmonary and systemic blood flows, the eventual development of failure of the systemic ventricle (morphologic right ventricle) is common and frequently becomes the dominant prognostic factor.

The natural history of patients with syncope and complete heart block arising in the His-Purkinje system depends to some extent on the mechanism of syncope and on the underlying state of the myocardium. In the early 1940s, Parkinson and colleagues noted that the natural history was more benign and survival was longer

in patients with AV block and syncope due to ventricular standstill, as compared with patients with syncope due to ventricular tachycardia or ventricular fibrillation, in whom the death rate was higher.[19] Although this is an interesting epidemiologic observation from the prepacing era, it should be emphasized that both groups of patients now should receive permanent pacemaker therapy.

The natural history of individuals with isolated chronic fascicular conduction disturbances and intact AV conduction remains unclear. Asymptomatic patients without associated clinical heart disease have a generally benign natural history over many years.[20] The incidence of complete heart block is low in patients with varying combinations of fascicular block, and no study has yet identified a group that is at a sufficiently high risk for high-degree AV block to justify prophylactic pacemaker insertion. In general, the type and severity of associated cardiac and other diseases exert the dominant influence on natural history and prognosis.

Methods of Treatment

The clinical context of the AV conduction disturbance is the primary determinant of treatment. Key factors include symptomatic status, the type of associated cardiac disease, and the site of AV block. Available modalities for treatment include (1) anticholinergic agents such as atropine, (2) sympathetic agents such as isoproterenol, and (3) temporary and permanent pacing.

DRUG THERAPY

Atropine, an anticholinergic or vagal blocking agent, enhances conduction through the AV node as well as the escape pacemaker function. It is administered either by intravenous or intramuscular injection. In the acutely ill patient, the former route is preferred. Its onset of action is rapid and its duration brief, making it particularly useful in the acute setting, where any adverse effects are short-lived and the medication can be titrated to a desired response. The usual dose for significant AV block is 0.5 mg given at 10-minute intervals, up to a total dose of 2.0 mg. For asystole in the setting of AV block, the recommended initial dose is 1.0 mg. Doses smaller than 0.4 mg have been associated with a paradoxical worsening of the bradyarrhythmia, presumably due to a centrally mediated enhancement of parasympathetic tone. Other adverse effects occurring with all doses to some degree include dry mouth, pupillary dilation, paralysis of accommodation with blurred vision, urinary retention, and gastrointestinal symptoms such as constipation.

Isoproterenol is a β-specific sympathomimetic amine that improves AV nodal conduction, increases the rate of escape junctional and ventricular pacemakers, and enhances myocardial contractility. It may cause increased ventricular irritability and must be used with caution in the setting of myocardial ischemia. It is given by continuous intravenous infusion (2 to 20 μg per minute), beginning with a low dose and titrated to the desired heart rate and blood pressure.

Either atropine or isoproterenol can be used as interim therapy for symptomatic bradycardias due to AV block until the dysfunction is reversed or pacing can be started. Other important clinical features such as hypovolemia or electrolyte imbalance should also be evaluated and, if necessary, corrected. The role of drugs in causing the AV block should be considered and, if present, corrected by stopping the responsible drug.

PACEMAKER THERAPY

Various types of temporary pacing (for example, Zoll precordial electrodes[21] and transvenous temporary pacing) can provide definitive interim therapy for patients who are at high risk for infranodal AV block (but who have not yet developed it); for patients who develop symptomatic AV nodal block unresponsive to pharmacologic management; and for patients with significant, potentially reversible AV block who are at risk for or have had severe bradyarrhythmias. In some instances, the use of temporary pacing is an interim step pending the placement of a permanent pacemaker. Whether to use precordial electrodes or a transvenous wire is often a matter of weighing factors related to both. With precordial electrode pacing, instability of ventricular capture, the degree of patient discomfort, and the hemodynamic significance of less reliable capture in the event of a severe bradyarrhythmia are potential disadvantages. In comparison, transvenous pacing typically provides pacing that is reliable and painless but is more invasive.

Permanent pacemaker implantation provides definitive treatment for the bradyarrhythmias of AV block. Frequently, concomitant factors such as the need for coordinated atrial systole or rate responsiveness, or both, to help maintain cardiac output are important considerations in choosing the specific variety of pacemaker (see Chapter 16).

First-degree AV block does not require treatment. These patients with inferior myocardial infarction but no bundle branch block should be carefully monitored for the progressive development of higher degrees of AV block. If first-degree AV block coexists with bundle branch block, bilateral involvement is possible, and "prophylactic" temporary pacing may be indicated, depending on the chronicity of the conduction disturbances and other aspects of the clinical setting.[17]

Second- or third-degree AV *nodal* block in the asymptomatic patient, regardless of cause, does not require treatment. With acute infarction, prophylactic temporary ventricular pacing should be carried out if the patient has complications secondary to bradycardia, such as heart failure, hypotension, slowing of the ventricular rate to less than 50 beats per minute, or significant PVCs necessitating treatment that may further suppress AV conduction or escape pacemakers.

Second- or third-degree *infranodal* AV block, regardless of the clinical status, should be treated with permanent pacing. The clinical status of the patient dictates the emergent need for temporizing with isoproterenol or temporary pacing prior to the insertion of the permanent pacemaker.

The patient with an acute myocardial infarction and bundle branch block who satisfies criteria for the high-risk group[17] (see pages 339 to 340) should have either prophylactic temporary transvenous pacemaking or the application of Zoll precordial pacing electrodes. If high-degree AV block develops, a permanent pacemaker should probably be inserted prior to discharge from the hospital.

In patients with bundle branch block who are asymptomatic, no treatment is indicated, but they should be carefully observed and evaluated for symptoms of intermittent bradycardia. Those who present with bundle branch block and intermittent symptoms of cardiac or central nervous system dysfunction should be evaluated thoroughly in a monitored setting. If second-degree or third-degree AV block is observed, permanent pacing is the treatment of choice. If other reasons for syncope have been ruled out and no progression in AV block is documented, the clinical decision regarding pacing needs to be based on the individual patient situation. As mentioned, an EPS evaluation is rarely helpful, but the absence of prolongation of the H-V interval (greater than 70 milliseconds) or the development of His-Purkinje block on incremental atrial pacing may be a reason for temporizing with periodic reevaluations. When the clinical history is highly suggestive of a symptomatic bradyarrhythmia, on the other hand, empiric placement of a pacemaker even without any documentation of AV block may be indicated as a therapeutic (and diagnostic) trial.

A cautionary note is necessary regarding the use of many of the antiarrhythmic agents in the setting of bundle branch block. They can slow conduction in the bundle branch system, thereby causing AV block, and suppress automatic escape pacemaker function; therefore, their use is contraindicated in the presence of second-degree or third-degree AV block.[22]

REFERENCES

1. Katz LN and Pick A: Clinical Electrocardiography. The Arrhythmias. Lea & Febiger, Philadelphia, 1956.
2. Langendorf R and Pick A: Atrioventricular block, type II (Mobitz)—Its nature and clinical significance. Circulation 38:819–821, 1968.
3. Lenegre J: Etiology and pathology of bilateral bundle branch block in relation to complete heart block. Prog Cardiovasc Dis 6:409–444, 1964.
4. Chung EK: Clinical value of ambulatory rhythm monitoring. In Castellanos A (ed): Cardiac Arrhythmias: Mechanisms and Management. FA Davis, Philadelphia, 1980, pp 113–126.
5. Rosenbaum MB: The hemiblocks: Diagnostic criteria and clinical significance. Mod Concepts Cardiovasc Dis 39:141–146, 1970.
6. Rotman M, Wagner GS, and Wallace AG: Bradyarrhythmias in acute myocardial infarction. Circulation 45:703–722, 1973.
7. Langendorf R, Cohen H, and Gozo EG: Observations on second degree atrio-ventricular block, including new criteria for the differential diagnosis between type I and type II block. Am J Cardiol 29:111–119, 1972.
8. Vadde PS, Caracta AR, and Damato AN: Indications for His bundle recordings. In Castellanos A (ed): Cardiac Arrhythmias: Mechanisms and Management. FA Davis, Philadelphia, 1980, pp 1–6.
9. Dhringa R, Palileo E, Strasberg B, et al: Significance of the HV interval in

517 patients with chronic bifascicular block. Circulation 64:1265, 1981.

10. Scheinman MM, Peters RW, Morady F, Sauve MJ, Malone T, and Modin G: Electrophysiologic studies in patients with bundle branch block. PACE 6:1157–1165, 1983.

11. Perloff JK: The Clinical Recognition of Congenital Heart Disease, ed 2. WB Saunders, Philadelphia, 1978, pp 43–56, 69–73, 357–361.

12. Lev M: Anatomic basis for atrioventricular block. Am J Med 37:741–748, 1964.

13. Hindman MC and Wagner GS: Arrhythmias during myocardial infarction: Mechanisms, significance, and therapy. In Castellanos A (ed): Cardiac Arrhythmias: Mechanisms and Management. FA Davis, Philadelphia, 1980, pp 81–102.

14. Rotman M, Wagner GS, and Waugh RA: The significance of high degree atrioventricular block in acute posterior myocardial infarction. Circulation 47:257–262, 1973.

15. Berger PB, Ruocco NA, Ryan TJ, Frederick MM, Jacobs AK, and Faxon DP: Incidence and prognostic implications of heart block complicating inferior myocardial infarction treated with thrombolytic therapy: Results from TIMI II. J Am Coll Cardiol 20:533–540, 1992.

16. Hindman MC, Wagner GS, Jaro M, et al: The clinical significance of bundle branch block complicating acute myocardial infarction. I. Clinical characteristics, hospital mortality, and one year follow up. Circulation 58:679–688, 1978.

17. Hindman MC, Wagner GS, Jaro M, et al: The clinical significance of bundle branch block complicating acute myocardial infarction. II. Indications for temporary and permanent pacemaker therapy. Circulation 58:689–699, 1978.

18. Strasberg B, Amat-y-Leon F, Dhingra RC, et al: Natural history of chronic second-degree atrioventricular nodal block. Circulation 63:1043–1049, 1981.

19. Parkinson J, Papp C, and Evans W: The electrocardiogram of the Stokes-Adams attack. Br Heart J 3:171–199, 1941.

20. Rotman M and Triebwasser JH: A clinical and follow up study of right and left bundle branch block. Circulation 51:477–484, 1975.

21. Zoll PM, Zoll RH, Falk RH, Clinton JE, Eitel DR, and Antman EM: External noninvasive temporary cardiac pacing: Clinical trials. Circulation 71:937–944, 1985.

22. Scheinman MN, Goldschlager NF, and Peters RW: Bundle branch block. In Castellanos A (ed): Cardiac Arrhythmias: Mechanisms and Management. FA Davis, Philadelphia, 1980, pp 57–80.

DRUGS AND DEVICES IN THE TREATMENT OF CARDIAC ARRHYTHMIAS

CHAPTER 15

Clinical Pharmacology and Use of Antiarrhythmic Drugs

KATHERINE T. MURRAY, MD,
BARRY W. RAMO, MD, and
JODIE L. HURWITZ, MD

OUTLINE

The pharmacologic treatment of cardiac arrhythmias remains one of the most challenging areas of modern clinical medicine. The goals of antiarrhythmic therapy are to reduce symptoms and to prevent sudden cardiac death, which is usually due to ventricular tachycardia or ventricular fibrillation. Conventional agents, however, have been shown to reduce mortality only in patients with recurrent life-threatening ventricular tachyarrhythmias. The benefit of treating patients with other arrhythmias that produce few or no symptoms remains unproven; in some cases such treatment is actually harmful.

Most antiarrhythmic drugs have a narrow therapeutic ratio (ratio of toxic-to-effective doses), as well as the potential for serious cardiac side effects such as aggravation of arrhythmia (proarrhythmia) and congestive heart failure. Recently, a number of new agents have been marketed in the United States, giving clinicians a bewildering array of drugs from which to choose. Once the decision is made to treat an individual patient, the selection of an appropriate therapeutic regimen requires a basic understanding of the electrophysiology and pharmacokinetics of antiarrhythmic drugs. The discussion that follows reviews these principles and important features of individual drugs.

BASIC ELECTROPHYSIOLOGY

The basic electrophysiology of cardiac arrhythmias was discussed in detail in Chapter 1. This section reviews some of the principles relevant to the electrophysiologic effects of pharmacologic agents. Under normal resting conditions, the interior of cardiac cells is negatively charged with respect to the exterior. The maintenance of this transmembrane potential depends on the concentrations of several ions such as sodium, calcium, potassium, and chloride on either side of the cellular membrane; these in turn are influenced by both electrical and chemical gradients. After delivery of a stimulus, an action potential results, composed of various phases arising from changes in ion conductance and subsequent ion movement across the cell membrane. Figure 15–1 is a simplified diagram of the phases of the cardiac action potential and the principal ion currents.

During phase 0 depolarization, conductance for sodium increases with its rapid inward movement into the cell, and the transmembrane potential rises to more positive values. The maximum rate of rise of the phase 0 upstroke slope is often termed $\dot{V}_{max}$ for maximum dV/dt. The early rapid repolarization that follows constitutes phase 1. The action potential is then prolonged by phase 2 (the plateau), which results from a slow inward current carried mainly by calcium. Rapid repolarization back to the resting potential defines phase 3, resulting from a reduction in the slow inward current and with an increase in the conductance of potassium with efflux from the cell. Phase 4 is characterized by a return of the resting membrane potential to its most negative values. Spontaneous diastolic depolarization occurs in pacemaker cells, while in working cells, phase 4 remains at a constant, resting level.

Potassium is the primary ion that determines the resting membrane potential, so that diastolic depolarization results largely from a decrease in outward potassium current. Two membrane-bound "pumps" also function during the cardiac cycle to promote ion movement. The sodium-potassium exchange (ATPase) pump moves sodium out of the cell and potassium into it to help restore ionic balance, whereas the sodium-calcium exchange pump operates in a bidirectional fashion. Cells in the sinoatrial (SA) and atrioventricular (AV) nodes, as well as in the His-Purkinje system, display phase-4 depolarization with spontaneous generation of action potentials and hence are termed *automatic* or *pacemaker cells*. Normally, cells in the SA node discharge most rapidly and function as the dominant pacemaker in the heart.

The speed of impulse conduction

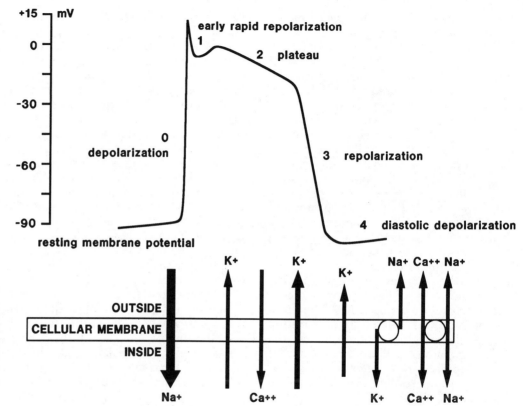

FIGURE 15–1. The top of the figure shows the cardiac action potential with its five phases: depolarization (phase 0), early rapid repolarization (phase 1), plateau (phase 2), repolarization (phase 3), and diastolic depolarization (phase 4). At the bottom are shown the principal ion currents during the cardiac cycle, with the sodium-potassium (Na^+–K^+) pump and the bidirectional sodium-calcium (Na^+–Ca^{++}) exchanger.

through cardiac tissue depends largely on resting membrane potential and $\dot{V}_{max}$. Conduction can be slowed by either a depressed (less negative) resting membrane potential or a reduction in $\dot{V}_{max}$. Slow conduction is normally seen in the SA and AV nodes, where the resting membrane potential is less negative and the upstroke during phase 0 more gradual, but diseased tissues can show similar properties. As described above, fast-channel current leading to rapid conduction velocity throughout the rest of the heart is carried primarily by the inward movement of sodium, whereas slow-current tissue is depolarized primarily by the inward movement of calcium during phase 0.

Refractoriness is a term used to describe the property of relative or total inexcitability that normally follows the generation of an action potential. In practical terms, it is determined by the introduction of a progressively more premature stimulus after an action potential. Initially, the action potential generated by the premature stimulus is normal in configuration. As this stimulus begins to encroach on phase 3 of the first action potential, however, the resulting premature action potential becomes abnormal, with depression of $\dot{V}_{max}$ until a point is reached where no response is possible. The time from the beginning of a given action potential to the first premature stimulus that generates any response is termed the *effective refractory period (ERP)*. The duration of the ERP is related to the duration of the given action potential and the changing state of sodium channels after initial depolarization. After opening during phase 0, the sodium channels remain inactivated for a period of time before finally returning to a resting or quiescent state, ready to open again. If the duration of the ERP is increased with respect to action potential duration (APD), the likelihood of generating abnormal, slow responses that can lead to arrhythmia initiation is reduced. As such, the ratio of effective refractory period to action potential duration (ERP/APD) describes one

important index of antiarrhythmic drug action.

It is currently believed that cardiac tachyarrhythmias can be generated by three mechanisms: abnormal or enhanced automaticity, reentry, and triggered activity.[1] These mechanisms were discussed in detail in Chapter 1. Enhanced automaticity can occur in cells that normally do not function as pacemaker cells. *Reentry* is a term used to describe abnormal circular or "circus" movement of an impulse in cardiac tissue which can lead to rapid arrhythmias. *Triggered activity* is spontaneous depolarization that occurs during or after an action potential. Its occurrence depends on one or more preceding impulses, whereas automaticity is activity that can arise in previously quiescent tissue.

Before beginning antiarrhythmic drug therapy in a patient, it is important to remember that certain conditions (e.g., hypoxia, acidosis, hypokalemia), diseases (ischemia, heart failure), and drugs (digitalis, catecholamines) are frequently reversible causes of cardiac arrhythmias, and their elimination can lead to complete resolution of the rhythm disturbance. Such factors should always be vigorously sought and corrected and the patient's rhythm reassessed before starting drug treatment.

Vaughan Williams has described a classification scheme that groups together antiarrhythmic drugs with similar cellular

electrophysiologic actions (Table 15–1). Although the effects of these drugs are more complex than originally thought and considerable overlap exists,[2] the classification is still a useful one from a clinical standpoint.

Class I drugs have local anesthetic activity in that they depress fast inward current by reducing sodium conductance. They are further subgrouped according to their effects on repolarization and their kinetics of interaction with the sodium channel. Class Ia drugs prolong APD and, as a consequence, lengthen the QT interval on the electrocardiogram (ECG). Their speed of dissociation from the sodium channel is intermediate, generally between 5 and 10 seconds, resulting in conduction slowing evidenced by mild QRS prolongation during normal sinus rhythm. Class Ib drugs shorten APD, with either a reduction or no change in the QT interval. These drugs display rapid kinetics in their interaction with sodium channels, with time constants of dissociation less than 1 second. For this reason, they do not cause apparent prolongation of the QRS interval on the ECG during normal sinus rhythm. Class Ic drugs have very potent effects on $\dot{V}_{max}$, to produce prominent conduction slowing with little change in repolarization. These drugs dissociate slowly from the sodium channel, with time constants ranging up to 30 seconds. Significant QRS prolongation can be seen during sinus rhythm, and the PR interval also is typi-

Table 15–1. ELECTROPHYSIOLOGIC PROPERTIES OF ANTIARRHYTHMIC DRUGS*

CLASSIFICATION	SPEED OF DISSOCIATION FROM SODIUM CHANNELS	EFFECTS ON REPOLARIZATION	EFFECTS ON THE ELECTROCARDIOGRAM
I. Fast sodium-channel blockers			

a. Quinidine
     Procainamide
     Disopyramide
	Intermediate	↑ APD, ERP
		↑ ERP/APD
			↑ QT
			Slight ↑ QRS

b. Lidocaine
     Tocainide
     Mexiletine
     Phenytoin
	Rapid	↓ APD, ERP
		↑ ERP/APD
			Slight ↓ QT
			QRS unchanged

c. Flecainide
     Encainide
     Propafenone
	Slow	APD unchanged
		↑ ERP
		↑ ERP/APD
			↑ PR
			↑ QRS
			↑ QT (due to ↑ QRS)

Moricizine	Rapid-intermediate	↓ APD, ERP	↑ PR, ↑ QRS
II. β-Adrenergic receptor blockers			± ↑ PR

III. Drugs that mainly prolong repolarization
     Bretylium
     Amiodarone
		↑ APD, ERP	↑ QT

IV. Calcium-channel blockers			± ↑ PR

APD = action potential duration; ERP = effective refractory period; ERP/APD = ratio of ERP to APD.

*Some drugs have multiple actions (e.g., amiodarone blocks sodium channels).

Source: Modified from Roden and Woosley,[16] page 37.

cally prolonged because of slowing of AV nodal conduction.

Class II drugs, the β-adrenergic–receptor blockers, may also prolong the PR interval due to slowing of AV nodal conduction. At higher concentrations of drugs with *membrane stabilizing* or local anesthetic (class I) activity, slight increases in the QRS interval can occasionally be seen.

The primary electrophysiologic effect of class III drugs is prolongation of APD and therefore of the QT interval. Amiodarone also displays sodium-channel blocking activity and can slow conduction through the AV node.

Finally, class IV drugs are the calcium-channel blockers. Their principal effect is to slow AV nodal conduction, although, like other antiarrhythmic drugs, they also depress automaticity.

PHARMACOKINETIC PRINCIPLES

The pharmacokinetics of a drug describe its disposition in the body over time and include the processes of absorption, distribution, metabolism, and excretion. Each of these processes has important ramifications for the use of antiarrhythmic drugs and are discussed in turn.

After oral administration, absorption of a drug generally depends on the physical characteristics of both the pharmaceutical preparation and the gastrointestinal tract. Slow-released preparations are designed to delay drug absorption over time to maintain more constant plasma concentrations. Other drugs and pathologic processes can affect absorption by altering factors such as pH (e.g., antacids) and gut motility (narcotics, diabetes mellitus).

The term *bioavailability* describes the amount of orally administered drug that reaches the systemic circulation as compared with intravenous (IV) administration (when bioavailability is 100%). As such, it reflects both absorption as well as any presystemic elimination. After absorption by the gastrointestinal tract, a drug can be metabolized before reaching the systemic circulation. This process can occur in either the gut wall or liver and is termed *presystemic* or *first-pass metabolism*. Drugs subjected to this phenomenon may require much higher doses by the oral rather than by the IV route (e.g., pro-

pranolol, verapamil), or they may be unsuitable altogether for oral administration (e.g., lidocaine).

Once a drug has entered the systemic circulation, its plasma concentration falls because of both distribution into various tissues and elimination from the body.[3] The distribution of most antiarrhythmic drugs follows a two-compartment model. The drug initially enters a central compartment comprising plasma and highly perfused organs such as the heart, lungs, and kidneys. This equilibrates with a deeper or peripheral compartment that involves binding of the drug to various tissues. The physiologic effects of the drug can arise from its accumulation in either or both compartments.

Generally, "free" or unbound drug in plasma interacts with target tissues to produce an effect, rather than drug bound to plasma proteins. Commercial assays routinely measure total plasma concentration of a drug, including both bound and free drug. It is important to remember that in certain situations, plasma protein binding, and thus the concentration of free drug can change without an alteration in total drug concentration. (For example, the protein binding of phenytoin decreases in renal failure.)

The volume of distribution (Vd) for a drug is the apparent or theoretic volume into which it is distributed. It does not correlate with any specific anatomic space and, because of tissue binding, may exceed the total volume of the body. During

a constant infusion, Vd can be determined from the amount of drug in the body (*dose*) and from the plasma concentration (Cp):

$$Vd = \frac{dose}{Cp}$$

Most antiarrhythmic drugs are metabolized to some extent in the body, usually in the liver. The generation of active metabolites is important in producing an antiarrhythmic response with some drugs (e.g., encainide), whereas with other drugs, the accumulation of metabolic products can contribute to side effects (e.g., lidocaine). *Clearance* is a term that describes the activity of the elimination process; for most antiarrhythmic drugs, it is a first-order process with a constant *proportion* of drug removed per unit time. For certain drugs, however (e.g., phenytoin, propafenone), clearance is saturable, and at high plasma concentrations the elimination is a zero-order process in that a certain *amount* of drug is removed per unit time.

The time course of drug elimination from the body is described by the elimination half-life, or the time required for the plasma concentration to fall to one half its initial value. After two elimination half-lives, 75% of the drug has been removed, and so forth. Thus after four to five elimination half-lives, over 90% of drug has been eliminated from the body. Because the process of drug accumulation mirrors that of elimination, plasma concentrations rise to steady-state values after four to five elimination half-lives have elapsed from time of drug initiation. This is an important concept to remember when escalating drug dosage, to avoid toxic plasma concentrations. As shown, elimination half-life ($t\frac{1}{2}$) is a function of both Vd and clearance (Cl):

$$t_{1/2} = \frac{0.693 \times Vd}{Cl}$$

Conditions that lower both Vd and clearance generally do not change the elimination half-life of a drug that is mainly eliminated through the liver (e.g., lidocaine in the setting of congestive heart failure). Disease states that reduce clearance alone, however, can be expected to prolong elimination half-life (e.g., lidocaine in hepatic disease).

During an IV infusion, the concentration of a drug at steady state ($CpSS$) depends only on clearance and dosage or infusion rate (I):

$$CpSS = \frac{I}{Cl}$$

Doubling the infusion rate doubles the final plasma concentration but does not alter the amount of time required to reach steady state. To achieve a therapeutic plasma concentration quickly during the IV infusion of antiarrhythmic drugs, it is often necessary to administer one or more loading doses followed by a constant infusion. Volume of distribution alone determines the plasma concentration achieved immediately after a loading dose.

The pharmacokinetic properties of the various classes of antiarrhythmic drugs are summarized in tables throughout the chapter.

PROARRHYTHMIA

Digitalis has long been known for its ability to produce arrhythmias while being used to treat arrhythmias, but the frequency with which other antiarrhythmic agents induce arrhythmias has only more recently been recognized. The exacerbation or precipitation of a new tachyarrhythmia by a drug is termed a *proarrhythmic effect* and can occur with virtually all of the antiarrhythmic agents. New bradyarrhythmias can also occur, especially in the setting of toxic plasma drug concentrations.

Certain conditions render patients more susceptible to either type of adverse effect. For example, patients with congestive heart failure and recurrent sustained ventricular arrhythmias are more likely to experience arrhythmia aggravation during treatment with some class Ic antiarrhythmic drugs. Similarly, patients with preexisting conduction system disease (e.g., sinus node dysfunction, trifascicular block) are at higher risk of serious bradyarrhythmias such as sinus arrest and complete heart block, despite therapeutic drug levels.

Proarrhythmia may assume a variety of appearances in different clinical situations. Prompt recognition is important, given its life-threatening nature and the specific measures that are often necessary for successful treatment.

Torsades de Pointes

Torsades de pointes is a rapid polymorphic ventricular tachycardia associated with marked QT prolongation.[4] It is seen most commonly with class Ia drugs (particularly quinidine, with an incidence of 2% to 10%), although other agents such as amiodarone (class III) can also cause a prolonged QT interval and torsades. Predisposing factors include hypokalemia, hypomagnesemia, bradycardia, concomitant tricyclic antidepressant drug therapy, and liquid-protein diets. A number of authorities have recommended that the initial institution of class Ia agents be effected with in-hospital monitoring because of the risk of this potentially lethal arrhythmia. Torsades de pointes is most likely to occur during the first few days of therapy, or it may arise during chronic therapy if one of the predisposing factors noted previously should develop. Treatment is discussed later in the section on quinidine.

Sustained Ventricular Tachycardia–Ventricular Fibrillation

In patients who have never had a sustained ventricular arrhythmia, its development may be precipitated by starting an antiarrhythmic drug or by increasing the drug dose. This is most likely to occur with class I or class III drugs and can happen very early during treatment. The appropriate therapy is to stop the antiarrhythmic drug immediately. In some situations, the ventricular tachycardia may be incessant and refractory to cardioversion. This is most often seen when certain class Ic drugs are used to treat patients with a history of sustained ventricular tachyarrhythmias and reduced left ventricular function. Treatment for this arrhythmia is discussed later, in the section on flecainide.

Increased Frequency of Premature Ventricular Complexes and Ventricular Tachycardia

This category of proarrhythmia is most difficult to recognize because of the marked day-to-day variation in the frequency ectopy that can exist in patients with sustained ventricular tachycardia. However, a dramatic increase in ambient ventricular ectopy and nonsustained ventricular tachycardia with the initiation of a new drug could herald a more serious event.

Proarrhythmia During Electrophysiologic Testing

What constitutes proarrhythmia during electrophysiologic testing is controversial, and criteria are still in the developmental stage. Factors being considered include the ease of induction of the sustained ventricular arrhythmia, its rate, and associated symptoms during an electrophysiologic study. A major difficulty in developing criteria is the variability in the ease of inducing the arrhythmia in patients taking no antiarrhythmic drugs. On one occasion it may be inducible with two extra stimuli, yet at another time it may not be inducible at all even though there has been no measurable change in the patient's condition or therapy. At the very least, this variation makes data from electrophysiologic studies difficult to use in judging a proarrhythmic drug effect.

The Cardiac Arrhythmia Suppression Trial

It is well known that the presence of ventricular ectopy and nonsustained ventricular tachycardia increases the risk of sudden cardiac death after myocardial infarction. More recently, patients treated for asymptomatic ventricular arrhythmias after acute myocardial infarction were found in the Cardiac Arrhythmia Suppression Trial (CAST) to have a higher mortality due to arrhythmia and cardiac arrest when treated with flecainide or encainide than during treatment with placebo. The excessive mortality occurred despite suppression of ambient ventricular ectopy by flecainide and encainide. Furthermore, the deaths that occurred on these two drugs were not clustered at the beginning of drug treatment, as typically occurs with proarrhythmia, but were spread out over the 1 to 2 years of follow-up. Treatment with moricizine, the third antiarrhythmic drug in the trial, was not associated with a definite increase in mortality, but unfavorable trends during early therapy and subsequently with randomized treatment have led to the termination of this arm of the trial as well. The clinical implications of these alarming data are discussed more fully in the section on flecainide. At a minimum, they suggest that suppressing nonsustained ventricular arrhythmias, at least with some drugs, does not reduce the risk of a serious arrhythmia and mortality, but actually increases it.

SPECIFIC ANTIARRHYTHMIC AGENTS

Proper use of antiarrhythmic agents requires a thorough knowledge of their important pharmacologic properties.[5] Each of the available antiarrhythmic agents is discussed according to its electrophysiology, hemodynamic effects, pharmacokinetics, clinical administration, adverse effects, and clinical use.

Class I: Fast Sodium-Channel Blockers

CLASS IA DRUGS

Quinidine. In the 1920s, quinidine was reported to be effective in the treatment of atrial fibrillation, making it the first of the standard antiarrhythmic drugs to become available. It is an alkaloid extracted from the bark of the cinchona tree and structurally is the *d*-stereoisomer of quinine.

ELECTROPHYSIOLOGY

The principal electrophysiologic effect of quinidine *in vitro* is depression of the maximal rate of rise of the phase-0 upstroke or $\dot{V}_{max}$, with conduction slowing in atrial and ventricular muscle, Purkinje fibers, AV node, and accessory pathways. This effect is due to blockade of the fast inward sodium current in a frequency-dependent manner, with a dissociation time constant of 4 to 8 seconds. Depression of $\dot{V}_{max}$ is also voltage dependent, because it is enhanced at more positive membrane potentials. At low concentrations, quinidine also prolongs repolarization by blocking potassium channels, and it increases refractoriness with an increase in the ratio ERP/APD (see Table 15–1). It de-

presses automaticity, especially at high concentrations. In cellular preparations, quinidine can lead to the production of triggered activity. Its predominant effects on the ECG include prolongation of the QRS and QT intervals. Typically, the resting heart rate is unchanged or slightly increased due to reflex sympathetic activity associated with hemodynamic effects.

HEMODYNAMIC EFFECTS

In tissue preparations, quinidine causes mild negative inotropic effects. It is an α-adrenergic receptor blocker and causes vasodilation. When given intravenously, the drug can cause hypotension because of this reduction in systemic vascular resistance and perhaps contractility. Such hypotension is rarely seen when quinidine is used orally. Its vasodilator properties may be the reason that it is well tolerated in the setting of poor ventricular function and congestive heart failure. The vasodilation also causes a sympathetically mediated reflex rise in heart rate that may counteract the depressant effects of quinidine on automaticity. In addition to its vasodilator properties, the drug has significant anticholinergic effects that counterbalance its direct effect on the AV node and, in concert with enhanced sympathetic activity, can speed conduction through the AV node.

PHARMACOKINETICS

Quinidine is marketed as various salts (sulfate, gluconate, polygalacturonate).

The quinidine base content is 83% for the sulfate salt and 62% for the gluconate salt, so that a 324-mg tablet of quinidine gluconate contains the same amount of base as 240 mg of quinidine sulfate. Quinidine sulfate is rapidly absorbed, with peak levels achieved in 60 to 90 minutes after oral administration (Table 15–2). Its bioavailability can vary but averages 80%. The other salts are more slowly absorbed; peak levels following the administration of quinidine gluconate are achieved in 3 to 4 hours. Quinidine is extensively metabolized in the liver, and several of its metabolic products are pharmacologically active. Unbound or free plasma concentrations of some of these metabolites can exceed free plasma concentrations of quinidine, and they probably contribute to its electrophysiologic effects. Roughly 10% to 27% of quinidine is excreted by the kidneys, as are many of its metabolites. Renal excretion of quinidine can be reduced by urinary alkalinization. The elimination half-life ranges from 4 to 17 hours, with a mean value of 6 hours. Thus, 2 to 3 days may be required to achieve steady-state plasma concentrations after initiation of quinidine therapy. The therapeutic range with current quinidine-specific assay methods is 2 to 5 μg/ml.

CLINICAL ADMINISTRATION

The initial dose is 200 mg orally of quinidine sulfate every 6 hours, or 324 mg (one tablet) of quinidine gluconate every 8 hours. Under closely monitored condi-

**Table 15–2 PHARMACOLOGIC PROPERTIES OF CLASS Ia AND CLASS Ib
ANTIARRHYTHMIC DRUGS**

DRUG	ROUTE OF ADMINISTRATION	DOSAGE	THERAPEUTIC RANGE	ELIMINATION HALF-LIFE	ROUTE OF EXCRETION
Class Ia					
Quinidine	PO	Quinidine sulfate: 200 mg q 6 hr Maximal: 2400 mg/d	2–5 μg/ml	4–17 hr	Hepatic
Procainamide	PO	SR: 500 mg q 6 h Maximal: 8000 mg/d	4–10 μg/ml	2–5 hr	Hepatic + renal (50%–70%)
	IV	Loading: 20–50 mg/min for a total of 1 g Maintenance: 1–4 mg/min			
Disopyramide	PO	150 mg q 6–8 hr Maximal: 1200 mg/d	2–5 μg/ml	6–15 hr	Hepatic + renal (35%–75%)
Class Ib					
Lidocaine	IV	Loading: 3–4 mg/kg over 20–30 min (see text) Maintenance: 1–4 mg/min	1.5–5.0 μg/ml	1.5–2 hrs	Hepatic
Tocainide	PO	200–400 mg q 8 hr Maximal: 2400 mg/d	3–10 μg/ml	9–18 hr	Hepatic + renal (40%–50%)
Mexiletine	PO	150 mg q 8 hr Maximal: 1200 mg/d	0.75–2.00 μg/ml	8–15 hr	Hepatic
Phenytoin	IV or PO PO	Loading: 10–15 mg/kg 50–100 mg q 8 hr Maximal: 450 mg/d	10–20 μg/ml (total) 1–2 μg/ml (free)	16–24 hr	Hepatic

IV = intravenous; PO = orally; SR = sustained release.

tions, the drug can be administered intravenously at a dose of 6 to 10 mg per kg given slowly over 30 to 45 minutes. Intramuscular administration is not advised due to the danger of muscle necrosis.

Drugs that induce hepatic enzymes, such as phenytoin and phenobarbital, accelerate the metabolism of quinidine so that higher dosages may be necessary. In addition, quinidine can increase the di-

goxin concentration by up to 100%, apparently from a combination of reduced elimination of digoxin and its displacement from tissue-binding sites. A similar interaction has been reported with digi-

Table 15-3. DOSAGE MODIFICATIONS FOR CLASS Ia ANTIARRHYTHMIC DRUGS

DRUG	DISEASE STATES REQUIRING DOSAGE REDUCTION	DRUG INTERACTIONS	CAUTION
Quinidine	Hepatic disease, elderly	Hepatic enzyme inducers: ↑ total dose Digoxin levels ↑ Cimetidine, propranolol, amiodarone: ↓ clearance Caution with vasodilators, neuromuscular blockers Quinidine may ↓ warfarin requirements	Long QT interval, hypokalemia, hypomagnesemia, bradycardia, myasthenia gravis
Procainamide	Renal disease, acute MI, LV dysfunction	Amiodarone reduces clearance Caution with other antiarrhythmics, neuromuscular blockers	Long QT interval, hypokalemia, hypomagnesemia, bradycardia, myasthenia gravis
Disopyramide	Renal disease, hepatic disease, elderly	Hepatic enzyme inducers: ↑ total dose Disopyramide may potentiate warfarin Caution with verapamil, β-blockers, flecainide Amiodarone reduces clearance	Long QT interval, hypokalemia, hypomagnesemia, bradycardia, prostatism, glaucoma, LV dysfunction

LV = left ventricular; MI = myocardial infarction.

toxin. Caution should be used when administering other vasodilators such as nitroglycerin with quinidine, because excessive hypotension can result. Cimetidine and propranolol may decrease drug clearance, and quinidine itself may decrease warfarin requirements. Possible additive effects require caution during anesthesia with succinylcholine and other neuromuscular-blocking drugs.

Renal insufficiency and congestive heart failure do not significantly alter quinidine pharmacokinetics. In patients with hepatic disease, plasma protein binding is reduced, and lower doses may be effective (Table 15–3). Elderly patients may also respond to lower doses, because of a reduction in clearance and Vd. The drug should be avoided in patients with myasthenia gravis, because it can precipitate or aggravate symptoms of neuromuscular blockade.

ADVERSE EFFECTS

Noncardiovascular side effects are common with quinidine; over 50% of pa-tients cannot tolerate its use long term. The most common symptoms are gastrointestinal and include diarrhea, nausea, vomiting, abdominal pain, and anorexia. These symptoms may improve with changing base preparations (e.g., from quinidine sulfate to quinidine gluconate). A syndrome known as *cinchonism* can also occur; it includes tinnitus, visual disturbances, and mental status changes. Other important adverse effects include fever, hepatitis, antibody-mediated thrombocytopenia, leukopenia, a lupus-like syndrome, hemolytic anemia, and reactive lymphadenopathy. Anaphylaxis is rarely seen.

The most important cardiovascular side effect, which occurs in 2% to 10% of patients, is syncope or sudden cardiac death as a result of torsades de pointes. This arrhythmia can occur early during quinidine therapy, at a time when plasma concentrations are low.[6] The patients at greatest risk appear to be those with concomitant hypokalemia, hypomagnesemia, bradycardia, a long QT interval at baseline, or some combination. Cellular data suggest the arrhythmia may be due to triggered activity. Treatment involves discontinuation of quinidine, administration of potassium or magnesium or both, and measures to increase resting heart rate, such as isoproterenol or pacing. Great caution should be used in combining quinidine with other drugs that also prolong the QT interval.

Other electrophysiologic side effects include sinus node depression, AV block, and bundle branch block, especially in patients with preexisting conduction disturbances. In addition, when used as single therapy for atrial flutter or fibrillation, the drug can actually accelerate the ventricular response by slowing the atrial rate and speeding conduction through the AV node with resulting 1:1 AV conduction (see Chapter 10, page 226 and Fig. 10–13). As with all standard antiarrhythmic agents, the drug can also cause proar-

rhythmia (e.g., new sustained ventricular tachycardia or ventricular fibrillation) unrelated to QT prolongation. Presyncope or syncope due to vasodilation with postural hypotension is rare but is more commonly seen in the older age group.

CLINICAL USE

Quinidine is effective in a wide variety of atrial and ventricular arrhythmias. In the past, it was successfully used in converting over 50% of cases of atrial flutter–fibrillation to normal sinus rhythm by pushing the dose to achieve cardioversion, QRS widening, or other toxic symptoms or side effects. In addition, the drug is effective in prophylaxis of these arrhythmias. Quinidine also appears to be useful in the treatment of automatic atrial tachycardias, as well as more common forms of supraventricular tachycardia such as AV node reentry and AV reciprocating tachycardias (see Chapter 9, page 200, and Chapter 11, pages 260 to 261). It slows the ventricular response in patients with the combination of atrial fibrillation and ventricular preexcitation by slowing antegrade accessory pathway conduction. Quinidine is also effective in suppressing frequent PVCs and nonsustained ventricular tachycardia. It should be emphasized, however, that there is no evidence that suppression of these ventricular arrhythmias by any drug improves survival rates, although intolerable symptoms may mandate therapy. Because it is unlikely to

cause congestive heart failure, quinidine is a useful agent in treating these arrhythmias as well as sustained ventricular tachyarrhythmias in patients with poor left ventricular function.

The recent demonstration of the frequent proarrhythmic effects of quinidine dictates caution in its use. The potential for producing torsades de pointes, in particular, should force the clinician to examine the indications for all the class Ia drugs. Patients with either atrial or ventricular arrhythmias who are starting quinidine therapy for the first time should be hospitalized for a brief (several days) period of monitoring. The treatment criteria outlined in Chapters 7, 9–12 for the specific arrhythmias should be carefully adhered to. The past practices, for example, of suppressing PVCs because they are a nuisance, or because it seemed logical to suppress them, is not tenable in the light of our understanding of the potentially lethal nature of these drugs. The need for hospitalization before the institution of such drugs with serious proarrhythmic potential has forced clinicians to become much more circumspect regarding the indications for treatment of possibly benign arrhythmias.

Procainamide. Procainamide is a structural analogue of procaine, which in the 1930s was found to elevate the threshold for myocardial excitability. It has been used as an antiarrhythmic agent since the 1950s.

ELECTROPHYSIOLOGY

Procainamide is very similar to quinidine in that it depresses $\dot{V}_{max}$ in a frequency-dependent fashion and prolongs repolarization and refractoriness (see Table 15–1). As with quinidine, the ERP/APD ratio rises. Procainamide also directly slows conduction in the AV node and AV accessory pathways and decreases automaticity. It has some vagolytic effects, but these are rarely seen clinically. During clinical use, the QRS and QT intervals typically are prolonged, although the QT interval is usually lengthened less than with quinidine. The major metabolite of procainamide, N-acetylprocainamide (NAPA), has electrophysiologic properties that are somewhat different from the parent compound.[7] N-acetylprocainamide appears to prolong repolarization and refractoriness without affecting $\dot{V}_{max}$, and is probably best classified as a class III drug. Like quinidine, NAPA can produce triggered activity *in vitro*.

HEMODYNAMIC EFFECTS

Procainamide has mild negative inotropic effects and, when given rapidly by the IV route, can cause hypotension and bradycardia owing to ganglionic blockade. Congestive heart failure can be precipitated in patients with significant left ventricular dysfunction, although generally this is not a major problem. The resting heart rate with therapy is usually unchanged.

PHARMACOKINETICS.

After oral administration, procainamide is rapidly and completely absorbed (see Table 15–2). Peak levels occur from 30 minutes to 4 hours after a dose. This variable time is related to the onset of the drug's rapid elimination from the body. Renal excretion accounts for 50% to 70% of the drug, while the remainder is metabolized in the liver, with a major portion converted to NAPA. N-acetylprocainamide is primarily eliminated by the kidneys. The enzyme that converts procainamide to NAPA is N-acetyltransferase; its activity is genetically determined. Roughly half of the North American population are slow acetylators of procainamide and accumulate less NAPA than do rapid acetylators. During chronic oral dosing (with normal renal function), if the ratio of the plasma concentration of NAPA to that of procainamide exceeds 1, the patient is probably a rapid acetylator. The elimination half-life of procainamide ranges from 2 to 5 hours, with a mean value of 3.5 hours, whereas that of NAPA is 6 to 11 hours. The therapeutic range is 4 to 10 $\mu g/ml$, although plasma concentrations up to 20 $\mu g/ml$ have been used to treat malignant ventricular tachyarrhythmias. *N*-acetylprocainamide appears to have antiarrhythmic effects at concentrations greater than 5 $\mu g/ml$, with a high incidence of side effects above 15 to 20 $\mu g/ml$.[8] The ranges of plasma concentrations of NAPA that produce beneficial and toxic effects overlap considerably, which has limited its use as an antiarrhythmic drug in its own right. For optimal treatment, plasma concentrations of both procainamide and NAPA should be monitored during therapy.

CLINICAL ADMINISTRATION

The newer sustained-release (SR) form has essentially replaced the use of regular procainamide. The initial dose is 500 mg every 6 hours, with maximum doses of 6000 to 8000 mg per day. The wax matrix of the SR preparation can be seen in the stool despite adequate gastrointestinal absorption of the drug, and patients noting this should be reassured.

During the IV administration of procainamide, the ECG and blood pressure should always be monitored closely no matter what regimen is used. One regimen calls for 275 $\mu g/kg$ per minute for 30 minutes, repeated as necessary; another uses 25 to 50 mg per minute, to a total dose of 1 g. Should hypotension occur or the QRS interval be prolonged by more than 25%, IV administration should be suspended and, if necessary, restarted at a slower rate. If hypotension develops in a patient receiving procainamide to terminate sustained ventricular tachycardia, the drug should be stopped immediately and the patient cardioverted. Some patients may respond to smaller doses. Maintenance infusion ranges from 1 to 4 mg per minute, although higher doses have been used. When switching from IV to oral procainamide, 1 to 2 hours should elapse from discontinuation of the IV form to administration of the first oral dose, because of rapid oral absorption.

Relatively few drug interactions have been described with procainamide (see Table 15–3). One concern is synergistic depression of left ventricular contractility when procainamide is used in combination with other antiarrhythmic drugs, especially lidocaine. The administration of amiodarone has been known to elevate procainamide levels. As with quinidine, caution should be used when procainamide is administered with other neuromuscular-blocking agents. During chronic renal failure, the clearance of both procainamide and NAPA fall, and NAPA levels can rise dramatically. In patients with chronic renal failure, the drug generally should be administered every 12 hours, with lower total daily dosages. After myocardial infarction and in the presence of congestive heart failure, both Vd and clearance are reduced, and therefore smaller loading and maintenance doses should be used. The dosage adjustment required, if any, for coexisting liver dysfunction is not known.

ADVERSE EFFECTS

Therapy with procainamide is associated with the frequent occurrence of non-cardiovascular side effects that limit its use in long-term therapy. Higher plasma concentrations are typically associated with nausea, vomiting, and anorexia. Other side effects include fever, rash, agranulocytosis, thrombocytopenia, granulomatous hepatitis, altered mental status (hallucinations, psychosis), and insomnia. Importantly, about 80% of treated patients develop a positive antinuclear antibody (ANA) test within 1 year. This appears to occur more rapidly in slow acetylators, suggesting that other metabolites besides NAPA may be involved in the development of procainamide-induced lupus. The development of a positive ANA test does not warrant discontinuation of therapy if the patient is asymptomatic. A syndrome similar to systemic lupus erythematosus can develop, however, with arthralgias, arthritis, rash, pleuritis, and pericarditis, although central nervous system (CNS) and renal involvement are rare and anti-DNA antibodies are negative. Symptoms resolve with discontinuation of the drug, although the positive ANA resolves much more slowly.

The cardiovascular side effects of procainamide include clinically significant depression of left ventricular function, especially if additional antiarrhythmic drugs are being used. This is an infrequent problem. Torsades de pointes can occur but is generally less common than with quinidine. A small percentage of patients may also experience other types of proar-rhythmic events. Finally, as with all class I drugs, sinus node dysfunction, AV block, and intraventricular conduction disturbances can occur, especially in the setting of preexisting disease.

CLINICAL USE

The clinical indications for procainamide are virtually identical to those for quinidine. Because the drug can be administered intravenously, it is frequently used for the emergency treatment of arrhythmias. For rapid treatment of sustained or nonsustained ventricular tachycardia, it is the second-line drug of choice if lidocaine is ineffective. Intravenous procainamide is the drug of choice for nonhypotensive patients with ventricular preexcitation and atrial fibrillation with rapid conduction down the accessory pathway, because it slows conduction over the accessory pathway and sometimes also converts the atrial fibrillation to sinus rhythm.

The drug is used in the electrophysiology laboratory (see also Chapters 6 and 12) to test its ability to suppress inducible ventricular tachycardia. Demonstrated ability to suppress the arrhythmia in this setting implies that the patient may respond to oral procainamide (although this is somewhat controversial), and perhaps to other class Ia drugs with a low chance for arrhythmia recurrence.

Because of the high incidence of toxic side effects with procainamide, long-term use of the drug is becoming less common, as clinicians turn to other, better-tolerated drugs for chronic use.

Disopyramide. Disopyramide was synthesized 20 years ago in a search for new antiarrhythmic drugs and was marketed in the United States in 1977. The commercial preparation is a racemic mixture of *d*- and *l*-stereoisomers.

ELECTROPHYSIOLOGY

The electrophysiologic effects of disopyramide are similar to those of quinidine and procainamide[9] in that it causes a reduction in $\dot{V}_{max}$ with prolongation of APD and refractoriness, and increases the ERP/APD ratio (see Table 15–1). The *d*-isomer is principally responsible for changes in repolarization. Disopyramide also slows conduction in accessory pathways, but does not affect slow-response tissue. As with other fast sodium-channel blockers, it suppresses automaticity by reducing the slope of phase-4 depolarization. On the surface ECG, the principal effect of therapy is prolongation of the QRS and QT intervals.

HEMODYNAMIC EFFECTS

Disopyramide differs from quinidine and procainamide in that it produces significant negative inotropic effects in a concentration-dependent fashion when administered to patients with either normal or abnormal left ventricular function. An important contributing factor is its vasoconstrictor properties, which can increase blood pressure and afterload and, consequently, myocardial oxygen consumption. The drug also has important anticholinergic effects which appear to be principally mediated by the *l*-isomer and a metabolic product with similar stereochemistry. This vagolytic action facilitates conduction through the AV node and increases the sinus node rate. The resting heart rate typically does not change during therapy, however, because of the counterbalanced direct depressant effects on phase-4 depolarization of the SA node.

PHARMACOKINETICS

Disopyramide is well absorbed after oral administration (see Table 15–2). Peak plasma concentrations occur 0.5 to 3.0 hours following a dose. A controlled-released (CR) preparation of disopyramide has been developed which allows twice daily oral dosing with peak plasma concentrations in 3 to 4 hours. Interestingly, the drug is protein bound in a saturable fashion; a progressive rise in total plasma concentration increases the percentage of the drug in plasma that is free. This may result in a greater-than-expected response to increased drug dosing. Such swings in free plasma concentration with dosing are less apparent with the CR preparation. Routine clinical measurement of free plasma concentrations of disopyramide has been advocated by some investigators. A major metabolite, mono-N-desisopropyldisopyramide, has electrophysiologic properties and can accumulate to plasma concentrations that are 30% of plasma disopyramide concentrations. Its protein binding is also saturable and it probably contributes to the pharmacologic effects of disopyramide therapy.

Approximately two thirds of a given dose of disopyramide is excreted unchanged, primarily in the urine, while one third is excreted as the major metabolite in both urine and feces. The elimination half-life ranges from 4 to 8 hours in normal volunteers but is 6 to 15 hours in patients. The therapeutic range for total plasma concentration is 2 to 5 μg/mL.

CLINICAL ADMINISTRATION

The initial dose of regular disopyramide is 150 mg orally at 6 to 8 hour intervals, with a maximum dose of 1200 mg. The CR preparation is administered every 8 to 12 hours, with a starting dose of 150 mg. When switching from the regular to the CR preparation, the total daily dose in milligrams should be equivalent.

Caution should be used when disopyramide is administered in conjunction with calcium-channel blockers, β-blockers, or flecainide, owing to combined depressant effects on left ventricular function (see Table 15–3). Drugs that induce hepatic enzymes accelerate the metabolism of disopyramide, reducing its plasma concentration and elimination half-life; higher doses are frequently required. There have been rare reports that the drug may also increase warfarin levels. The clearances of disopyramide and its major metabolite correlate well with creatinine clearance, and renal failure increases the elimination half-life. In addition, disopyramide is principally bound in plasma to α_1-acid glycoprotein; its elevation in uremia can cause a reduction in the free concentration of disopyramide so that higher plasma concentrations are required for a given effect. Overall, it is recommended that in renal insufficiency, low initial doses be used, with careful titration. The decreased renal function of the elderly dictates the need for care in treating this patient group. The drug typically is not removed with hemodialysis except by resin hemoperfusion. Dosage also should probably be reduced in patients with hepatic insufficiency.

ADVERSE EFFECTS

The anticholinergic actions of disopyramide lead to its most frequent noncardiovascular adverse effects, including blurred vision, constipation, urinary retention, dry mouth, and worsening of glaucoma. Other more unusual side effects include hypoglycemia, nausea, cholestasis, psychosis, anaphylaxis, and the initiation of uterine contractions.

The most important cardiovascular side effect is the exacerbation of congestive heart failure.[10] Approximately 50% of patients with a history of heart failure develop worsening of symptoms, and in this setting, disopyramide is contraindicated. The same proarrhythmic effects seen with quinidine and procainamide can occur

with disopyramide. The drug may produce torsades de pointes, although this side effect occurs less commonly with disopyramide than it does with quinidine. Because of its vagolytic properties in combination with slowing of the atrial rate, disopyramide can accelerate the ventricular response in atrial flutter–fibrillation. Conduction disturbances such as sinus slowing and AV block have been observed, especially with preexisting disease.

CLINICAL USE

The spectrum of arrhythmias that respond to disopyramide is similar to that of quinidine and procainamide. Because of its negative inotropic effects, disopyramide is used less often in patients with sustained ventricular tachyarrhythmias, who frequently have poor left ventricular function. The drug may be effectively used with EPS-guided therapy for life-threatening or refractory ventricular and supraventricular arrhythmias, including the various arrhythmias associated with ventricular preexcitation.

CLASS IB DRUGS

Lidocaine. Lidocaine is a tertiary amine synthesized in 1946[11] in an attempt to create an anesthetic agent with a longer duration of action than procaine. It was first used as an antiarrhythmic in the 1950s and achieved great popularity in the 1960s for the treatment of ventricular arrhythmias.

ELECTROPHYSIOLOGY

Lidocaine depresses $\dot{V}_{max}$ in ventricular muscle and Purkinje fibers in a rate- and voltage-dependent fashion. In its interaction with the sodium channel, lidocaine displays very rapid kinetics, with time constants of onset and offset of block of less than 1 second. Its sodium-channel blocking effects are more marked when resting potentials are elevated, as in diseased or ischemic tissue. It is the prototype of the class Ib drugs, as it shortens APD as well as refractoriness (see Table 15–1). The ERP/APD ratio increases, however.

The drug appears to have little, if any, effect on atrial tissue. In accessory pathways, conduction may either slow or accelerate. Lidocaine raises the ventricular fibrillation threshold and depresses both automaticity and triggered activity.[12] On the surface ECG, QT shortening may be observed, but otherwise typically there is no change.

HEMODYNAMIC EFFECTS

Lidocaine can depress contractility to some degree, especially in patients with poor left ventricular function. Usually, however, it is well tolerated even in the setting of congestive heart failure.

PHARMACOKINETICS

Because of extensive first-pass metabolism and the generation of toxic metabolites when lidocaine is given by the oral route, lidocaine has been restricted to IV or intramuscular administration (see Table 15–2). Its kinetics follow a two-compartment model, with a distribution half-life of 8 minutes for movement between the central and peripheral compartments. Plasma concentrations in the central compartment correlate well with antiarrhythmic activity. The elimination half-life is 1.5 to 2 hours, so that steady-state levels are not achieved until approximately 8 to 10 hours after starting a maintenance infusion. The same is true for the elimination process, so there is no reason to taper lidocaine before discontinuation. The drug is extensively metabolized in the liver; its clearance there approximates liver blood flow. The two major metabolites, glycinexylidide and monoethylglycinexylidide, have both antiarrhythmic activity and CNS toxicity. They are excreted via the kidneys. During prolonged infusions, clearance decreases and the elimination half-life of lidocaine can be prolonged to 3 to 7 hours, with a rise in plasma concentration. The therapeutic range is 1.5 to 5.0 μg/mL, although higher levels can be used to achieve arrhythmia control in the absence of adverse effects.

CLINICAL ADMINISTRATION

Various dosing regimens have been devised to obtain therapeutic concentrations rapidly without toxicity. A popular method is to administer 75 to 100 mg of lidocaine intravenously over 2 minutes, followed by three boluses of 50 mg given every 5 minutes, with subsequent initiation of a maintenance infusion. The total loading dose should be roughly 3 to 4 mg/kg over the first 30 minutes; maintenance infusions are 1 to 4 mg per minute. If the arrhythmia recurs during the maintenance infusion, a lidocaine level should be drawn, a small supplemental IV loading dose administered (e.g., 50 mg), and the maintenance infusion rate increased. Lidocaine can be given intramuscularly if necessary. Because lidocaine clearance decreases with time, the infusion rate may need to be decreased after 24 hours.

Drugs that decrease liver blood flow, such as norepinephrine and β-adrenergic–receptor blockers, also decrease clearance of lidocaine and prolong its elimination half-life, so that lower doses might be required if these drugs are used (Table 15–4). Cimetidine also reduces clearance of lidocaine. Hepatic enzyme inducers, on the other hand, accelerate elimination and may necessitate higher doses. Left ventricular function may be synergistically depressed when lidocaine is administered intravenously with other antiarrhythmic agents. In patients with congestive heart failure, the Vd and clearance are both reduced, so that lower loading doses and maintenance infusions should be used. As already discussed, however, significant changes in elimination half-life do not occur. Hepatic insufficiency leads to a reduction in clearance without a change in volume of distribution. In this setting, normal loading doses are administered but the maintenance infusion should be lowered. Elimination half-life can be prolonged up to 6 hours (mean 4 hours). With acute myocardial infarction, clearance may be reduced and elimination half-life can be prolonged up to 4 hours. Because the associated rise in α_1-acid glycoprotein may lead to a decrease in free plasma concentration, however, higher *total* plasma concentrations of lidocaine may be required for effect. Maintenance infusion may need to be reduced in elderly patients, whose liver blood flow is often diminished. The kinetics of lidocaine do not change in the presence of renal insufficiency, although the metabolites mentioned above may accumulate to toxic levels and, in conjunction with lidocaine, lead to early CNS effects such as coma.

ADVERSE EFFECTS

The adverse effects of lidocaine are primarily related to the CNS. These include the development of paresthesias, slurred speech, mental status changes, tremor, and agitation. Nausea and vomiting are also commonly seen. The drug should be administered over 2 to 3 minutes with each bolus. More rapid administration can lead to seizures or hypotension with depression of left ventricular contractility. Similarly, seizures, respiratory depression, and coma may result from high plasma concentrations.

Cardiovascular side effects include lidocaine's negative inotropic properties,

Table 15–4. DOSAGE MODIFICATION FOR CLASS Ib ANTIARRHYTHMIC DRUGS

DRUG	DISEASE STATES REQUIRING DOSAGE REDUCTION	DRUG INTERACTIONS	CAUTION
Lidocaine	LV dysfunction, hepatic disease, elderly	Hepatic enzyme inducers: ↑ total dose Norepinephrine, β-blockers, cimetidine:↓ clearance Caution with other antiarrhythmics Additive CNS toxicity with tocainide and mexiletine	Ventricular preexcitation with atrial fibrillation
Tocainide	Renal disease	Additive CNS toxicity with lidocaine	
Mexiletine	Hepatic disease	Hepatic enzyme inducers: ↑ total dose Additive CNS toxicity with lidocaine Amiodarone reduces clearance	
Phenytoin	Renal disease, hyperbilirubinemia	Antacids impair absorption Isoniazid, sulfonamides, barbiturates, chloramphenicol, carbamazepine, disulfiram, cimetidine, amiodarone reduce clearance Levels of quinidine, disopyramide, theophylline, thyroxine, mexiletine, lidocaine ↓	Pregnancy (teratogenic)

CNS = central nervous system; LV = left ventricular.

as noted above. In addition, the drug can increase the ventricular response during atrial flutter–fibrillation in patients with or without an accessory pathway. It can also cause conduction system disturbances such as sinus slowing and AV block, especially with preexisting disease. It rarely has a proarrhythmic effect.

CLINICAL USE

The principal role for lidocaine is in the suppression of ventricular arrhythmias that require rapid control. The drug is effective in suppressing PVCs in all settings and has proved useful in preventing ventricular fibrillation when used prophylactically in the setting of acute myocardial infarction. In the past, a lidocaine infusion was typically maintained for 24 to 48 hours after the infarction. This procedure may not reduce mortality rates from acute myocardial infarction; therefore its use for this indication is controversial, and generally not recommended, although it does reduce the morbidity associated with the cardiac arrest scenario and defibrillation. The drug can be used to terminate sustained ventricular tachycardia, whereas bretylium may be more effective in the treatment of ventricular fibrillation, although this is also controversial. In general, lidocaine is not effective in the treatment of supraventricular arrhythmias. It has been used in the electrophysiology laboratory to attempt to predict responsiveness to the other class Ib drugs, but has not proved very reliable in this regard.

Tocainide. Although lidocaine is an effective antiarrhythmic drug in the treatment of ventricular arrhythmias, significant first-pass metabolism and the generation of toxic metabolites have limited its use during oral administration. Tocainide is a primary amine analogue of lidocaine which emerged as a result of a systematic search for structurally similar compounds suitable for oral administration. The commercial preparation is a racemic mixture of *d*- and *l*-stereoisomers.

ELECTROPHYSIOLOGY

The electrophysiologic and ECG effects of tocainide are similar to those of lidocaine, with either no change or slight shortening of the QT interval (see Table 15–1). Tocainide also reduces automaticity *in vitro* and causes mild slowing of conduction in the AV node in a concentration-dependent fashion.

HEMODYNAMIC EFFECTS

When it is given orally, tocainide appears to have minimal hemodynamic effects in humans. Intravenous bolus therapy has been associated with a reduction in cardiac index and systemic vascular resistance. The incidence of congestive heart failure during compassionate-use trials in the United States was low (1% to 2%).

PHARMACOKINETICS

Tocainide is a relatively simple drug with few drug interactions.[13] After oral administration, it is rapidly and completely absorbed (see Table 15–2). This process is delayed by concomitant food administration; peak plasma concentrations are reduced by approximately 40%, but there is no change in overall bioavailability. Peak plasma levels are achieved in approximately 60 to 90 minutes. Tocainide does not appear to generate active metabolites.

Approximately 40% to 50% of the drug is excreted unchanged in the urine, while the rest undergoes glucuronidation in the liver. Renal clearance is reduced following urinary alkalinization. The elimination half-life ranges from 8 to 20 hours, averaging 9 to 18 hours, or even longer in the presence of left ventricular dysfunction. Thus, steady-state plasma concentrations would be achieved within approximately 3 to 4 days of initiating a maintenance dose of tocainide. The therapeutic range is 3 to 10 μg/mL; the incidence of side effects increases with doses above 10 μg/mL.

CLINICAL ADMINISTRATION

The usual initial dose is 200 to 400 mg orally every 8 hours, with a maximum of 2400 mg orally per day. Side effects are frequently seen at total daily doses greater than 1800 mg per day. The drug is usually administered at 6- to 8-hour intervals.

Tocainide does not appear to have significant pharmacokinetic interactions with other drugs, notably digoxin. When administered concomitantly with lidocaine, however, low doses should be used and caution taken, because adverse effects may occur synergistically (see Table 15–4). Significant renal disease is associated with reduced clearance and prolongation of the elimination half-life up to 22 hours, so that total daily dose, frequency of administration, or both may need to be reduced. With hemodialysis, approximately 25% of the drug is cleared. Hepatic disease probably does not require significant dosage adjustments, although data regarding this point are lacking.

ADVERSE EFFECTS

During dose ranging, adverse effects may occur in up to 50% of patients. The most common symptoms include nausea, vomiting, dizziness, tremor, and paresthesias. Mental changes can range from confusion to psychosis. The incidence of adverse effects is minimized by administering tocainide with food, which results in a reduction in peak plasma concentrations. The incidence of arrhythmia aggravation appears similar to that seen with most standard antiarrhythmic drugs, probably on the order of a few percent.

An important side effect is agranulocytosis, with an incidence of 0.18% in some initial series. It is recommended that leukocyte counts be obtained frequently, especially early during therapy. Rash and fever can also occur; more unusual side effects include systemic lupus erythematosus, pneumonitis or pulmonary fibrosis, and hepatitis. This toxicity profile, in particular the occurrence of agranulocytosis, limits the usefulness of this drug.

CLINICAL USE

The efficacy of tocainide in suppressing chronic, stable, frequent PVCs and nonsustained ventricular tachycardia appears to be similar to that of quinidine; arrhythmias are effectively suppressed in roughly one half to two thirds of patients. Some data suggest that lidocaine sensitivity may predict success with tocainide therapy, although these responses are not totally concordant. It does appear that arrhythmias that are lidocaine resistant are unlikely to respond to tocainide. As with most antiarrhythmic drugs, tocainide is less effective in suppressing sustained ventricular tachyarrhythmias, doing so in only about 10% to 20% of patients. The drug appears to be safe in the treatment of ventricular arrhythmias associated with a long QT interval. It appears that response or tolerance (or both) to tocainide therapy in suppressing ventricular arrhythmias is not synonymous with response or tolerance to mexiletine. Success during treatment of ventricular arrhythmias with tocainide may be improved by combination therapy with a class Ia agent. The drug is rarely effective in the treatment of supraventricular tachyarrhythmias and is not useful in the treatment of atrial flutter–fibrillation.

Mexiletine. Mexiletine was originally developed as an anticonvulsive agent. Once its structural resemblance to lidocaine was recognized, investigation of its antiarrhythmic properties began. It was marketed in the United States in 1986, approximately 2 years after tocainide.

ELECTROPHYSIOLOGY

Mexiletine's electrophysiologic effects *in vitro* are similar to those of lidocaine and tocainide,[14] with little effect or shortening of the QT interval (see Table 15–1). It may depress automaticity and, like tocainide, produces mild slowing of AV nodal conduction.

HEMODYNAMICS

As with tocainide, oral therapy with mexiletine produces minimal hemodynamic effects in humans, although rare episodes of hypotension have been reported.

PHARMACOKINETICS

After oral administration, rapid and complete absorption occurs, primarily in the small intestine, with peak plasma concentrations in approximately 2 to 4 hours. Absorption is slowed in the setting of delayed gastric emptying (e.g. narcotic therapy), following acute myocardial infarction, and with concomitant administration of food. There is no evidence that active metabolites are generated.

The primary route of excretion is hepatic metabolism; renal excretion generally is less than 10%. In the presence of urinary acidification, however, renal excretion can increase several fold. The elimination half-life averages 8 to 15 hours, with values up to 24 hours occa-

sionally observed. Therefore, as with tocainide, steady-state plasma concentrations may not be achieved for 3 to 4 days. The therapeutic range is 0.75 to 2.00 $\mu g/mL$.

CLINICAL ADMINISTRATION

The recommended initial dose is 150 mg orally every 8 hours, with a maximum dose of 1200 mg per day, although higher doses have been used (see Table 15–2). The drug is generally administered at 6- to 8-hour intervals.

Drugs that activate or induce hepatic enzymes (such as phenytoin, phenobarbital, and ethanol) increase the clearance of mexiletine and shorten elimination half-life, so that higher daily doses and more frequent dosing may be required (see Table 15–4). There does not appear to be a significant pharmacokinetic interaction between mexiletine and digoxin or anticoagulant drugs. Like tocainide, mexiletine may display synergism in the occurrence of toxic effects during concomitant administration with lidocaine.

The disposition of the drug is not altered in the setting of advanced renal insufficiency with a creatinine clearance as low as 10 cc per minute. Hepatic disease (particularly cirrhosis), however, can be associated with a marked increase in elimination half-life, generally requiring reduced doses. As the extraction of mexiletine is generally low in the liver and not related to liver blood flow, its pharmacokinetics do not seem to change significantly in the presence of congestive heart failure, although elimination half-life may be prolonged.

ADVERSE EFFECTS

Mexiletine has a more favorable toxicity profile than tocainide, in that agranulocytosis is not a problem with this drug. Adverse effects may be common during dose ranging and include tremor, nausea, vomiting, diplopia, constipation or diarrhea, and dizziness. Once again, the occurrence of these adverse effects can be minimized by giving mexiletine with a snack or meal. Fever, rash, and mental changes can also occur. Rarely, thrombocytopenia, hepatitis, and the induction of a positive ANA test have been reported. The incidence of proarrhythmic effects is low, similar to that seen with tocainide. Depression of the conduction system leading to sinus arrest or heart block is rare, except with preexisting disease.

CLINICAL USE

Mexiletine is effective in the treatment of ventricular arrhythmias. Its efficacy against frequent PVCs and nonsustained ventricular tachycardia is similar to that of procainamide and quinidine. Although it is less effective in the treatment of sustained ventricular tachycardia and ventricular fibrillation, combination therapy with quinidine-like agents, propranolol, or amiodarone may increase success. The drug is useful in the treatment of arrhythmias associated with a long QT interval. Response or tolerance (or both) to tocainide is not predictive of response to mexiletine. The drug is generally less effective in supraventricular tachyarrhythmias, although some response in the treatment of arrhythmias associated with ventricular preexcitation has been reported.

Phenytoin. Phenytoin is an anticonvulsant drug that is structurally similar to barbiturates. It was reported to have antiarrhythmic properties in 1950.[15]

ELECTROPHYSIOLOGY

Phenytoin's electrophysiologic effects are similar to those of lidocaine (see Table 15–1). The drug also depresses digitalis-induced sympathetic activity and may depress vagal stimulation, as well, by CNS-mediated mechanisms. Automaticity is also inhibited by phenytoin.

HEMODYNAMIC EFFECTS

During oral therapy, phenytoin may depress left ventricular contractility, but only in patients with severe left ventricular dysfunction. When phenytoin is administered intravenously, the drug can cause hypotension if given more rapidly than 25 to 50 mg per minute. In this setting, the ECG and blood pressure should be continuously monitored.

PHARMACOKINETICS

Phenytoin is slowly and unpredictably absorbed after oral administration (see Table 15–2). It is extensively protein bound and is metabolized in the liver in a saturable fashion. Thus, during therapy, a small increase in dosage can lead to a dramatic rise in plasma concentration, as with disopyramide. There are no known active metabolites. The elimination half-life ranges from 16 to 24 hours, so that 3 to 4 days may be required to achieve steady-state plasma concentrations. The therapeutic range for total plasma concentration is 10 to 20 $\mu g/ml$, and for the free plasma concentration, 1 to 2 $\mu g/ml$.

CLINICAL ADMINISTRATION

The drug can be loaded orally or intravenously at a dose of 10 to 15 mg/kg. It can be given by mouth in three divided doses over 12 hours, with a maintenance dose of roughly 5 mg/kg per day. It is soluble only at a very high pH, and the IV preparations can cause venous sclerosis. When phenytoin is given intravenously, the drug should be administered via slow bolus injections with a syringe through a large-caliber vein to avoid the crystallization that occurs when the drug is mixed in saline or dripped slowly through intravenous lines. Constant IV infusion is not recommended, both because of the difficulties in keeping the drug in solution and because of the risk of venous sclerosis, thrombosis, and pain. Also, as mentioned, rapid IV administration can lead to hypotension and high-grade heart block.

As might be expected, cimetidine inhibits the metabolism of phenytoin, so that lower doses may be required (see Table 15–4). Drugs reducing the clearance of phenytoin include isoniazid, sulfonamides, barbiturates, disulfiram, chloramphenicol, and carbamazepine. The absorption of phenytoin may be impaired by the concomitant administration of antacids. The drug itself increases requirements for quinidine, disopyramide, theophylline, mexiletine, lidocaine, and thyroxine. It is important to remember that the protein binding of phenytoin can decrease significantly with uremia or hyperbilirubinemia. In these settings, one must guide therapy by monitoring the free plasma concentration of the drug.

ADVERSE EFFECTS

As with other class Ib drugs, adverse effects due to phenytoin are typically related to CNS toxicity. Symptoms most commonly observed include nystagmus, ataxia, and drowsiness. Other, more unusual side effects include gingival hypertrophy, psychosis, lymphoid hyperplasia, peripheral neuropathy, microcytic anemia, rash, Stevens-Johnson syndrome, the lupus syndrome, and cytopenias. Phenytoin is known to be teratogenic; multiple congenital abnormalities such as cranial-facial deformities and digital hypoplasia may be seen.

CLINICAL USE

Phenytoin is generally less effective than other agents in the treatment of ventricular arrhythmias. It is useful in the treatment of digoxin toxicity, although lidocaine is also effective and much easier to administer. Phenytoin is effective for ventricular arrhythmias in the congenital long QT syndrome. It can have a synergistic effect with propranolol and class Ia drugs such as procainamide in the treatment of chronic ventricular arrhythmias. The drug is also useful in patients with tetralogy of Fallot and ventricular arrhythmias, although newer agents such as mexiletine are also effective. Phenytoin has not been found effective in suppressing supraventricular arrhythmias unless they are due to digitalis intoxication.

CLASS IC DRUGS

Class Ic drugs depress $\dot{V}_{max}$ and slow conduction much more than other class I agents; in general, they are more effective against both ventricular and supraventricular arrhythmias.[16] Although a lower incidence of noncardiac side effects occurs with these drugs as compared with standard antiarrhythmic agents, a higher incidence of proarrhythmia may be seen.

Flecainide. Flecainide is the first class Ic drug to be marketed in the United States.[16] Structurally, it is an analogue of procainamide. However, recent data from CAST have demonstrated an increased mortality in patients treated with flecainide or encainide for nonsustained ventricular arrhythmias after myocardial infarction, prompting relabeling by the Food and Drug Administration (FDA) (see later sections).[17]

ELECTROPHYSIOLOGY

At the cellular level, the drug produces a marked, frequency-dependent depression of $\dot{V}_{max}$ at low concentrations, with a long dissociation time constant. This effect may explain the marked prolongation of the QRS interval that can occur in normal sinus rhythm (see Table 15–1). Action potential duration and ERP are typically shortened in Purkinje fibers, but can lengthen in ventricular muscle. High concentrations of flecainide may also depress the slow inward current. Therapy is usually associated with significant increases in the PR and QRS intervals, but repolarization typically is not affected. Thus, any increase in the QT or QT_c interval usually is due to QRS prolongation; the JT interval (J point to end of T wave) is unchanged. Depression of sinus node automaticity and of conduction in the AV node and accessory pathways is common. Flecainide can elevate the pacing threshold by as much as 200%; therefore, caution should be exercised in treating patients with permanent pacemakers.

Table 15–5. PHARMACOLOGIC PROPERTIES OF CLASS Ic, MORICIZINE, AND CLASS III ANTIARRHYTHMIC DRUGS

DRUG	ROUTE OF ADMINISTRATION	DOSAGE	THERAPEUTIC RANGE	ELIMINATION HALF-LIFE	ROUTE OF EXCRETION
Class Ic					
Flecainide	PO	50–100 mg q 12 hr Maximal: 400 mg/d	0.2–1.0 μg/ml	7–23 hr	Hepatic + renal (10%–50%)
Encainide	PO	25 mg q 8 hr Maximal: 200 mg/d	—	EMs: 2–3hr* PMs: 8–12 hr	Hepatic
Propafenone	PO	150 mg q 8 hr Maximal: 900 mg/d	EMs: 0.05–1.4 μg/ml†	EMs: 1–9 hr PMs: 10–32 hr	Hepatic
Moricizine	PO	200 mg q 8 hr Maximal: 900 mg/d	—	6–13 hr	Hepatic
Class III					
Bretylium	IV	5 mg/kg Maximal: 30 mg/kg or 4 mg/min by continuous infusion	—	4–17 hr	Renal
Amiodarone	PO	Loading: 10–15 g in first wk Maintenance: 200–600 mg/d	— (1.0–2.5 μg/ml?)	8–107 days	Hepatic

EMs = extensive metabolizers; IV = intravenous; PMs = poor metabolizers; PO = orally.

*The elimination half-life of the active metabolites of encainide can be considerably longer than that of encainide.

†For poor metabolizers, plasma concentrations for effect are 1.4 to 1.8 μg/ml (see text).

HEMODYNAMIC EFFECTS

In both normal volunteers and patients with coronary artery disease, IV administration of flecainide reduced the cardiac index and elevated the pulmonary capillary wedge pressure. Significant negative inotropic effects may occur, so that up to 16% of patients with a history of congestive heart failure may experience aggra-

vation of symptoms while taking flecainide. Therefore, the drug should be used with caution, if at all, in patients with poor left ventricular function.

PHARMACOKINETICS

After oral administration, complete absorption is achieved; peak plasma concentrations occur in approximately 3 hours (Table 15–5). Small amounts of active me-

tabolites are generated, but it is unlikely that they contribute to the electrophysiologic effects. Urinary alkalinization reduces the normal 10% to 50% (mean 27%) of the drug that is excreted unchanged in the urine. The elimination half-life in normal volunteers ranges from 7 to 23 hours, with a mean value of 14 hours, but this parameter may be higher in patients. Steady-state plasma concentrations can be expected after 3 to 4 days of therapy. The drug is usually given at intervals of 8 or 12 hours. The therapeutic range is 0.2 to 1.0 μg/mL, although lower concentrations may be effective. Levels over 1.0 μg/mL are associated with proarrhythmia and should be avoided (see later section).

CLINICAL ADMINISTRATION

The initial starting dose is 100 mg orally every 12 hours, with a maximum dose of 400 mg per day. Drug levels should be carefully monitored in patients with poor left ventricular function or sustained ventricular arrhythmias, who are most likely to manifest a proarrhythmic response. In patients with evidence of left ventricular dysfunction or conduction system disturbances, a starting dose of 50 mg orally every 12 hours is recommended.

Cimetidine can reduce the clearance of flecainide by up to 27%, and prolongs elimination half-life in normal volunteers. Thus, lower doses may be effective (Table 15–6). Flecainide raises trough digoxin plasma concentrations by an average of 25%, and adjustments in the digoxin dosage may be required. Because of depressant effects on electrophysiologic and hemodynamic parameters, great caution should be exercised if flecainide is administered with calcium-channel blockers, β-blockers, and other antiarrhythmic agents. The initiation of amiodarone during flecainide therapy raises its plasma concentrations. In the presence of end-stage renal insufficiency, flecainide clearance can be reduced by up to 40%, prolonging elimination half-life up to 58 hours. Thus, smaller daily doses are required, and the time to achieve steady-state plasma drug concentrations may be markedly prolonged. In the setting of congestive heart failure, clearance is reduced by approximately 20%, and elimination half-life averages 19 hours. No data are available about the effect of hepatic dysfunction.

ADVERSE EFFECTS

During dose ranging with flecainide, noncardiovascular side effects are often mild, transient, and better tolerated than with class Ia or class Ib drugs. Transient CNS symptoms, including dizziness, visual disturbances, and headache, may necessitate discontinuation of the drug. Other side effects include fatigue, nervousness, nausea, abdominal pain, constipation, dysgeusia, and impotence. These side effects may diminish or resolve if smaller amounts of the drug are given at more frequent intervals.

During effective therapy, the PR and QRS intervals can increase by 20% to 30% without sequelae. Second- or third-degree AV block, as well as sinus node depression, can occur. The risks of these side effects increases with underlying disease of the sinus node or AV conduction system. Importantly, the incidence of proarrhythmia can be as high as 20% in patients with severe left ventricular dysfunction and sustained ventricular tachyarrhythmias. This effect is most likely to occur when daily oral doses are greater than 400 mg and plasma concentrations exceed 1.0 μg/ml. Flecainide toxicity may cause an incessant ventricular tachycardia that cannot be suppressed or electrically cardioverted. Some patients with such an event cannot be resuscitated despite appropriate measures. Marked prolongation of the PR and QRS intervals are not necessarily a consistent premonitory feature. Initial data suggest that sodium loading (e.g., $NaHCO_3$) and β-adrenergic–receptor blockade may be useful in treating this form of proarrhythmia. In other groups of patients, however, the incidence of proarrhythmia has been similar to that seen with standard antiarrhythmic agents, generally less than 10%. Nevertheless, because of its potentially toxic effects, the drug should probably be started in the hospital in most patients with structural heart disease.

CLINICAL USE

Flecainide is highly effective in the treatment of frequent PVCs and nonsustained ventricular tachycardia; arrhythmia suppression and virtual abolition of complex arrhythmias is achieved in up to

**Table 15–6. DOSAGE MODIFICATIONS FOR CLASS Ic, MORICIZINE,
AND CLASS III ANTIARRHYTHMIC DRUGS**

DRUG	DISEASE STATES REQUIRING DOSAGE REDUCTION	DRUG INTERACTIONS	CAUTION
Class Ic			
Flecainide	Renal disease	Caution with other antiarrhythmic drugs, β-blockers, calcium-channel blockers Cimetidine can reduce clearance Digoxin levels ↑ by 25% ·	LV dysfunction; conduction system disturbances; sustained VT/VF
Encainide	Renal disease, (hepatic disease?)	Caution with other antiarrhythmic drugs, β-blockers, calcium-channel blockers Cimetidine may reduce clearance	Conduction system disturbances; sustained VT/VF
Propafenone	Hepatic disease (renal disease?)	Caution with other antiarrhythmic agents, β-blockers, calcium-channel blockers Digoxin levels ↑ by 30%–85% Propafenone potentiates warfarin Cimetidine inhibits metabolism	LV dysfunction; conduction system disease; bronchospasm
Moricizine	Hepatic disease, renal disease	Moricizine induces its own hepatic metabolism Cimetidine can reduce clearance Moricizine ↑ clearance of theophylline	Conduction system disturbances
Class III			
Bretylium	Renal disease	Caution with pressor agents Tricyclic antidepressants block uptake by amine pump and reduce hypotension	Pulmonary hypertension; states with fixed cardiac output; digitalis-related arrhythmias
Amiodarone	Hepatic disease	Amiodarone ↑ levels of digoxin, warfarin, most antiarrhythmic drugs Caution with antiarrhythmic drugs (especially ones that ↑ QT interval), β-blockers, calcium-channel blockers, anesthesia	Preexisting pulmonary disease; conduction system disease

LV = left ventricular; VF = ventricular fibrillation; VT = ventricular tachycardia.

90% of patients at dosages up to 600 mg orally per day. In this respect, it is more effective than any of the class Ia drugs. The results are less impressive with recurrent, sustained ventricular tachyarrhythmias, although patients with good ventricular function experience a greater likelihood of success. Flecainide is also an effective antiarrhythmic drug for a variety of supraventricular arrhythmias, including the AV junctional reentry tachycardias (see Chapter 11, page 261). It slows the ventricular rate during atrial fibrillation with ventricular preexcitation. The drug is also effective in the termination and prophylaxis of atrial flutter–fibrillation, as well as focal reentry and automatic atrial tachycardias.

As reported in CAST,[17] however, patients taking flecainide or encainide for treatment of nonsustained ventricular arrhythmias after myocardial infarction died more often from arrhythmia and cardiac arrest than did patients randomized to placebo. For this reason, flecainide is now indicated only for treatment of life-threatening (sustained) ventricular arrhythmias. Of interest, the FDA subsequently approved flecainide for use in supraventricular tachycardia and atrial fibrillation/flutter in patients without structural heart disease. This approval was based on data showing virtually no risk of proarrhythmia or sudden death in patients with supraventricular tachycardia who had structurally normal hearts and no evidence of ventricular arrhythmias.

Encainide. Encainide, the second class Ic drug released in the United States, is also a structural analogue of procainamide. Very recently, as a result of CAST, encainide was removed from the market in the United States. Nevertheless, its use is discussed here because the pharmaceutical sponsor continues to provide the drug to patients who already require it for life-threatening arrhythmias.

ELECTROPHYSIOLOGY

Encainide's electrophysiologic effects are similar to those of flecainide (see Table 15–1). The metabolic products O-demethylencainide (ODE) and 3-methoxy-O-demethylencainide (MODE) have pharmacologic activity *in vitro* and likely mediate the effects of encainide therapy in most patients.[18] Among the three compounds, ODE is the most potent; it causes more prominent effects on refractoriness of the heart than does encainide. Like flecainide, encainide appears to dissociate from the sodium channels in a slow fashion, with a time constant usually greater than 20 seconds. Oral therapy with encainide is typically associated with prolongation of PR and QRS intervals, with an occasional increase in the QT interval unrelated to QRS prolongation. Encainide slows conduction through the AV node and accessory pathways but does not appear to affect sinus node function.

HEMODYNAMIC EFFECTS

The ejection fraction generally does not change with oral therapy. Heart failure may develop in patients with severe left ventricular dysfunction, but this occurs much less frequently than with flecainide.

PHARMACOKINETICS

After oral administration, absorption is rapid and complete, with peak plasma concentrations occurring in the first 1 to 2 hours (see Table 15–5). In over 90% of patients, encainide is rapidly transformed in the liver to ODE and MODE.[19] Because of this significant first-pass metabolism, oral bioavailability is generally low, at 30%. O-demethylencainide and MODE achieve higher plasma concentrations and have longer elimination half-lives than encainide and, as noted, appear to mediate the electrophysiologic effects of encainide therapy in most patients. Less than 10% of patients are termed *poor metabolizers* of encainide; in these patients, a genetic defect prevents expression of the enzyme responsible for converting encainide to its primary metabolic products. Also in these patients, there is little first-pass metabolism and oral bioavailability is high (85%); clearance is 10-fold lower than in *extensive metabolizers*. In poor metabolizers, higher plasma concentrations of encainide are achieved, whereas the plasma concentration of ODE is relatively low and MODE is absent. Encainide therapy at the usual dosages can suppress arrhythmias in these patients, however, and the incidence of side effects does not appear higher. The primary route of excretion for encainide is hepatic elimination, although the metabolites are excreted to some extent by the kidneys. The elimination half-life of encainide is 2 to 3 hours in extensive metabolizers and 8 to 12 hours in poor metabolizers. It is somewhat longer for the metabolites, averaging 5 to 10 hours for ODE and 17 hours for MODE, with values that can rise to over 24 hours. Thus, steady-state plasma concentrations after starting encainide may not be achieved for approximately 3 to 4 days. As might be expected, there is little correlation in most patients between plasma encainide concentration and antiarrhythmic response, so routine monitoring of plasma concentrations is not helpful. A better correlation exists for the metabolites, with effective plasma concentrations of 50 to 100 ng/mL for ODE and 100 to 150 ng/mL for MODE.

CLINICAL ADMINISTRATION

The initial starting dose is 25 mg orally every 8 hours, with a maximum dose of 200 mg per day. The dose should be increased no more frequently than every fourth day. The drug can be given at intervals of 8 to 12 hours and comes in capsules of 25, 35, and 50 mg.

Encainide does not appear to interact significantly with digoxin or oral anticoagulants. The hepatic enzyme inhibitor cimetidine can raise the plasma concentration of encainide and its metabolites by 30% to 45%, so that caution should be used during concomitant dosing with this drug or any other agent that might inhibit cytochrome P-450 enzymes (see Table 15–6). As with flecainide, great care should be taken if encainide is to be administered concomitantly with β-blockers, calcium-channel blockers, or other antiarrhythmic agents, because of additive effects on AV nodal and His-Purkinje conduction. Moderate to severe renal insufficiency reduces clearance of encainide and its metabolites and elevates their plasma concentrations. Total daily dose and frequency of administration should be reduced; a starting dose of 25 mg orally per day is recommended. Although concentrations of encainide can rise in patients with hepatic disease, no definite changes in dosage are recommended, although caution should be exercised. The kinetics of encainide are not altered by the presence of congestive heart failure.

ADVERSE EFFECTS

As with flecainide, the incidence of side effects during dose ranging with encainide is lower than with older antiarrhythmic drugs. The most frequent symptoms include dizziness, visual disturbances, and headache, followed by abdominal pain, nausea, and diarrhea or constipation. Rare cases of elevated liver function tests and frank hepatitis, as well as hyperglycemia, have been reported. As with flecainide, the incidence of proarrhythmia is higher within certain patient populations receiving encainide than it is for standard antiarrhythmic drugs. Patients at risk include those with depression of left ventricular function and sustained ventricular tachyarrhythmias. Associated clinical situations include higher doses of encainide, higher plasma concentrations of the metabolites, and the presence of congestive heart failure symptoms. Careful dose titration has decreased this incidence of proarrhythmia, however. Because excessive prolongation of the PR and QRS intervals may not be present to herald proarrhythmia, however, and because encainide markedly depresses conduction throughout the heart, it should be administered with caution in patients with pre-existing conduction system disturbances. Bundle branch block and other abnormalities occasionally have been reported. Based on the CAST findings,[17] encainide should not be used to treat nonsustained ventricular arrhythmias after recent myocardial infarction.

CLINICAL USE

Encainide is effective in treating frequent PVCs and nonsustained ventricular tachycardia, with successful therapy achieved in approximately 80% of patients with these arrhythmias. Like flecainide, it is more effective than quinidine or procainamide. With sustained ventricular tachyarrhythmias, the response rate appears to average about 25% to 30%, although the drug is more effective if the left ventricular ejection fraction is greater than 35%. Because of its effects on the AV node and AV accessory pathways, encainide also is effective in treating reentrant AV junctional tachycardia, and slows the ventricular response during rapid atrial fibrillation in patients with ventricular preexcitation. Like flecainide, it also appears to be effective in the treatment of atrial flutter–fibrillation and automatic atrial tachycardias, although these data are preliminary. Because of data from CAST (see also the section on flecainide earlier in this chapter),[17] however, encainide has been removed from the market and is now available only to patients previously taking it for serious arrhythmias.

Propafenone. Propafenone is the newest class Ic antiarrhythmic agent to be marketed in the United States. Its structure resembles that of propranolol, and like many β-blockers, the commercial preparation is a racemic mixture of *d*- and *l*-stereoisomers.

ELECTROPHYSIOLOGY

Propafenone depresses $\dot{V}_{max}$ in a potent fashion, especially in ischemic tissue, with no consistent change in APD.[20] In addition, it has mild β-adrenergic–receptor blocking effects (in this respect approximately 1/40th as potent as propranolol). The drug also has slight calcium-channel blocking effects, 1/100th as potent as those of verapamil. One metabolic product, 5-hydroxypropafenone, has electrophysiologic properties similar to the parent compound; another metabolite, N-depropylpropafenone, is less active. As with other class Ic drugs, oral therapy with propafenone prolongs the PR and QRS intervals, with little change in the QT interval (see Table 15–1). Propafenone depresses the SA node and slows conduction through the AV node and accessory pathways.

HEMODYNAMICS

During oral therapy, the drug may precipitate congestive heart failure, especially in patients with reduced left ventricular function. However, this adverse effect is not as common as with flecainide or disopyramide.

PHARMACOKINETICS

After oral administration, the drug is slowly but completely absorbed. In most patients, first-pass clearance is extensive and saturable. Because of saturable clearance, a threefold increase in dose can be associated with a 10-fold increase in plasma concentration. Peak plasma concentrations occur 2 to 3 hours after an oral dose. As with encainide (see Table 15–5), the capacity to metabolize propafenone appears to be genetically determined.[21] The principal enzyme, which can be deficient in up to 10% of patients, appears to be the same enzyme responsible for the metabolic transformation of encainide. In patients who are poor metabolizers of propafenone, clearance is markedly reduced and the plasma propafenone concentration and elimination half-life are increased. Little or no 5-hydroxypropafenone is generated in these patients. Poor metabolizers appear more likely to suffer CNS side effects during the administration of propafenone, probably due to higher plasma concentrations, but the efficacy of the drug is similar to that in extensive metabolizers, and equivalent dosages are required. As expected, the primary route of excretion is through hepatic metabolism. The elimination half-life of the drug is 1 to 9 hours (mean 5.5) in extensive metabolizers and 10 to 32 hours (mean 17.2) in poor metabolizers. Thus, the time required to achieve steady-state plasma concentrations after starting a given dose of propafenone varies in the two patient populations. Perhaps due to the generation of active metabolites in extensive metabolizers, different plasma concentrations are associated with an antiarrhythmic response in the two groups. For extensive metabolizers, this range is 50 to 1400 ng/ml (mean 350 ng/ml), whereas in poor metabolizers it is 1400 to 1800 ng/ml (mean 1600ng/ml). In both groups, side effects are generally associated with plasma concentrations greater than 1000 ng/ml.

CLINICAL ADMINISTRATION

The initial dose is 150 mg orally every 8 hours, with a maximum dose of 900 mg per day. The drug can be given every 8 to 12 hours.

Propafenone can increase plasma digoxin concentrations in a dose-related fashion, with increases of 30% to 40% at a total daily dose of 450 mg orally per day (see Table 15–6). At dosages of 900 mg per day, the digoxin level can rise by an average of 83%. Thus, the dose of digoxin initially should be reduced by 50% when propafenone is begun. A digoxin plasma level should be obtained after steady-state with propafenone is achieved and the digoxin dose adjusted as necessary. Propafenone also appears to potentiate the effects of warfarin; in normal volunteers, prothrombin time may rise and should therefore be followed closely. Cimetidine can increase propafenone plasma concentrations by approximately 20%, with small but significant increases in the QRS interval. In patients with severe hepatic disease, oral bioavailability can increase with reduced clearance and protein binding. These patients should receive 50% of the usual propafenone dosage. As significant amounts of metabolic products are excreted by the kidneys, caution should

be used when propafenone is administered to patients with moderate to severe renal insufficiency.

ADVERSE EFFECTS

Noncardiovascular side effects from propafenone are usually mild. Most commonly these include a metallic or bitter taste, constipation, nausea and vomiting, and dizziness. Diplopia, paresthesias, fatigue, and headache can also be seen. Rarely, psychosis, rise in liver function tests, cholestatic jaundice, and reduction in spermiogenesis have been reported. In addition, some degree of β-blockade can be expected, especially at higher doses, and bronchospasm has been reported. The potential to precipitate congestive heart failure has been mentioned, and conduction system disturbances including bundle branch block can also be seen. The incidence of proarrhythmia is probably lower with propafenone than with flecainide and encainide, although incessant ventricular tachycardia has occurred.

CLINICAL USE

Propafenone can effectively suppress frequent PVCs and nonsustained ventricular tachycardia in roughly 65% to 85% of patients with these arrhythmias. The likelihood of success in treating sustained ventricular tachyarrhythmias is less, but is improved in patients with preserved left

ventricular function. Some data suggest that the results of programmed ventricular stimulation during an electrophysiologic study do not predict patient responses to propafenone, in that patients with inducible arrhythmias during drug therapy may still do well and remain asymptomatic from a clinical standpoint. There are data to suggest that the incidence of proarrhythmia may be lower with propafenone than with flecainide and encainide, although incessant ventricular tachycardia can be seen. Propafenone currently is marketed solely for the treatment of life-threatening, sustained ventricular arrhythmias.

Moricizine. Moricizine is a phenothiazine derivative developed in Russia and recently approved by the FDA for clinical use in the United States. Although moricizine is a class I agent, its electrophysiologic characteristics at the cellular level are somewhat unique, so that it is not easily classified into one of the three previous subgroups. The drug does not appear to have significant dopaminergic-receptor antagonist activity.

ELECTROPHYSIOLOGY

Moricizine blocks sodium channels with a subsequent reduction in $\dot{V}_{max}$ and conduction slowing *in vitro* in a use-dependent fashion (see Table 15–1). In isolated canine Purkinje fibers, it also shortens APD, with an increase in the APD/ERP ratio. Recent data suggest that it primarily blocks inactivated sodium channels, with kinetics of exiting channels that are intermediate between class Ia and class Ib agents. The drug also suppresses abnormal automaticity and has little effect on sinus node and atrial tissue. In patients, moricizine slows AV nodal conduction, increasing the PR interval by 15% to 20%, and the QRS interval by 10% to 15% at dosages of 750 to 900 mg per day. The JT interval is slightly shortened.

HEMODYNAMIC EFFECTS

Moricizine may depress myocardial contractility to a mild degree. This is most apparent in patients with preexisting poor left ventricular function. Generally, the drug is well tolerated, but it can exacerbate congestive heart failure in patients with serious left ventricular dysfunction.

PHARMACOKINETICS

Moricizine is rapidly absorbed following oral administration, with peak plasma concentrations in 0.5 to 2.0 hours (see Table 15–5). Oral absorption is slowed when there is food in the stomach, but overall bioavailability is not altered. First-pass hepatic metabolism is significant, making oral bioavailability roughly 38%. Moricizine undergoes extensive metabolism in the liver, with less than 1% excreted unchanged in the urine. Numerous metabolites appear to be present in small quantities, and some have apparent electrophysiologic activity. The elimination half-life of the parent compound in patients is on the order of 6 to 13 hours but can be quite variable. The elimination half-life of total radioactivity following a dose of radioactive moricizine has been found to be considerably longer, suggesting the prolonged excretion of metabolites with time. The antiarrhythmic drug effect does not appear to correlate with the plasma concentration of the parent compound or with any specific metabolite. Suppression of PVCs starts to occur within two hours of an oral dose, with a full effect in 10 to 14 hours. This effect may persist in its full extent for up to 10 hours following discontinuation of the drug, suggesting either an unknown metabolite with a relatively long elimination half-life, or distribution of the drug into a deep tissue compartment that communicates slowly with plasma. For all of these reasons, it is not clinically useful to specify a therapeutic range for the parent compound in plasma.

CLINICAL ADMINISTRATION

Moricizine is approved for oral administration in the United States. The initial starting dose is 200 mg orally every 8 hours. This dose can be increased after 3 days to 250 mg and subsequently to 300 mg orally every 8 hours (as necessary) for effect.

Moricizine induces cytochrome P450 activity and its own hepatic metabolism, with a reduction in plasma concentration over time without significant alteration in clinical effect (see Table 15–6). It also decreases the clearance of cimetidine by about 50%, but no clinically significant outcome of this interaction has been demonstrated. It is recommended that patients on cimetidine should start at low doses of moricizine (i.e., 600 mg or less per day). Moricizine also increases theophylline clearance by roughly 50%; it is recommended that plasma concentrations of theophylline be closely monitored. No interaction has been demonstrated with digoxin, warfarin, or other cardiovascular drugs. Caution should be used with other AV nodal–blocking drugs, however, as moricizine appears to slow AV nodal conduction.

The hepatic clearance of moricizine is reduced in patients with significant hepatic disease, and the elimination half-life is prolonged. It is recommended that such patients be started on dosages of 600 mg or less per day. Approximately 39% of metabolites of moricizine are excreted in the urine, and their elimination may be slowed in the presence of renal insufficiency. Therefore, lower doses (600 mg or less per day) are recommended for these patients as well. It does not appear that the pharmacokinetics of moricizine are altered in the presence of congestive heart failure.

ADVERSE EFFECTS

Generally, the drug is well tolerated, although CNS and gastrointestinal side effects have been reported, including dizziness, nausea and vomiting, headache, paresthesias, fatigue, and dyspnea. Rare episodes of documented drug-induced fever, hepatotoxicity, and thrombocytopenia have also been seen.

As with all class I antiarrhythmic drugs, moricizine has the potential to cause proarrhythmia, and this is more likely to occur in the setting of acute myocardial infarction and congestive heart failure with depressed left ventricular function. The actual incidence of proarrhythmia is somewhat unclear, but there are data to suggest that moricizine may be similar to class Ic drugs like encainide. In CAST, survival rates in the moricizine arm of therapy were no different than with placebo, although more patients died initially during early randomized therapy with the drug as compared with placebo. In addition, moricizine can cause disturbances of AV nodal and intraventricular conduction, leading to serious bradyarrhythmias as well as sinus pauses and asystole. Its ECG effects are somewhat similar to those of class Ic drugs, so caution should be used when administering it to patients with preexisting conduction disturbances.

CLINICAL USE

Administration of moricizine causes a reduction in PVCs related to dose. In this regard it is similar in efficacy to quinidine and disopyramide, reducing ectopy and nonsustained ventricular tachycardia by 75% in roughly two thirds of patients. It is less effective than flecainide and encainide in suppressing ambient PVCs. As noted above, a trend toward adverse effects in CAST has led recently to the termination of this arm of the trial and the drug is now approved by the FDA exclusively for the treatment of life-threatening ventricular arrhythmias such as recurrent sustained ventricular tachycardia and ventricular fibrillation. The success of moricizine in suppressing these arrhythmias during electrophysiologic testing is on the order of 25%.

The drug is not approved for the treatment of supraventricular arrhythmias, but early results using small numbers of patients suggest that it may be effective in treating both reentrant AV junctional tachycardia and arrhythmias related to the Wolff-Parkinson-White syndrome. The drug is also reported to be effective in a small number of pediatric patients for the treatment of ectopic atrial tachycardia.

Class II: β-Adrenergic–Receptor Blockers

Since the development of dichloroisoproterenol in the 1950s, 10 β-adrenergic–receptor blockers have been marketed in the United States at the time of this writing. In addition to their antiarrhythmic effects, these drugs have been widely used for angina pectoris, hypertension, and reduction of morbidity and mortality during and after acute myocardial infarction and for many noncardiac indications.

ELECTROPHYSIOLOGY

At low concentrations, these agents antagonize the effects of catecholamines on β-adrenergic receptors. This reduces automaticity and has variable effects on repolarization.[22] Thus they are effective in treating arrhythmias secondary to enhanced automaticity or excessive sympathetic stimulation (for example, digoxin toxicity, exercise, and acute myocardial infarction). At higher plasma concentrations, they may also have a membrane stabilizing effect, which results in local anesthetic activity with blockade of the fast inward sodium current.[23] *In vitro*, this effect reduces $\dot{V}_{max}$ and shortens APD. Preliminary data suggest that propranolol may work at least in part by the mechanism of membrane stabilization in suppressing ventricular arrhythmias. β-Blockers also slow conduction through

Table 15–7. COMPARATIVE PROPERTIES OF THE β-ADRENERGIC–RECEPTOR BLOCKERS

DRUG	POTENCY OF β-BLOCKADE (PROPRANOLOL = 1)	CARDIOSELECTIVITY	PARTIAL AGONIST ACTIVITY	MEMBRANE STABILIZING ACTIVITY	LIPID SOLUBILITY
Acebutolol	0.3	+	+	+	+
Atenolol	1.0	+	0	0	0
Esmolol	—	+	0	0	—
Labetolol	0.2	0	+ ?	+	+
Metoprolol	1.0	+	0	+	+
Nadolol	6.0	0	0	0	0
Oxprenolol	0.5–1.0	0	+	+	+
Pindolol	6.0	0	+	+	+
Propranolol	1.0	0	0	+	+
Timolol	6.0	0	0	0	+

the AV node and may affect conduction over accessory pathways. The predominant effects *in vivo* of therapy with these agents include a reduction in heart rate and, at times, prolongation of the PR interval (see Table 15–1). The QRS and QT intervals often do not change. An investigational β-adrenergic receptor blocker, sotalol, has additional class III effects, and thus prolongs APD and the QT interval.

HEMODYNAMIC EFFECTS

Stimulation of β_1-adrenergic receptors results in increases in heart rate, contractility, and lipolysis, whereas stimulation of β_2-adrenergic receptors primarily medi-ate bronchodilatation, vasodilatation, and glycogenolysis. Cardioselective β-blockers primarily block β_1 receptors at low doses, although at higher doses, blockade of both types is apparent. Cardioselective agents such as acebutolol, atenolol, esmolol, and metoprolol (Table 15–7) might be advantageous in patients with chronic obstructive pulmonary disease, asthma, peripheral vascular disease, or diabetes; however, untoward effects such as bronchospasm occasionally can occur with these agents, even at low doses.[24]

In addition to β-blockade, some of these agents (including acebutolol, pindolol, oxprenolol, and possibly labetolol) act as partial β-agonists at the receptor level. This agonist activity generally leads to less depression of resting heart rate and cardiac output, while maintaining the reduction in exercise-induced tachycardia that results from β-blockade. Whether partial agonist activity offers any particular advantage remains controversial.

As mentioned, some β-blockers (acebutolol, labetolol, metoprolol, oxprenolol, pindolol, and propranolol) are able to block fast sodium channels by what is termed membrane stabilizing activity. This property may also lead to antiaggregatory effects on platelets, as well as to additional physiologic changes. Most β-

Table 15–8. PHARMACOLOGIC CONSIDERATIONS FOR USE OF
β-ADRENERGIC–RECEPTOR BLOCKERS

DRUG	ROUTE OF ADMINISTRATION	INITIAL DOSE	MAXIMUM DOSE	ROUTE OF EXCRETION	ELIMINATION HALF-LIFE (HRS)
Acebutolol	PO	400 mg/day	1200 mg	Hepatic	3–4
Atenolol	PO	50 mg	200 mg	Renal	6–9
Esmolol	IV	500 μg/kg* followed by 50 μg/kg/min infusion	300 μg/kg/min	RBC esterase	9 min
Labetolol	PO, IV	200 mg PO 20 mg IV (2 mg/min)	2400 mg PO, 300 mg IV	Hepatic	6–8
Metoprolol	PO, IV	100 mg PO 5 mg IV	400 mg PO 15 mg IV	Hepatic	3–7
Nadolol	PO	40 mg	240 mg	Renal	14–24
Oxprenolol	PO	60 mg	480 mg	Hepatic	4–5
Pindolol	PO	10 mg	60 mg	Hepatic	3–4
Propranolol	PO, IV	20 mg PO 1 mg IV	640 mg PO —	Hepatic	3–4
Timolol	PO	10 mg	60 mg	Hepatic	4–5

*Loading dose may be omitted because of rapid pharmacokinetics such that time to steady state is rapidly achieved with a maintenance infusion alone.

blockers are fairly lipid-soluble, but some (including atenolol and nadolol) are more water-soluble and thus are less likely to enter the CNS. Central nervous system side effects such as insomnia and depression are reduced. These drugs are also primarily eliminated through the kidney, with longer elimination half-lives which allow once-a-day dosing.

PHARMACOKINETICS AND CLINICAL ADMINISTRATION

The pharmacokinetic features of the various β-adrenergic blockers are shown in Table 15–8. As can be seen, esmolol is available exclusively in the IV form, and three other agents can also be given by this route. As mentioned, atenolol and na-dolol can be administered once daily, as can the slow-released form of propranolol. For some uses, acebutolol and metoprolol can also be given once a day. As noted, the more water-soluble agents are primarily excreted through the kidney and have longer elimination half-lives. Acebutolol, pindolol, and labetolol also have significant renal excretion.

Because of depressant effects on SA and AV nodal function, as well as on ventricular function, caution should be exercised in administering β-adrenergic–receptor blockers concomitantly with calcium-channel blockers, class Ic antiarrhythmic agents, and amiodarone. Interactions of β-adrenergic blockers with other drugs are numerous and are best reviewed elsewhere.[21] In the presence of liver disease, drugs with significant hepatic metabolism (such as metoprolol, propranolol, and oxprenolol) should be avoided. Conversely, it would seem reasonable to avoid the water-soluble β-blockers for patients with renal insufficiency.

ADVERSE EFFECTS

The adverse effects of these agents are primarily a result of β-adrenergic receptor blockade. Side effects can be especially prominent in patients dependent on adrenergic stimulation. Most frequent are bronchospasm, precipitation of congestive heart failure, bradycardia or AV block or both, claudication, and Raynaud's phenomenon. Abrupt discontinuation of β-blockers has been associated with ventricular arrhythmias, angina, myocardial infarction, and death. For these reasons, it is best to taper off over 4 to 7 days. In diabetics who are hypoglycemic, β-blockers may mask important symptoms such as diaphoresis and tachycardia, delaying the recovery from hypoglycemia. A rise in

blood pressure may also occur. Other side effects from β-blockers include CNS symptoms such as vivid dreams, insomnia, hallucinations, and depression, as well as nausea, abdominal pain, diarrhea, constipation, hair loss, and rarely, agranulocytosis. Fatigue is a common problem and is aggravated by bradycardia.

CLINICAL USE

β-Blockers can be useful in the treatment of unwanted sinus tachycardia as long as it is not due to congestive heart failure. In addition, these drugs can be effective in treating AV junctional reentry tachycardias. In atrial flutter–fibrillation, they effectively slow the ventricular response and are useful either in place of digoxin therapy or as an adjunct to it. They can also slow the ventricular response to sinus node reentry and intra-atrial reentry tachycardias, as well as to automatic atrial tachycardias. In the treatment of ventricular arrhythmias, various β-blockers are effective in suppressing frequent PVCs in 50% to 60% of patients.[25] They have been considerably less successful in treating sustained ventricular tachycardia, and are often avoided because such patients typically have poor left ventricular function. An investigational β-blocker, sotalol, however, which has class III activity, has been reported to be modestly effective in treating sustained ventricular tachyarrhythmias. In several major trials, certain β-adrenergic receptor blockers have been

effective in reducing the incidence of sudden cardiac death in the 1 to 2 years after acute myocardial infarction, but the mechanism of this protection is unclear.

Class III: Drugs That Primarily Prolong Repolarization

BRETYLIUM

Bretylium is a quaternary ammonium compound that was originally developed as an antihypertensive agent in the 1950s. In 1978, it was approved for use as an antiarrhythmic agent in the United States.

ELECTROPHYSIOLOGY

Its electrophysiologic effects place bretylium in the class III category, in that its principal action is to increase APD and ERP in vitro (see Table 15–1).[26] The ratio of ERP/APD does not change. The effects on APD are most pronounced in areas of short APD, and as such, the drug reduces disparity in repolarization and thus decreases the likelihood for reentry. In low concentrations, it causes early transient effects that probably result from norepinephrine release, with increases in the resting membrane potential, $\dot{V}_{max}$, phase-4 depolarization, and conduction velocity. At high doses (probably not achieved clinically), $\dot{V}_{max}$ can be reduced. The drug increases the ventricular fibrillation threshold in vivo to a significant degree. On the surface ECG, the primary effect of bretylium therapy is prolongation of the QT interval without a change in the QRS duration.

HEMODYNAMIC EFFECTS

Bretylium is selectively concentrated in postganglionic adrenergic nerve terminals and produces an initial release of norepinephrine without causing catecholamine depletion.[27] The drug subsequently prevents further norepinephrine release. Thus during the first 15 minutes of IV therapy, norepinephrine release can cause transient hemodynamic effects, including an increase in heart rate, blood pressure, and peripheral vascular resistance, as well as an increase in the occurrence of arrhythmias. This phase is then followed by a reduction in heart rate and systemic vascular resistance that is primarily characterized by postural hypotension. Pulmonary vascular resistance can be increased. Overall, there is usually little change in cardiac output and left ventricular end-diastolic pressure.

PHARMACOKINETICS

Bretylium can be administered intramuscularly, but its absorption by this route is uncertain. Therefore, the primary route of administration is IV (see Table 15–5). The onset of effect is approximately 10 to 20 minutes after an IV bolus, although it can be delayed up to 2 hours when the drug is given more slowly. It is concentrated in the myocardium, with peak levels occurring in approximately 3 to 6 hours. There do not appear to be any active metabolites of bretylium. It is primarily excreted unchanged through the kidney, with 70% to 80% eliminated in the first 24 hours. The drug is also significantly removed during hemodialysis. The elimination half-life ranges from 4 to 17 hours (mean 10 hours). Because the effects parallel the myocardial concentration rather than the plasma concentration, a therapeutic range is not used to monitor therapy.

CLINICAL ADMINISTRATION

The dosage for life-threatening ventricular tachycardia or ventricular fibrillation is 5 mg/kg intravenously as a rapid bolus. This can be repeated in a dose of 5 to 10 mg/kg every 10 to 30 minutes until a maximum value of 30 mg/kg has been reached. The intramuscular dose is 5 to 10 mg/kg. For therapy of hemodynamically stable arrhythmias, a 5 mg/kg dose can be diluted in at least 50 mL of IV fluid and administered over 10 to 30 minutes to decrease the incidence of nausea and vomiting that occurs with a rapid IV bolus. A continuous drip can then be instituted, at a dose of 1 to 4 mg per minute.

Patients receiving bretylium may be very sensitive to sympathomimetic pressor agents, which should thus be used with caution if at all (see Table 15–6). Tricyclic antidepressants, however, which block uptake of bretylium by the amine pump, minimize hypotension without apparently affecting its antiarrhythmic action. In patients with renal insufficiency, clearance of bretylium is decreased proportional to the reduction in creatinine clearance. Elimination half-life can be markedly prolonged in these patients, who generally require reduced doses. It is not known whether congestive heart failure or liver disease alter the drug's kinetics. Because of changes in pulmonary and systemic vascular resistances, bretylium should be avoided in patients with pulmonary hypertension or fixed cardiac output (for example, aortic stenosis).

ADVERSE EFFECTS

The initial adverse effects of bretylium therapy include a rise in heart rate and blood pressure, as well as the potential for worsening arrhythmias. Rapid IV administration can also be associated with nausea and vomiting. After these effects, the most common complication of therapy is hypotension, typically orthostatic. This can be dramatic in patients with reduced left ventricular function or preexisting volume depletion; to avoid using pressor agents, the hypotension is best treated by placing patients in the Trendelenburg position and administering intravenous fluids. The patient should be kept supine even after discontinuation of bretylium, as the hypotension can last up to a week after therapy. Less common adverse effects include bradycardia, abdominal cramps, diarrhea, parotitis, rash, and mental status changes. Due to the initial catecholamine release, it is theoretically contraindicated in digitalis-toxic arrhythmias.

CLINICAL USE

Bretylium has been used almost exclusively in the emergency treatment of life-threatening ventricular tachycardia and ventricular fibrillation. With ventricular fibrillation, normal sinus rhythm can be restored in over 50% of patients, so that many investigators believe that it is the drug of choice for this arrhythmia. A recent study has demonstrated that lidocaine may be equally effective for ventricular fibrillation, however, and some controversy exists as to which is the best drug in this situation. On occasion, bretylium can even achieve chemical defibrillation, without the use of DC countershock. It also can be especially useful for arrhythmias after acute myocardial infarction, but it is generally not effective in treating supraventricular arrhythmias.

AMIODARONE

Amiodarone is a benzofuran derivative with two iodines per molecule which was developed in Belgium as part of a systematic search for coronary vasodilators. Its antiarrhythmic effects in patients were reported in 1974, and it was approved for clinical use in the United States in 1985.

ELECTROPHYSIOLOGY

The electrophysiologic effects of amiodarone have been difficult to characterize, largely because it is poorly soluble in water. In addition, the vehicle used for the IV preparation (Tween 80) has electrophysiologic effects. The principal effects of amiodarone are prolongation of APD and ERP throughout the heart (see Table 15–1). It also depresses $\dot{V}_{max}$ in a frequency-dependent fashion by blocking sodium channels, primarily in their inactivated state.[28] The drug elevates the ventricular fibrillation threshold and reduces automaticity by depressing the phase 4 diastolic slope. The mechanism of its effects are unknown, but two hypotheses have been popularized: (1) the iodine in amiodarone may alter thyroid function and induce a hypothyroid-like state, or (2) it may alter the metabolism of high-energy phosphate compounds. In humans, the predominant effects of therapy include slowing of sinus rhythm from depression of SA node automaticity, an occasional increase in the PR interval due to slowing of AV nodal conduction, and prolongation of the QT interval, often with large U waves.

HEMODYNAMIC EFFECTS

Amiodarone is a complicated drug from a pharmacologic standpoint. It is a vasodilator and blocks both α- and β-receptors in a noncompetitive manner. Acute intravenous dosing is associated with reduced blood pressure and peripheral vascular resistance; coronary blood flow increases. At doses greater than 5 mg/kg, cardiac output may drop, with an elevation in left ventricular end-diastolic pressure. These negative inotropic effects may occur at a lower dose in patients with left ventricular dysfunction. Oral therapy is much less likely to cause negative inotropic effects, even in patients with severe left ventricular dysfunction. Indeed, because of its vasodilator properties, ejection fraction and congestive heart failure symptoms may actually improve. The drug is an effective antianginal agent and appears to be particularly beneficial in Prinzmetal angina.

PHARMACOKINETICS

After oral administration, bioavailability is variable. It ranges from 20% to 55%, with peak plasma concentrations occurring approximately 4 to 5 hours following a dose (see Table 15–5). The drug is highly protein bound and binds extensively with most tissues throughout the body. Specifically, it is taken up, to a large extent, in adipose tissue, liver, lung, myocardium, and red blood cells. Concentrations in tissue can be about 10 to 50 times those in plasma. The onset of action is distinctly delayed, probably because of its extensive tissue distribution, so that a loading dose is usually administered to speed the onset of antiarrhythmic effects. Even with loading regimens, however, the onset of response follows the initiation of therapy by 2 to 10 days.

The drug is almost totally metabolized in the liver. At least two metabolites are known to occur—desethylamiodarone and didesethylamiodarone. Desethylamiodarone accumulates to high concentrations during therapy in humans, and its levels can even exceed those of amiodarone. In animal models, it is electrophysiologically active, is taken up in various tissues extensively (like amiodarone), and has a longer elimination half-life than the parent compound. Renal excretion of amiodarone is minimal, and the drug is not removed by hemodialysis. The elimination half-life ranges from 8 to 107 days (mean 52 days). Thus, it may be *months* before steady state is achieved after dosage initiation or change. Its distribution follows that of a three-compartment model, and elimination is biphasic, with an initial drop of about 50% in the plasma concentration, followed by a much slower terminal elimination phase. The therapeutic range is not clearly determined, although it appears that the onset of antiarrhythmic response occurs at plasma concentrations of 0.5 to 1.0 μg/mL, and that most side effects occur at plasma concentrations greater than 2.0 to 2.5 μg/mL.

CLINICAL ADMINISTRATION

Most oral loading regimens involve the administration of 10 to 15 g of amiodarone during the first week of therapy, with a gradual reduction in total daily dose thereafter. Many patients with ventricular arrhythmias require 400 to 600 mg for long-term therapy, although attempts should be made to achieve the lowest possible maintenance dose. The IV form is currently investigational.

Amiodarone interferes with the clearance of most drugs that have been examined (see Table 15–6). It can notably elevate levels of digoxin and warfarin, but these effects are somewhat unpredictable and can vary over time. It is generally recommended that the dosage of both drugs be reduced by approximately 50% during the initiation of amiodarone therapy, with close observation. The drug also elevates the plasma concentration of numerous antiarrhythmic agents, including quinidine, procainamide, disopyramide, phenytoin, flecainide, mexiletine, and propafenone. Particular caution should be used when the drug is combined with antiarrhythmic agents that prolong the QT interval, because of the risk of torsades de pointes. With the coadministration of anesthetic agents during surgery, excessive hypotension and bradycardia can occur; there have been numerous reports of difficulty weaning patients from cardiopulmonary bypass. Because of additive depressant effects on SA and AV nodal conduction, the drug should be used with extreme caution, if at all, in the presence of β-blockers or calcium-channel blockers. It is also important to remember that the effects of amiodarone may persist for many months after discontinuation of therapy.

ADVERSE EFFECTS

Clinical use of amiodarone has been complicated by a variable incidence of important side effects, some of which can be serious.[29] Various studies have documented an incidence of adverse effects ranging from 30% to 93%, with the likelihood of serious effects from 9% to 26%. Potentially fatal complications include hepatitis and proarrhythmia, congestive heart failure, and pneumonitis. The first three are probably low in incidence, but pneumonitis can occur in 1% to 13% of cases, depending on the duration of therapy and the dosage, and 10% to 20% of patients with overt pulmonary involvement may die. It is recommended that baseline pulmonary function testing with diffusion capacity for carbon monoxide (DLCO) be obtained prior to initiation of amiodarone therapy, as an abnormal initial DLCO or a falling DLCO may predict toxicity. Baseline reductions in forced vital capacity and total lung capacity also may predict patients at greater risk for pulmonary complications. The symptoms typically include cough, weight loss, pleuritic chest pain, shortness of breath, and fever, with either unilateral or bilateral infiltrates. The diagnosis can be made with pulmonary function testing, diffuse uptake on gallium scanning, and a hypersensitivity picture on bronchoalveolar lavage. Symptoms usually respond to the discontinuation of amiodarone but occasionally may require steroids. The mechanism of this adverse effect is unknown. Cardiac side effects include depressant effects on the sinus and AV nodes, an occasional increase in defibrillation thresholds, an increase in pacemaker threshold, and rarely, precipitation of congestive heart failure.

A number of other peculiar effects probably result from its accumulation in tissues. Almost all patients develop corneal microdeposits after about 3 months of therapy. Photophobia, halos around lights, diplopia, and rarely, macular degeneration may occur. Other common side effects include photosensitivity (which can be prevented by topical sun blocks and protective clothing), a bluish discoloration of the skin (typical with higher doses and prolonged therapy), and various neurologic symptoms including muscle weakness, tremor, ataxia, paresthesias, insomnia, and headaches. In addition, amiodarone appears to inhibit the conversion of T_4 to T_3 and can cause either hyperthyroidism or hypothyroidism. During loading, amiodarone rarely causes anorexia and nausea and can be associated with renal insufficiency. Disposition of the drug does not appear to be altered in the presence of preexisting renal insuffi-

ciency or congestive heart failure. No data are available as regards hepatic disease, but probably reduced doses are required.

CLINICAL USE

Amiodarone is effective in the treatment of life-threatening ventricular tachycardia and ventricular fibrillation; up to 50% to 70% of patients respond with control of their arrhythmias during the first year. It should only be used if the patient is refractory to less toxic drugs, however. As treatment is continued, the dropout rate rises owing to side effects and arrhythmia recurrence. The drug should be started at a specialized arrhythmia center where treatment modalities such as programmed electrical stimulation, implantable defibrillators, and surgical therapy are available. An electrophysiologic study is probably useful several weeks following the initiation of therapy, especially to identify patients who may be at risk for potentially fatal recurrences of their arrhythmia on the drug. Although amiodarone is also effective in treating various types of supraventricular tachyarrhythmias, including those due to intra-atrial and AV junctional reentry, automatic atrial tachycardia, and atrial flutter–fibrillation with or without preexcitation, it is generally not recommended for the treatment of these nonlethal arrhythmias, due to its serious side effects.

Class IV: Calcium-Channel Blockers

Of the calcium blockers available in the United States, verapamil and diltiazem have electrophysiologic activity, whereas nifedipine is essentially devoid of these effects. As verapamil is the most potent and most extensively used, our discussion centers exclusively on this agent.

Verapamil is a papaverine derivative and the commercial preparation is a racemic mixture of d- and l-stereoisomers. Although the drug was initially developed as an antianginal agent, its electrophysiologic properties were investigated after negative chronotropic effects were noted during therapy.

ELECTROPHYSIOLOGY

Verapamil effectively blocks calcium channels that lead to the generation of the slow-response action potentials typical of the SA and AV nodes.[30] These calcium channels are also important in the slow inward current that prolongs the plateau phase of the action potential in fast-channel tissue.[31] In slow-response tissue, verapamil depresses $\dot{V}_{max}$ in a frequency-dependent fashion, but it has no significant effects on phase 0 in fast sodium-channel tissue. The drug can also abolish triggered activity (when associated with intracellular calcium overload). Because of these effects, it reduces automaticity of the SA node and slows conduction consistently through the AV node. Its direct effects on accessory pathways are somewhat unpredictable but usually minimal. Changes in the surface ECG include occasional prolongation of the PR interval and slowing of the resting heart rate (see Table 15–1).

HEMODYNAMIC EFFECTS

Verapamil causes relaxation of vascular smooth muscle by blockade of voltage-dependent calcium channels. This leads to a reduction in blood pressure and afterload. As a vasodilator, verapamil is less potent than nifedipine.[32] Coronary blood flow is increased, whereas little effect occurs in venous beds. The drug also possesses potent direct negative inotropic effects on cardiac tissue, but its vasodilator properties typically lead to reflex sympathetic stimulation, and these effects combine to offset the negative chronotropic and inotropic actions.

PHARMACOKINETICS

Verapamil is well absorbed after oral administration and undergoes extensive first-pass metabolism in the liver, leading to low bioavailability. For this reason, the oral dose is considerably greater than the IV dose (Table 15–9). After oral administration, peak effects occur in approximately 5 hours. When administered intravenously, peak effects on AV nodal conduction can be seen in 1 to 2 minutes and persist for 15 to 20 minutes. The major metabolite, norverapamil, is pharmacologically active but somewhat less so than the parent compound. It can achieve concentrations similar to those of verapamil during chronic administration and undergoes renal excretion. The elimination half-life of verapamil is 3 to 7 hours (mean 5 hours), whereas that of norverapamil is 8 to 10 hours. For both com-

Table 15–9. PHARMACOLOGIC PROPERTIES OF VERAPAMIL (CLASS IV DRUG), DIGOXIN, AND ADENOSINE

DRUG	ROUTE OF ADMINISTRATION	DOSAGE	THERAPEUTIC RANGE	ELIMINATION HALF-LIFE	ROUTE OF EXCRETION
Verapamil	IV	0.15 mg/kg	—	3–7 hr	Hepatic
	PO	80 mg q 8 hr			
		Maximal: 720 mg/d			
Digoxin		Loading dose:	0.5–2.0 μg/ml	1–2 days	Renal
	IV	0.50–1.0 mg			
	PO	0.75–1.5 mg			
	PO	Maximal: 0.5 mg/d			
Adenosine	IV	Initial dose: 6 mg or 30–40 μg/kg	—	<10 sec	Cellular uptake
		Subsequent dosages: 12 mg or 37.5 μg/kg			

IV = intravenous; PO = orally.

Table 15-10. DOSAGE MODIFICATIONS FOR VERAPAMIL (CLASS IV DRUG), DIGOXIN, AND ADENOSINE

DRUG	DISEASE STATES REQUIRING DOSAGE REDUCTION	DRUG INTERACTIONS	CAUTION
Verapamil	Hepatic disease	Digoxin levels ↑ Caution with β-blockers, disopyramide, flecainide	Ventricular preexcitation with atrial fibrillation; LV dysfunction.
Digoxin	Renal disease (elderly)	Levels ↑ with quinidine, flecainide, propafenone, amiodarone (see text)	Ventricular preexcitation with atrial fibrillation; hypokalemia, hypercalcemia, hypomagnesemia; hypothyroidism; states of sympathetic hyperactivity
Adenosine	None known	Methylxanthines block effects; dipyridamole potentiates effects	Bronchospasm; preexisting conduction-system disease

LV = left ventricular

pounds, the elimination half-life can increase with chronic administration. Plasma concentrations of verapamil are generally not monitored during clinical therapy.

CLINICAL ADMINISTRATION

The initial oral dose is 80 mg administered at 8-hour intervals; the dose is increased every 2 to 3 days to a maximum of 720 mg per day. The slow-release preparation allows once or twice daily dosing. For acute treatment, verapamil can be administered intravenously at a dose of 0.15 mg/kg (5 to 10 mg) over 1 to 2 minutes. A second dose can be given 30 minutes later. Verapamil can also be administered by continuous IV infusion (for example, to decrease the ventricular response in atrial fibrillation) at a dose of 0.005 mg/kg per minute.

Verapamil should be administered cautiously with β-adrenergic blockers or any other agents known to depress left ventricular function (Table 15–10). Many clinicians believe that concomitant administration of verapamil and β-blockers is contraindicated, but precise data to this point are lacking. Verapamil is also known to increase digoxin levels by an average of 50%. Hepatic insufficiency reduces elimination, requiring lower doses. Similarly, norverapamil can accumulate excessively during chronic renal failure.

ADVERSE EFFECTS

In general, verapamil is extremely well tolerated. Only 1% of patients taking the drug discontinue it due to noncardiac adverse affects. Most commonly, these include constipation, headaches, pruritus, and vertigo. Rarely, hyperprolactinemia and galactorrhea may be seen. The most important limitation to verapamil usage is its tendency to precipitate or worsen congestive heart failure. Hypotension during intravenous administration can be prevented or reversed by concomitant calcium administration. The drug can also lead to significant sinus node dysfunction and AV conduction disturbances, particularly in the presence of underlying disease.

CLINICAL USE

Verapamil is extremely effective in the acute treatment of reentry supraventricular tachycardias that require the AV node as part of the tachycardia circuit (that is, the AV junctional reentry tachycardias; see Chapter 11, page 257). The drug can terminate such arrhythmias in 80% or more of patients and is also effective in their prophylaxis. It should not be used for wide-QRS tachycardias unless they are unequivocally known to be supraventricular with aberration. In addition, verapamil is useful in slowing the ventricular response during atrial flutter–fibrillation, and it occasionally converts these arrhythmias to normal sinus rhythm. Intravenous verapamil is contraindicated in the treatment of atrial fibrillation in patients with ventricular preexcitation, because it can both accelerate conduction over the accessory pathway and cause vasodilation. These effects can combine to produce severe hypotension and cardiovascular collapse in this clinical setting. Verapamil has been reported effective in treating multifocal atrial tachycardia. It is generally less effective in the treatment of ventricular tachycardias, although it can be effective for exercise-induced ventricular tachycardia and the ventricular tachycardia that can occur in younger patients having a right bundle branch block and left axis deviation morphology.

Digitalis

Digitalis was first recognized to improve symptoms in patients with congestive heart failure in the 18th century, when William Withering reported on the effects of the leaf from the foxglove plant. Since then, digitalis has been used most frequently for the treatment of congestive heart failure, but it is also important in the treatment of certain arrhythmias. Cardiac glycosides, collectively referred to here as *digitalis*, have a steroid nucleus in their structure. Our discussion specifically involves digoxin, the most frequently and widely used of these agents.

ELECTROPHYSIOLOGY

Digitalis inhibits the sodium-potassium ATPase, leading to an increase in intracellular sodium and, through sodium-calcium exchange, ultimately to an increase in intracellular calcium. It also increases the slow inward current during the plateau phase of the action potential. The increase in intracellular calcium is thought to be vital for the positive inotropic action of the drug.

Electrophysiologically, the drug affects the conduction system both directly and indirectly. In Purkinje fibers, atrial muscle, and ventricular muscle, it reduces APD, mainly by shortening the plateau phase (with shortening of the QT interval and ST-T wave changes). The slope of phase 4 depolarization increases, especially in the setting of low extracellular potassium, and resting membrane potential rises. The drug can also induce a form of triggered activity known as *delayed afterdepolarizations*. These are transient depolarizations occurring after termination of an action potential, and may be the mechanism responsible for some digitalis-toxic tachycardias (see Chapter 1, page 8).

The indirect effects of digitalis are predominant in the SA and AV nodes and atrial tissue. They include enhancement of vagal tone with reduced automaticity in the SA node (slowing of heart rate) and slowing of AV nodal conduction (slower ventricular response in atrial flutter-fibrillation, increased PR interval). The effects of digitalis on the sympathetic nervous system are probably more important at toxic plasma concentrations, when increased efferent sympathetic activity may abnormally enhance automaticity, leading to arrhythmias. Digitalis may decrease refractoriness in AV accessory pathways, thereby increasing the ventricular rate during atrial fibrillation in patients with ventricular preexcitation.

In summary, during digitalis therapy the surface ECG may show shortening of the QT interval with an increase in the PR interval. The QRS complex is typically not affected even at toxic plasma concentrations. The T wave is diminished or inverted, with ST segment depression. With exercise, ST segment depression may mimic ischemia.

HEMODYNAMIC EFFECTS

Digitalis possesses important direct positive inotropic effects in man. In normal volunteers, it is associated with an increase in systemic vascular resistance and arterial blood pressure, as well as venous constriction. Generally, cardiac output remains unchanged and heart rate may diminish. In patients with congestive heart failure, however, the positive inotropic effects are associated with a reduction in efferent sympathetic activity, leading to decreased systemic vascular resistance and venous tone. Typically, heart rate falls, cardiac output rises, renal perfusion improves, and edema is reduced.

PHARMACOKINETICS

After oral administration of digoxin, absorption from the gastrointestinal tract is variable, ranging from 40% to 90%, largely due to differences in pharmaceutical preparations. Absorption of the encapsulated gel preparation is predictably higher (greater than 90%). Because of this variability, only one type of commercial preparation should be administered to an individual patient. Absorption is retarded by concomitant administration of food.

Peak plasma concentrations after an oral dose occur in 2 to 3 hours, with a maximum effect in 4 to 6 hours. Following IV administration, the peak effect is seen at 1.5 to 3 hours. Elimination half-life is 1 to 2 days (average 1.6) (see Table 15–9). The significant tissue uptake of digoxin means that concentrations in cardiac tissue are 15 to 30 times greater than those seen in plasma. In most patients, the drug is mainly eliminated through the kidneys, where it is both filtered and secreted. In 10% of patients, digoxin is metabolized to inactive products in the gut lumen by bacteria; higher doses are necessary to achieve a given plasma concentration in these cases. Monitoring plasma concentrations of digoxin is important in reducing toxicity. Because of the distribution phase that occurs for up to 6 hours after oral administration, samples are best obtained just before a dose. For treatment of congestive heart failure, the therapeutic range is 0.5 to 2.0 ng/mL. Patients with atrial fibrillation may require higher doses and plasma concentrations, although there is considerable overlap. In general, requirements during atrial fibrillation are best assessed by gauging the patient's ventricular response rather than a given plasma level.

CLINICAL ADMINISTRATION

For rapid effect, a digitalizing dose can be given either orally (0.75 to 1.5 mg) or intravenously (0.5 to 1.0 mg). These are generally administered in divided doses over 12 to 24 hours. The maximal maintenance oral dose is usually 0.5 mg per day. During the treatment of atrial fibrillation, children may require higher doses. Intramuscular administration is not recommended, owing to pain and necrosis at the site of injection as well as the more unpredictable pharmacokinetics, particularly in acutely ill patients.

Digoxin is known to have multiple drug interactions that are important to consider during clinical therapy (see Table 15–10). It should be used with caution in conjunction with calcium-channel blockers or β-adrenergic–receptor blockers, owing to synergistic effects on AV nodal conduction. During quinidine administration, plasma concentrations of digoxin rise by an average of 100%, with a steady state occurring roughly 4 days after quinidine is begun. Plasma concentrations can also rise following the administration of verapamil, flecainide, propafenone, and amiodarone. Diuretics should be used with caution in conjunction with digoxin, owing to their propensity to cause hypokalemia. The absorption of digoxin is inhibited by small bowel disease and the use of antacids, kaolin pectin, cholestyramine, neomycin, and sulfasalazine. In those patients whose intestinal bacteria metabolize digoxin, the concomitant use of oral antibiotics can increase oral bioavailability by up to 40%. The dose of digoxin should be reduced for patients with chronic renal insufficiency, as well as for the elderly, who frequently have a reduced creatinine clearance.

ADVERSE EFFECTS

In the past, adverse effects due to digitalis therapy were frequent and often life-threatening. Better understanding of the drug's pharmacokinetics and increased monitoring of plasma digoxin concentrations have reduced the incidence of toxicity. Noncardiac symptoms most frequently involve the gastrointestinal and neurologic systems and include nausea, vomiting, anorexia, diarrhea, abdominal pain, mental status changes, headache, fatigue, malaise, visual disturbances, paresthesias, and convulsions. Gynecomastia has also been seen.

Cardiac toxicity of digoxin can be emergent and includes many types of arrhythmias. It is important to note that cardiac toxicity sometimes occurs when the plasma concentration is within the *therapeutic range*. That is, the range of plasma concentrations associated with toxicity shows considerable overlap with therapeutically effective concentrations. The most frequent arrhythmias observed include sinus bradycardia with SA block, supraventricular tachycardias (particularly atrial tachycardia due to accelerated pacemakers, typically with AV block, and accelerated junctional rhythms), AV nodal block (type I second-degree AV block), PVCs, and ventricular tachycardia–fibrillation. Arrhythmias are more likely in patients with underlying heart and lung disease with hypoxia and diuretic use, hypokalemia, hypercalcemia, hypomagnesemia, hypothyroidism, and with increased activity of the sympathetic nervous system. Treatment includes discontinuing digoxin and correcting electrolyte disturbances. Ventricular arrhythmias can be treated with phenytoin or lidocaine; atropine can be useful in bradyarrhythmias. In life-threatening situations, digoxin antibodies effectively bind the drug and promote rapid excretion.

CLINICAL USE

The principal antiarrhythmic use of digitalis is to slow the ventricular response during atrial flutter–fibrillation, especially in patients with poor left ventricular function who are not good candidates for verapamil or β-blockers. In some cases, it may be effective as prophylaxis against recurrence of these arrhythmias. Because it can decrease AV nodal conduction, digitalis is also useful in reentry AV junctional tachycardias. It can also slow the ventricular response to intra-atrial reentry and automatic atrial tachycardias. Because of its propensity to speed the ventricular response during atrial fibrillation in patients with ventricular preexcitation, however, digitalis should not be used as single-drug therapy in such patients unless antegrade conduction over the accessory pathway is either poor or absent.

Adenosine

Adenosine is an endogenous nucleoside with potent depressant effects on AV nodal conduction.[33] It has been marketed recently in the United States in IV form for the acute treatment of supraventricular tachycardia.

ELECTROPHYSIOLOGY

Adenosine depresses automaticity in the SA node and in Purkinje fibers, as well as depressing AV nodal conduction. It causes hyperpolarization of the atrial action potential and depression of catecholamine-stimulated triggered activity. It also antagonizes the effects of isoproterenol on the action potential of ventricular muscle. Adenosine produces these effects in part by enhancing certain potassium currents while blocking the calcium current in cardiac muscle.

HEMODYNAMIC EFFECTS

Adenosine is a coronary vasodilator with minimal effects on blood pressure and contractility. Because it depresses the SA node, it may also reduce heart rate.

PHARMACOKINETICS

Adenosine is rapidly taken up by cellular elements in the blood and vascular endothelium and is metabolized to inosine and ultimately adenosine monophosphate (see Table 15–9). Elimination half-life in the plasma is less than 10 seconds, with total clearance in 30 seconds.

CLINICAL ADMINISTRATION

The drug should be administered as a rapid IV injection over 1 to 2 seconds. If it is given more slowly, systemic vasodilation and reflex tachycardia may result. The initial dose is 6 mg, with subsequent doses of 12 mg every 1 to 3 minutes. Alternatively, an initial dose of 30 to 40 μg/kg can be given, with subsequent doses of 37.5 μg/kg. The total effective dose is variable, but in adults ranges from 80 to 90 μg/kg. Arrhythmia termination generally occurs within 20 to 30 seconds.

Methylxanthines such as theophylline are antagonists and block the effects of adenosine (see Table 15–10). Dipyridamole inhibits the uptake of adenosine into cells and thus potentiates its effects, so that patients who are taking dipyridamole require lower doses of adenosine for similar effect. No specific dosage adjustments are recommended at the present time for hepatic or renal insufficiency.

ADVERSE EFFECTS

The intravenous administration of adenosine frequently causes flushing, dyspnea, and angina-like chest pain. These effects are usually mild and very transient (typically less than a minute). Because the dyspnea may be due to mild bronchoconstriction, adenosine should be used with caution in patients with asthma or bronchospastic disease. Rarely, sinus arrest and AV block can occur, especially in patients with preexisting disease. Typically, adenosine causes minimal hypotension, even in the setting of ventricular tachycardia. In doses higher than those used to terminate supraventricular tachycardia, atrial fibrillation or flutter may develop following the administration of the drug.

CLINICAL USE

Adenosine is very effective in the acute termination of supraventricular tachycardias that employ the AV node as part of their reentrant circuit. It may also be valuable diagnostically in the setting of wide-complex tachycardia and other arrhythmias in which induction of AV block would be useful (for example, atrial flutter). Finally, because of its effects on the atrium, it may be helpful for certain atrial arrhythmias, such as ectopic atrial tachycardia.

ACKNOWLEDGMENTS

The authors wish to thank Drs. Dan Roden and Eric Prystowsky for their review and commentary during the preparation of this chapter.

REFERENCES

1. Zipes DP: Genesis of cardiac arrhythmias: Electrophysiological considerations. In Braunwald E (ed): Heart Disease: A Textbook of Cardiovascular Medicine, ed 3. WB Saunders, Philadelphia, 1988, pp 581–620.
2. Siddoway LA, Roden DM, and Woosley RL: Clinical pharmacology of old and new antiarrhythmic drugs. In Josephson ME (ed): Sudden Cardiac Death. FA Davis, Philadelphia, 1985, pp 199–248.
3. Woosley RL and Shand DG: Pharmacokinetics of antiarrhythmic drugs. Am J Cardiol 41:986–995, 1978.
4. Keren A, Tzivoni D, Gavish D, et al: Etiology, warning signs and therapy of torsade de pointes. Circulation 64:1167–1174, 1981.
5. Prystowsky EN and Zipes DP: Treatment of tachycardia. In Rakel RE (ed): Conn's Current Therapy. WB Saunders, Philadelphia, 1986, pp 188–197.
6. Reynolds EW and VanderArk, CR: Quinidine syncope and the delayed repolarization syndromes. Mod Concepts Cardiovasc Dis 45:117–122, 1976.
7. Jaillon P, Rubenson D, Peters F, Mason JW, and Winkle RA: Electrophysiologic effects of N-acetylprocainamide in human beings. Am J Cardiol 47:1134–1140, 1981.
8. Roden DM, Reele SB, Higgins SB, et al: Antiarrhythmic efficacy, pharmacokinetics and safety of N-acetylprocainamide in human subjects: Comparison with procainamide. Am J Cardiol 46:463–468, 1980.

9. Befeller B, Castellanos A, Wells D, Vaguenor MC, and Yeh BK: Electrophysiologic effects of the antiarrhythmic agent disopyramide phosphate. Am J Cardiol 35:282–287, 1975.

10. Leach AJ, Brown JE, and Armstrong, PW: Cardiac depression by intravenous disopyramide in patients with left ventricular dysfunction. Am J Med 68:839–844, 1980.

11. Rosen MR, Hoffman BF, and Wit AL: Electrophysiology and pharmacology of cardiac arrhythmias. V. Cardiac antiarrhythmic effects of lidocaine. Am Heart J 89:526–536, 1975.

12. Collingsworth K, Kalman S, and Harrison D: The clinical pharmacology of lidocaine as an antiarrhythmic drug. Circulation 50:1217–1230, 1974.

13. Roden DM and Woosley RL: Tocainide. N Engl J Med 315:41–45, 1986.

14. Campbell RWF: Mexiletine. N Engl J Med 316:29–34, 1987.

15. Atkinson AJ and Davisai R: Diphenylhydantoin as an antiarrhythmic drug. Annu Rev Med 25:99–113, 1974.

16. Roden DM and Woosley RL: Flecainide. N Engl J Med 315:36–41, 1986.

17. The Cardiac Arrhythmia Suppression Trial (CAST) Investigators: Preliminary report: Effect of encainide and flecainide on mortality in a randomized trial of arrhythmia suppression after myocardial infarction. N Engl J Med 321:406–412, 1989.

18. Mason JW: Basic and clinical cardiac electrophysiology of encainide. Am J Cardiol 58:18C–24C, 1986.

19. Roden DM and Woosley RL: Pharmacology and clinical use of encainide. Int Med Special 8:1–4, 1987.

20. Karagueuzian HS, Peter TC, and Mandel WJ: Propafenone. In Scriabine A (ed): New Cardiovascular Drugs. Raven Press, New York, 1985, pp 285–299.

21. Siddoway LA, Thompson KA, McAllister CB, et al: Polymorphism of propafenone metabolism and disposition in man: Clinical and pharmacokinetic consequences. Circulation 75:785–791, 1987.

22. Silverman R and Frishman WH: Drug treatment of cardiac arrhythmias: Propranolol and other beta-blockers. In Gould LA (ed): Drug Treatment of Cardiac Arrhythmias. Futura, Mount Kisco, NY, 1983, pp 249–272.

23. Shand DG: State of the art: Comparative pharmacology of the beta-adrenoreceptor blocking drugs. Drugs 25(Suppl 2):92–99, 1983.

24. Frishman WH: Clinical difference between beta-adrenergic blocking agents: Implications for therapeutic substitution. Am Heart J 113:1190–1198, 1987.

25. Morganroth J: Role of beta-blocking agents in the treatment of ventricular arrhythmias. In Morganroth J and Moore EN (eds): Cardiac Arrhythmias: New Therapeutic Drugs and Devices. Martinus Nijhoff, Boston, 1984, pp 132–141.

26. Anderson JL: Bretylium tosylate: Profile of the only available class III antiarrhythmic agent. Clin Ther 7:205–224, 1985.

27. Skale BT and Prystowsky EN: A practitioner's guide to bretylium tosylate. J Cardiovasc Med 9:79–87, 1984.

28. Heger JJ, Prystowsky EN, Miles WM, and Zipes DP: Clinical use and pharmacology of amiodarone. Med Clin North Am 68:1339–1366, 1984.

29. Mason JW: Amiodarone. N Engl J Med 316:455–466, 1987.

30. Singh BN and Nademanee K: Use of calcium antagonists for cardiac arrhythmias. Am J Cardiol 59:153B–162B, 1987.

31. Antman EM, Stone PH, Muller JE, and Braunwald E: Calcium channel blocking agents in the treatment of cardiovascular disorders. Part I: Basic and clinical electrophysiologic effects. Ann Intern Med 93:875–885, 1980.

32. Singh BN, Hecht HS, Nademanee K, and Chew CYC: Electrophysiologic and hemodynamic effects of slow-channel blocking drugs. Prog Cardiovasc Dis 25:103–132, 1982.

33. Bellardinelli L, Linden J, and Berne RM: The cardiac effects of adenosine. Prog Cardiovasc Dis 32:73–97, 1989.

CHAPTER 16

Cardiac Pacing for Bradycardia

LAWRENCE D. GERMAN, MD

OUTLINE

Electrical stimulation of the heart to prevent bradycardia was first developed in the late 1920s, but the first implantable pacemakers were not used until the late 1950s. Early pacemakers were very large and contained batteries that typically lasted less than 2 years before needing replacement. The electronic circuitry contained in early pacemakers was also very simple. Initial pacemakers were not able to sense the patient's spontaneous cardiac activity, and therefore paced asynchronously, competing with the patient's underlying rhythm. Until recently, most pacemakers were nonprogrammable, functioning at a fixed, preset rate. Limitations in transvenous lead design meant that many pacemakers were implanted using epicardial lead systems, requiring thoracotomy for placement. Single-chamber pacing was the rule.

Amazing advances have been made in the field of cardiac pacing in the past 30 years. Significant advances in pacemaker technology include the development of smaller, more reliable batteries that last 8 to 10 years and electronic circuitry that allows for a wide range of functions, most or all of which can be adjusted noninvasively after implantation by means of a special programmer. Pacemakers that pace and sense in both atria and ventricles are routinely used, and more recently, pacemakers have been developed that are capable of increasing their pacing rate in response to a variety of physiologic stimuli such as exercise, body temperature, and QT interval.[1]

Equally important have been improvements in pacing lead design. Transvenous leads that are smaller, more reliable, and less thrombogenic have been developed, with electrodes that provide lower pacing thresholds, requiring less energy and prolonging battery life.

Physicians have long recognized bradycardia as a cause of cardiac failure and death, whether due to conduction block (failure of impulse propagation; see Chapter 14) or due to a failure of normal impulse formation (see Chapter 13). Unlike tachycardias, for which medical therapy was developed centuries ago, there is no treatment for sustained bradycardia except cardiac pacing. Well into the 20th century, patients suffering from bradycardia due to complete heart block were doomed to progressive cardiac failure and sudden death while their physicians remained powerless to offer more than symptomatic treatment.

Despite the advances made in cardiac pacing, or perhaps because of the rapidity of these advances, many physicians are not familiar with the function of cardiac pacemakers or the indications for their use. The purpose of this chapter is to provide a general description of the fundamentals of pacemaker operation and to discuss the medical indications for pacemaker implantation for the treatment of bradyarrhythmias. Chapter 17 discusses the nonpharmacologic treatment of tachyarrhythmias, including implantable antitachycardia pacing and shocking devices.

BASIC CONCEPTS OF PACEMAKER FUNCTION

Components of the Pacing System

The pacing system is composed of the pulse generator (pacemaker) and the pacing lead. The pacing lead conducts the stimulus from the pulse generator to the myocardium and is composed of three parts: a wire conductor, an electrode which is in contact with the heart, and an insulating covering (Fig. 16–1). The pacing lead may contain one conductor (unipolar) or two conductors (bipolar). Each conductor is connected to an electrode at the distal end of the lead. These electrodes are engineered to provide optimal current density into the myocardium, lowering the energy required for cardiac stimulation. At the same time, the pacing lead must conduct the intrinsic cardiac activity to the pacemaker so that it can sense the patient's spontaneous rhythm. At the proximal end of the lead are connector pins for attaching the lead to the pacemaker.

Pacemakers are highly sophisticated devices which contain batteries to pro-

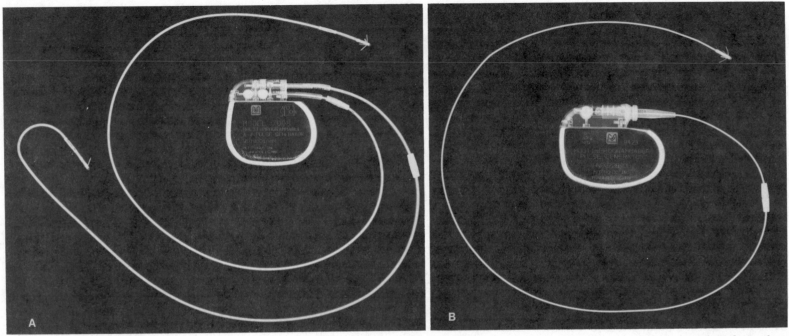

FIGURE 16–1. (*A*) A typical dual-chamber pacing system. There are two leads, atrial and ventricular. Each lead is bipolar. Note the preformed "J" shape of the atrial lead, for placement in the atrial appendage. (*B*) A single-chamber (atrial or ventricular) pacing system. The pulse generator and lead in this example are unipolar.

vide the energy for pacing and electronic circuitry to enable the pacemaker to function. The components of the pacemaker are enclosed in a metal case, usually made of titanium, which is sealed against fluid intrusion.

THE PULSE GENERATOR

The Reed Switch. This switch, found in most pacemakers, is made of two metal leaves (like the reed of a woodwind instrument) that come together when a strong magnet is placed near the pacemaker. Although the exact function of the reed switch varies from one pacemaker to another, the application of a magnet typically results in asynchronous pacemaker operation and may be associated with a operation and may be associated with a change in the pacing rate. Closing the reed switch may also prepare the pacemaker to receive coded instructions transmitted from a programmer. In some pacemakers, application of the external magnet activates specialized pacing functions, and in some devices, the response of the pacemaker to the magnet can actually be programmed off.

The Pacemaker Battery. Pacemaker batteries have been made from a variety of electrolytes and even from atomic fuel. Transcutaneously rechargeable batteries have been used in some pacemakers since the earliest days of pacing. Today, batteries using lithium iodide or lithium cupric sulfide are common. Early batteries were bulky, contributing significantly to the size of early pacemakers. Modern technology has developed relatively small, longer-life batteries which, when combined with modern leads and electronic circuitry, provide pacing and sensing for 8 to 10 years. As the battery is depleted, its voltage drops, and its internal impedance rises. Certain models can telemeter these values to the pacemaker programmer, providing an accurate means of following battery life and predicting replacement. In most pacemakers, battery depletion is accompanied by a gradual fall in the pacing rate, allowing pacemaker replacement to be scheduled electively and preventing unexpected pacing failure.

The Lead and Electrode

The pacing lead is a vitally important component of the pacing system; many pacemaker malfunctions (if not most) now are directly related to the lead rather than to the pulse generator. The lead must be thin, highly biocompatible, capable of active or passive fixation to the ventricular or atrial endocardium, and able to resist fracture from metal fatigue associated with the constant motion of the heart. The insulation around the conductor must be durable but not thrombogenic, and flexible enough to allow easy positioning. Present-day leads are insulated with either polyurethane or silicone. Electrodes are composed of polished platinum or alloys and are shaped, machined, and coated to reduce polarization during pacing and to deliver high current densities while maintaining a large effective surface area for sensing.

Fixation of the lead to the endocardium is either active or passive. Active-fixation leads use a screw which can be advanced into the endocardium after the lead is positioned. Passive-fixation leads use a variety of tines, fins, or other devices to engage the trabeculae of the endocardial surface until chronic scar formation occurs. As shown in Figure 16–1*A*, special atrial leads have preformed "J" shapes designed to fit into the right atrial appendage.

Unipolar Versus Bipolar Pacing

Pacing systems are either unipolar or bipolar, depending on whether the cathode and anode are both physically located within the heart on the pacing lead itself (*bipolar*) or only the cathode is located on the pacing lead and the anode is remote (*unipolar*). Because cathodal stimulation is associated with lower pacing thresholds, the negative terminal of the pacemaker is always connected to the electrode with the best pacing threshold. This is almost always the distal (tip) electrode of an endocardial lead. In a bipolar system, both terminals of the pacemaker are connected to electrodes on the pacing lead, and the proximal electrode is connected to the positive terminal (anode) of the bipolar pacemaker. The entire electrical circuit of the bipolar system involves only the relatively small distance between the distal and proximal electrodes on the bipolar lead.

Unipolar systems also employ the tip electrode as the cathode, but the anode is an indifferent electrode remote from the pacing lead, usually the pacemaker case itself. The much larger electrical circuit formed by the unipolar system makes it more susceptible to external interference. Furthermore, because the pacemaker itself is part of the electrical circuit and because it rests over a large muscle mass, the possibility of pectoral muscle pacing, or the sensing of myopotentials from the pectoral muscle, is present. Another consequence of the difference between unipolar and bipolar pacing circuits is that the pacing artifact of unipolar systems is much more obvious on the electrocardiogram (ECG) than that of bipolar systems. Otherwise there is no difference between the two configurations in terms of sensing or pacing efficiency.

Basic Pacing Functions: Definitions

PACING RATE

The rate of the pacemaker is the frequency with which it stimulates the heart in the absence of any sensed cardiac activity. In pacemakers that only function at one rate, this is referred to as the *backup* or *demand* rate. Pacemakers that have the capability of increasing their rate, either because of atrial synchronous pacing or in response to some other physiologic variable, may also have an upper rate that

the pacemaker does not exceed. In this case, the demand rate may also be referred to as the *lower* rate. Both the upper rate and the backup or demand rate are programmable in modern pacemakers.

HYSTERESIS

Many pacemakers also have a programmable function known as *hysteresis,* which allows the patient's heart rate to fall lower than the programmed demand rate for one cycle before the pacemaker begins pacing (Fig. 16–2). When pacing begins, however, it is at the faster demand rate. This allows patients who tolerate slow heart rates without symptoms, and in whom the pacemaker is intended to prevent only rare episodes of excessive bradycardia, to avoid pacing much of the time. Thus, a patient with a demand rate of 70 beats per minute and a hysteresis rate of 40 beats per minute would require a pause of 1.5 seconds (corresponding to a rate of 40 beats per minute for one cycle) before the pacemaker responded, but if such a pause occurred, the pacemaker would then begin to pace at the rate of 70

beats per minute. If the patient's heart rate only dropped to 60 beats per minute, the pacemaker would remain inhibited even though this is below the demand pacing rate.

PULSE AMPLITUDE, RESISTANCE, AND PULSE DURATION

Most pacemakers produce a constant voltage output with every stimulus. The voltage is governed by the battery and electronic circuitry, and is usually programmable. The voltage of most pacemakers is in the range of 2.5 to 5.0 V, although some can be programmed to deliver voltages of up to 10 V or as low as 1.6 V. The current that flows during each pacing stimulus is governed by Ohm's Law:

$$I = \frac{V}{R}$$

wherein the current in amperes (I) equals the voltage (V) divided by the resistance (R) in ohms. The resistance of the pacing

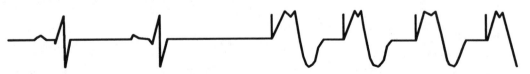

FIGURE 16–2. Hysteresis: The escape interval is longer than the automatic (pacing) interval. A pause that exceeds the hysteresis interval results in ventricular pacing at the programmed rate.

system is the resistance to current flow in the lead and across the electrode-tissue interface. Because there is a component of capacitance involved in this electrode-tissue interface, the resistance is more properly referred to as *impedance* (*Z*). A typical lead-tissue impedance is in the range of 500 ohms, so that with a 5-V battery, the current flow during each pacing stimulus would be 10 mA. Some pacemakers deliver a constant current rather than constant voltage.

The total *energy* used during each pacing stimulus is the product of voltage, current, and time. The time (t) during which current is flowing, or the duration of the pacing stimulus, is called the *pulse width*. Typical pacing pulse widths range from 0.3 to 1.5 milliseconds. Thus, the energy used per pacing pulse, assuming a 0.5-millisecond pulse width and the values given above, would be in the range of 25 µJ:

$$E = V \times I \times t$$

PACING THRESHOLD

The minimum energy required to stimulate the heart muscle is called the *pacing threshold. Threshold* can be defined in a number of ways, including the voltage, current, energy, pulse width, or pulse charge (the number of electrons flowing during each pacing stimulus) below which capture or myocardial pacing is lost. A goal of programming pacemakers is to use the minimum safe energy necessary for pacing, to prolong battery life as much as possible. This can be accomplished by programming voltage or pulse width. It can be seen from the equation for energy, and by substituting for current (*I*), that pacing energy is proportional to the square of the voltage, and directly proportional to the pulse width, whereas inversely proportional to impedance:

$$E = \frac{V^2 \times t}{R}$$

Thus, halving the voltage output from the pacemaker has a greater effect in prolonging battery life than halving the pulse width.

When the pacing lead is first implanted, the pacing threshold is measured by means of an external device known as a *pacing system analyzer*. This device functions in much the same way as the pacemaker itself. The lowest voltage required to produce capture at a given pulse width is determined. This is the *threshold voltage*. Acutely, the threshold is quite low, usually between 0.2 and 1.0 V at a pulse width of 0.5 millisecond. Over the next 10 to 14 days the threshold rises as the pacing lead becomes affixed to the ventricular or atrial endocardium, and localized edema and inflammation develop. This subacute rise in pacing threshold may double or triple the voltage required to pace at implant. Gradually, the pacing threshold falls as the lead becomes chronic and the initial tissue reaction subsides. A capsule of fibrous tissue is left around the electrode at the lead tip, however, so the chronic threshold usually is not as low as was the acute pacing threshold.

SENSITIVITY

The intracardiac electrogram transmitted to the pacemaker over the lead and electrode when spontaneous cardiac activity occurs is the *sensed electrogram*. The sensitivity of the pacemaker determines the amplitude of the intracardiac electrogram required for the pacemaker to sense the signal and inhibit its output. Sensitivity is also programmable, and although typical intracardiac electrograms range from 1 to 4 mV in the atrium, and from 4 to over 25 mV in the ventricle, pacemaker sensitivities are usually programmable over a wide range of from 0.6 to 2.0 mV in the atrium, and 1.25 to 5.0 mV in the ventricle. The greater the number, the larger the intracardiac signal required for sensing to take place. If sensing does not occur because of a high programmed sensitivity or a very low intracardiac electrogram amplitude, the pacemaker does not sense spontaneous cardiac activity and paces as though no spontaneous heartbeats had occurred. This is said to represent *asynchronous operation*. Asynchronous pacing is typical of most pacemakers when an external magnet is applied and, in this case, does not represent a true malfunction.

REFRACTORY PERIOD

Refractoriness refers to the inability of the pacemaker to sense spontaneous cardiac activity because the pacemaker's sensing circuits are temporarily disabled. The period of time during which this takes place is called the *refractory period* of the pacemaker. This typically occurs following a pacing stimulus and lasts for 200 to 400 milliseconds. In the simplest case of a fixed-rate ventricular demand pacemaker (VVI), a refractory period begins with the ventricular pacing stimulus and continues for about 250 milliseconds, to prevent the possibility that the pacemaker might sense ventricular repolarization and be inappropriately inhibited. Spontaneous events (such as premature ventricular complexes [PVCs]) that occur early in the cardiac cycle, during the refractory period of the pacemaker, are not sensed. This does not represent a malfunction of sensing and cannot be corrected by programming the pacemaker's sensitivity to a lower value; on the other hand, appropriate sensing may occur if the pacemaker's refractory period is shortened.

Dual-chamber pacemakers are somewhat more complex, because both atrial and ventricular channels have refractory periods. In these pacemakers, a special problem occurs with sensing. Because both atrial and ventricular channels have some part of the electronic circuitry in common, the potential exists for atrial pacing activity to be transmitted to the ventricular sensing circuit, resulting in inhibition of the ventricular pacing output. This is termed *crosstalk*, and is usually prevented by temporarily disabling the ventricular sensing circuitry during the atrial pacing pulse. This short ventricular refractory period, usually 12 to 30 milliseconds, begins with the atrial pacing output and is called a *blanking period*.

PROGRAMMING AND TELEMETRY

Programmability is the ability to make permanent but reversible changes in the function of the pacemaker noninvasively after it is implanted. Some early pacemakers had crude mechanisms for altering pacing parameters such as rate or voltage, but true programmability using a transmitted signal from an external device to the pacemaker was first developed in the early 1970s. Today, programmability usually implies the ability to alter at least three basic pacing functions, such as rate, output, sensitivity, or refractoriness. *Multiprogrammability* implies the ability to alter *many* of the functions of the pacemaker, including pacing mode, hysteresis, pulse width, voltage, and polarity. In the case of dual-chamber pacemakers, atrial and ventricular channels can be programmed independently, and atrioventricular (AV) delay, blanking period, and upper-rate limit can also be programmed. Programming instructions are sent to the pacemaker from a programmer in the form of either radio-frequency signals or coded electromagnetic pulses.

Programmability is an important feature of modern pacemakers, because the ability to change the basic pacing functions after implant often allows correction of pacing malfunctions. Pacing malfunctions such as loss of capture due to insufficient output may be corrected by increasing voltage or pulse width, both of which result in an increase in pacing energy. Likewise, the lowest safe energy needed to pace can be determined after the chronic pacing threshold is reached and the output accordingly is reduced to conserve power and increase battery longevity. Other common pacing malfunctions that can be corrected by reprogramming include oversensing and undersensing, as well as the sensing of T waves due to a short refractory period. The ability to correct these problems by reprogramming frequently prevents the necessity of reoperating to correct a suboptimal pacing lead location.

More important, the ability to adjust the pacing rate, or parameters of dual-chamber pacing function such as AV interval and upper rate, allows the pacemaker to be fitted to the individual patient's condition. A need for increasing heart rate or for the use of hysteresis to prevent pacing at lower heart rates may develop over time as the patient's underlying cardiac condition changes. Changes in pacing mode may also become necessary. At least two pacemaker models are able to convert a bipolar pacing system to unipolar, which may be of great help in distinguishing pacing stimuli on the ECG. As improved batteries permit current pacemakers to last for 10 years or more, it becomes increasingly important to have a pacemaker that can be made to adapt to the patient's changing condition.

A related function that has been incorporated into newer pacemakers is telemetry of data from the pacemaker to the programmer. Telemetered data may consist of the current programmed parameters, functional characteristics of the pacemaker such as lead impedance, battery voltage, pulse charge, pulse energy, and battery impedance, or actual intracardiac electrograms as sensed by the pacemaker leads. The advent of telemetry has been a significant improvement in the care of pacemaker patients, because without telemetry it is often impossible to verify certain programmable functions that cannot be readily observed during pacemaker operation. Although the programmed pacing rate and mode can usually be determined by simply obtaining a paced ECG tracing, other parameters are not as easily confirmed. Sensitivity, refractory period, output voltage, and pulse width are examples of programmable parameters that cannot be seen directly on the ECG, but all settings can easily be confirmed if the pacemaker can transmit its currently programmed settings. The ability to follow certain parameters such as battery voltage, battery impedance, and battery current noninvasively allows much more accurate estimates of pacemaker longevity after implantation. Finally, telemetry of the sensed electrograms from the pacing leads lets physicians see exactly what the pacemaker is sensing and is extremely useful in diagnosing possible sensing and pacing malfunctions, or in interpreting complicated paced rhythms, especially with dual-chamber pacemakers.

PACING MODES

Pacing Code

The *pacing mode* is the manner in which the pacemaker operates. Virtually all pacemakers are able to operate in more than one mode, and many may be programmed to one of several pacing modes; some dual-chamber pacemakers can be programmed to operate in almost a dozen modes. As pacemakers have become more complex, old nomenclature has become inadequate to describe their function. Terms such as *ventricular demand* and *AV sequential* often are not useful in describing the range of functions of modern pacemakers. To standardize pacemaker terminology and fully describe the function of a given pacemaker, or to specify a particular pacing modality, a code was devised by the Inter-Society Commission for Heart Disease Resources.[2] This code has recently been further modified to include newer pacemakers with previously unavailable pacing functions (Table 16–1).[3]

The pacemaker code, shown on the table, uses letters in each of five positions to summarize pacing functions. Position I describes the chamber(s) of the heart paced, position II describes the chamber(s) sensed, and position III describes the way in which the pacemaker responds to sensed events. Position IV describes programmability and rate responsiveness, and position V describes antitachycardia functions. The letter "O" in any position means *none* or *not applicable* and was added so the antitachyarrhythmia devices with no bradyarrhythmia pacing functions could be described.

Thus, a single-chamber pacemaker that paces the ventricle, senses in the ventricle, and is inhibited when spontaneous ventricular activity occurs would be designated as VVI. If the pacemaker is multiprogrammable (more than simply rate and output), the designation would be VVIM. Automatic implantable cardioverter-defibrillators (or ICDs; see Chapter 17, pages 419 to 420) which are multiprogrammable but have no standby antibradyarrhythmia pacing functions would be designated OOOMS. In common practice, the first three letters are used frequently, and the last two, more rarely.

TABLE 16–1. GENERIC PACEMAKER CODES NASPE/BPEG*

I (CHAMBER PACED)	II (CHAMBER SENSED)	III (RESPONSE TO SENSED EVENTS)	IV (PROGRAMMABILITY, RATE MODULATION)	V (ANTITACHYARRHYTHMIA FEATURES)
O = None	O	O	O	O
A = Atrium	A	I = Inhibited	C = Communicating (telemetry)	P = Pacing (antitachyarrhythmia)
V = Ventricle	V	T = Triggered	P = Programmable (simple)	S = Shock
D = Dual (A & V)	D	D = Atrial triggered & ventricular inhibited	M = Multiprogrammable	D = Dual (P & S)
			R = Rate Modulation	

*As proposed by the North American Society of Pacing and Electrophysiology and the British Pacing and Electrophysiology Group.

Single-Chamber Pacing Modes

With AAI pacing (see Fig. 16–3A), the pacing lead is positioned in the atrium and the pacemaker can pace only the atria and sense only atrial activity. When no atrial activity is sensed, atrial pacing occurs at the demand rate. Spontaneous P waves occurring during the interval between pacing stimuli are sensed, the pacer inhibited, and its timing reset from the sensed beat. The use of AAI pacing presumes normal AV conduction, because there is no provision for ventricular pacing if AV block develops. The advantage of atrial pacing over ventricular pacing is preservation of normal AV synchrony and normal ventricular activation. Atrial pacing is ineffective in the presence of atrial arrhythmias such as atrial fibrillation or atrial flutter, and even the intermittent occurrence of these arrhythmias in a given patient may render single-chamber atrial pacing impractical.

The most common pacing mode has been the VVI pacemaker (see Fig. 16–3B). In this mode, one lead (unipolar or bipolar) is placed in the ventricle. The pacemaker can only pace the ventricle and can sense only ventricular activity. The pacemaker is programmed to a basic pacing (demand) rate, and when no cardiac activity is sensed between pacing stimuli, the pacemaker paces the ventricle at the demand rate. When spontaneous cardiac activity occurs during the interval between pacing stimuli, the pacemaker is inhibited and resets its timing from the sensed beat.

In contrast to the demand or inhibited mode is the *asynchronous* pacing mode, in which no sensing takes place and pacing continues at a fixed rate regardless of spontaneous cardiac activity. This mode (VOO or AOO) is rarely used on a permanent basis, but is the usual pacing mode that occurs temporarily with application of an external magnet. In the "triggered" mode, the pacemaker responds to sensed events by pacing, rather than by inhibiting its output. This mode is also primarily

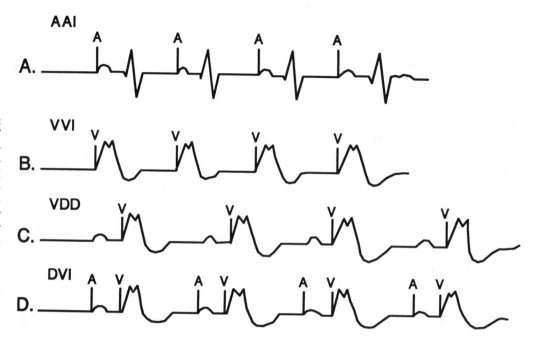

FIGURE 16–3. Pacing modes. (*A*) AAI pacing: Fixed-rate atrial pacing is followed by normal A-V conduction and a nonpaced QRS complex. Spontaneous atrial activity would inhibit the pacemaker. No ventricular pacing is possible. (*B*) VVI pacing: Only the ventricle is paced at the programmed rate. (*C*) VDD or atrial synchronous pacing: Spontaneous atrial activity is sensed, and after the programmed A-V delay elapses, ventricular pacing occurs. As the spontaneous atrial rate rises and falls, the paced ventricular rate changes accordingly. (*D*) DVI or fixed-rate A-V sequential pacing: Atrium and ventricle are paced at the programmed rate, separated by the programmed A-V interval. A = atrial pacing stimulus; V = ventricular pacing stimulus.

used on a temporary basis, and is useful to test sensing by the pacemaker.

Dual-Chamber Pacing Modes

The simplest of the dual-chamber modes of pacing is the fixed-rate, AV sequential pacemaker, designated DVI (see Fig. 16–3D) because, although pacing occurs in both atrium and ventricle, separated by a programmed AV interval, sensing occurs only in the ventricle. The chief disadvantage of the DVI pacemaker is that it functions at only one programmed rate, just as the VVI pacemaker does in the ventricle. If the patient's atrial rate is faster than the pacing rate, even if ventricular activity is slow (as in complete heart block), synchronization of atrial and ventricular activation may not occur owing to the asynchronous competition of the atrial pacing stimuli with the patient's P waves. To achieve effective AV synchronization during DVI pacing, the rate of the pacemaker must be set higher than the *atrial* rate. A useful modification of the DVI mode is the DDI mode, in which the pacemaker also functions at a fixed rate but atrial sensing is added. In the absence of spontaneous activity in either chamber, the pacemaker paces atrium and ventricle at the programmed rate, separated by the programmed AV delay. Unlike the DVI pacemaker, the DDI pacemaker senses both atrial and ventricular activity, and therefore does not compete with the patient's spontaneous atrial beats when sinus node activity exceeds the pacemaker's rate.

The most sophisticated form of pacing is the dual-chamber, atrial synchronous (DDD) mode, often referred to as AV *universal* pacing. The DDD pacemaker actually embodies two modes of pacing, depending on whether or not atrial activity is present at rates higher than the programmed low rate of the pacemaker. At its lower-rate limit, in the absence of sensed atrial activity, the pacemaker functions in the DVI mode, pacing AV sequentially. When atrial activity occurring faster than the low-rate limit is detected, the pacemaker functions in the VAT mode. Atrial activity is sensed, triggering ventricular pacing after a programmed AV delay. The pacemaker thus functions in an atrial synchronous mode, with varying rates up to the programmed upper-rate limit, above which the pacemaker does not continue to track atrial activity on a 1:1 basis.

The upper-rate–limited behavior of DDD pacemakers varies depending on the specific pacemaker in question.[4] In most models, an upper-rate limit can be programmed independently, but the upper tracking rate is also limited by the total atrial refractory period of the pacemaker. This is the sum of the AV interval during which no atrial sensing occurs and the postventricular atrial refractory period (PVARP). The PVARP is the period after a ventricular sensed or paced event during which the atrial sensing amplifiers are turned off. The purpose of the PVARP is to prevent the ventricular pacing artifact, "far-field" ventricular signals (e.g., T waves), or retrograde P waves from being sensed by the atrial channel of the pacemaker. During the time that atrial sensing cannot occur (the total atrial refractory period), however, spontaneous P waves also do not result in ventricular pacing. Therefore, the rate at which spontaneous P waves can result in ventricular pacing is effectively limited. This rate may actually be less than the programmed upper-rate limit, if long AV delays or long postventricular atrial refractory periods, or both, are programmed.

Rate-Responsive Pacing

The obvious advantage of the DDD pacemaker is the possibility of increasing heart rate to meet physiologic demand, assuming a normally functioning sinus node. If sinus node function is not normal, however, a physiologic increase in heart rate with exercise does not occur. In this situation, although AV synchrony is maintained at rest, the full advantage of DDD pacing is not realized because of *chronotropic incompetence*. The desire for a pacemaker that would increase its rate in response to exercise or other physiologic stimuli has led to the development of sensor-driven *rate-responsive* pacemakers.

Rate-responsive pacemakers respond to a sensed physiologic parameter with an increase in pacing rate. Parameters used to drive rate-responsive pacemakers should be easily detected by a bioelectrical sensor and should bear a constant and meaningful relationship to the body's demand for a higher cardiac output. Parameters that have been used include body motion, temperature, stroke volume, QT interval, respiratory rate, and mixed venous oxygen saturation. Rate-responsive pacemakers are available as both single-chamber and dual-chamber devices.

The advantage of rate-responsive pacing is the ability to increase heart rate with exercise if the sinus node fails to increase its rate normally. Single-chamber rate-responsive pacemakers are especially well suited to patients with atrial fibrillation, in whom dual-chamber pacing is not feasible to begin with. Dual-chamber rate-responsive pacing is expected to provide a major benefit to patients with severe sinus bradycardia, with or without AV conduction problems.

HEMODYNAMICS OF PACING
AV Synchrony

In the normal sequence of cardiac contraction, atrial systole occurs just prior to ventricular systole, providing a surge of blood into the left ventricle. Properly timed atrial systole provides several important functions. First, atrial systole plays a role in normal mitral valve function. Second, the end-diastolic filling provided by atrial systole allows for optimal left ventricular filling and stroke volume without requiring high mean left atrial pressures that would result in pulmonary congestion. Finally, the stretch of left ventricular myofibers that results just prior to ventricular systole augments left ventricular contractility. Numerous studies have investigated the contribution of atrial systole to cardiac output.[5] Properly timed atrial systole can augment stroke volume by as much as 25% compared with a ventricular contraction without preceding atrial systole. The primary importance of this augmentation occurs at rest. With a chronic loss of AV mechanical synchrony, stroke volume may be preserved at the expense of a higher mean left atrial pressure.

The contribution of atrial systole depends on the timing of atrial contraction. The importance of the PR interval in this timing has been demonstrated, with optimal PR intervals usually 100 to 200 milliseconds preceding ventricular systole.[6] When atrial systole falls during the QRS complex, after the QRS complex, or more than 250 to 300 milliseconds before the QRS complex, stroke volume is often reduced. The ability to program the AV in-

terval in DDD pacemakers allows some regulation of the timing of atrial and ventricular systole. The optimal AV interval for any given patient is unpredictable, however, and "fine-tuning" of the AV interval is seldom done for purposes of optimizing cardiac output.

Rate Responsiveness

The importance of the timing of atrial systole becomes relatively insignificant in comparison to the increases in cardiac output achieved by increasing heart rate during exercise. Whereas properly timed atrial systole may increase stroke volume by 25% at rest, tripling the heart rate during exercise may result in a 300% increase in cardiac output. In many patients, the increase in heart rate is the only mechanism available to increase cardiac output to meet the peripheral demands of exercise. The patient whose heart rate fails to increase, either because of sinus node dysfunction (*sick sinus syndrome* or chronotropic incompetence; see Chapter 13) or because of complete AV block with a VVI pacemaker, may display severe symptoms of exercise intolerance. It is generally assumed that the normally functioning sinus node is the best determinant of proper rate responsiveness. Therefore, in patients with AV block but normal sinus node function, DDD pacing is recommended. The patient with stable sinus rhythm that fails to increase in rate with

exercise, or the patient with atrial fibrillation and a slow ventricular response during exercise may benefit from rate-responsive pacing.

The Pacemaker Syndrome

Whereas often lifesaving in the patient with severe, chronic bradycardia or complete heart block without a reliable escape rhythm, cardiac pacing rarely provides completely normal cardiac function. It may be associated with mild to severe adverse hemodynamic effects if an inappropriate pacing mode is chosen or if the pacemaker is programmed injudiciously.

The most widely recognized complication of single-chamber ventricular pacing is referred to as the *pacemaker syndrome*, a constellation of symptoms consisting of fatigue, exercise intolerance, pulsations in the neck, dyspnea, cold extremities, and other manifestations of low cardiac output. The pacemaker syndrome is usually due to the hemodynamic effects of ventricular pacing without AV synchrony or to the lack of rate responsiveness, or due to both factors. Its worst manifestations occur when retrograde conduction from the ventricular paced beat results in atrial contraction following ventricular systole. Besides the effects of the loss of AV synchronization, atrial contraction against closed mitral and tricuspid valves also contributes to the pacemaker syndrome by creating the sensation of pulsations in the neck and by activating vasomotor reflexes. The pacemaker syndrome can be prevented by proper use of dual-chamber pacing and by the proper programming of ventricular pacemakers to allow sinus rhythm to suppress pacemaker activity at rest through the use of low programmed rates and hysteresis.

Even the paced ventricular beat that occurs in dual-chamber pacing systems in response to a normal or paced atrial systole may be felt by some patients as uncomfortable. The abnormal ventricular contraction that occurs with paced beats results in higher myocardial oxygen consumption and less effective contraction than does normally conducted ventricular activation. Although insignificant in most pacemaker patients, in some patients with dual-chamber pacing systems it may be advantageous to program the AV interval wide enough to allow normal conduction to take place (if present at all). This also conserves battery longevity, but should not be done if it allows an overly long PR interval due to abnormal intrinsic AV conduction.

PACING AND SENSING MALFUNCTIONS

Abnormal Pacing

Pacing malfunctions may be considered in two categories: failure of a pacing stimulus to capture (depolarize) the myocardium, and failure of the pacemaker to emit a stimulus at the appropriate time. When a properly timed pacing stimulus fails to achieve cardiac pacing, it usually indicates that the pacing threshold is too high. This may occur shortly after implant because of lead dislodgement, or simply because of the expected rise in pacing threshold as edema and inflammation surround the electrode. The later development of an excessively thick fibrous capsule around the electrode may cause *exit block* of the pacing stimulus, with failure of pacing. Antiarrhythmic drugs and electrolyte imbalances may depress myocardial excitability and raise the pacing threshold above the pacemaker's output. Lastly, mechanical problems with the lead itself, such as insulation breaks and conductor fractures, may result in permanent or intermittent pacing failure.

Total absence of pacing artifacts usually signifies a lead fracture, or rarely, loss of pacemaker output due to component failure or a spent battery. Intermittent loss of pacing artifact may be due to oversensing rather than to any actual pacing malfunction. The use of telemetry to identify sensing and pacing events from the pacemaker itself is often helpful in distinguishing loss of output due to lead fracture from that due to oversensing. Likewise, telemetry of parameters such as pulse current and lead impedance is also useful in determining causes of failure to capture.

When failure to capture is due to elevated pacing thresholds, it may be possible to regain pacing by programming an increase in pacing energy, by increasing pulse width or pulse amplitude (voltage), or both. Transiently elevated pacing thresholds following implantation often return toward baseline values after 4 to 6 weeks, allowing a reduction in pacemaker output. Reversible causes of high pacing thresholds, such as drug effect or toxicity and hyperkalemia, should be sought and corrected.

Pacing failure due to fractured leads, lead dislodgement, or excessive scar formation around the electrode leads to high impedances and high pacing thresholds and usually requires reoperation to replace or reposition the lead. In a bipolar pacing system with fracture of one lead, reprogramming to a unipolar mode is sometimes possible and can restore pacing if the other pole of the electrode is intact (Fig. 16–4).

Abnormal Sensing

Sensing malfunctions are divided into those problems due to oversensing and those due to undersensing of intrinsic cardiac signals. Oversensing may involve inappropriate sensing of far-field cardiac events such as T waves, or may involve the sensing of extracardiac signals, including myopotentials; electromagnetic signals from nearby power sources; microwaves; and electrical interference from cautery, other biostimulation equipment (e.g.,

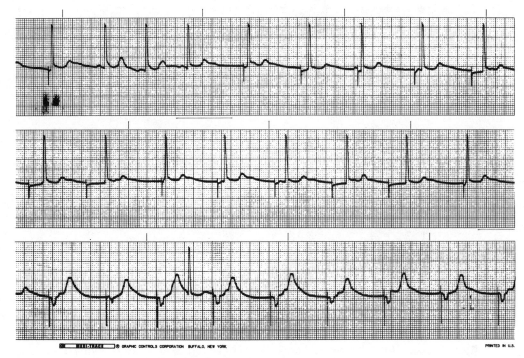

FIGURE 16-4. Pacing failure due to one faulty lead of a bipolar system. The top and middle traces show complete failure of pacing impulses to capture. When the pacemaker was converted to a unipolar system using the one good lead (bottom trace), normal pacing resumed, albeit with failure to sense (note the interpolated sinus beat between the third and fourth paced beats).

transcutaneous electrical nerve stimulation units), or partially fractured lead conductors.

Unipolar pacing systems are more susceptible to oversensing than are bipolar systems, especially myopotentials and far-field components of the ECG. Sensing of T waves, an example of the latter, usually is easily eliminated by prolonging the refractory period of the pacemaker to en-

compass the interval from stimulus to T wave. The sensing of myopotentials, the electrical signals generated by large masses of skeletal muscle lying adjacent to the pacemaker (i.e., the pectoralis muscles), can also result in inappropriate inhibition (Fig. 16–5). If myopotentials are sensed by the atrial lead of a dual-chamber pacemaker, the pacemaker may track the myopotentials as if it were tracking

atrial activity. Thus, in addition to inhibition of the pacemaker, false sensing may result in abnormal pacing as well. Most modern pacemakers are designed so that when continuous interference is sensed, the pacemaker reverts to a backup asynchronous mode of pacing rather than allowing itself to become totally inhibited.

Undersensing is a common problem, especially with atrial leads, where proper

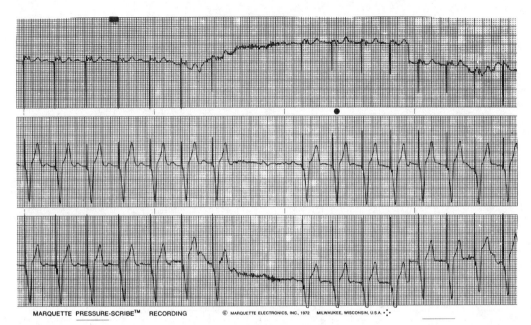

MARQUETTE PRESSURE-SCRIBE™ RECORDING   © MARQUETTE ELECTRONICS, INC., 1972   MILWAUKEE, WISCONSIN, U.S.A.

FIGURE 16–5. Oversensing due to myopotentials. Muscular activity is visible in the baseline of the electrocardiogram (ECG). Myopotentials sensed by the pacemaker result in inappropriate inhibition of pacing.

P-wave sensing is critical for normal atrial synchronous operation. When undersensing occurs in the ventricle, the pacemaker paces competitively with the patient's spontaneous rhythm. This may result in paced beats falling closer to spontaneous beats than the programmed pacing rate should allow for. The most common cause of ventricular undersensing is the external application of a magnet during pacemaker testing, which causes the pacemaker to revert to the VOO mode. Often, PVCs are not sensed,

whereas normal sinus beats are sensed properly. Two factors may cause this difference: first, the premature beat may be conducted in a direction relative to the electrode that results in a smaller R-wave amplitude than the normally conducted beats; and second, the premature beat may fall close to a paced or sensed beat, thereby occurring during the refractory period of the pacemaker. The failure to sense PVCs is not usually a significant problem, but it can be corrected either by programming the pacemaker to a more

sensitive setting (in the first case), or by shortening the refractory period.

Undersensing on the atrial lead in a dual chamber DDD pacing system results in the pacemaker pacing AV sequentially at its low rate limit, as a result of the pacemaker's failure to detect spontaneous atrial activity. The pacemaker assumes that no spontaneous cardiac rhythm is present. Spontaneous R waves may inhibit the ventricular output of the pacemaker, depending on its particular mode of operation.

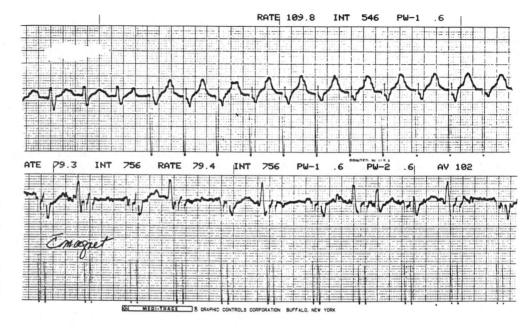

FIGURE 16–6. Pacemaker-mediated tachycardia (PMT). In the top tracing, a DDD pacemaker demonstrates atrial synchronous pacing at its upper rate limit (110 beats per minute) on a routine transtelephonic check. Application of the magnet (bottom trace) results in asynchronous DVI operation and demonstrates an underlying rhythm much slower than the artificially accelerated paced rhythm above.

Pacemaker-Mediated Tachycardia

Pacemaker-mediated tachycardia (PMT) is a complication of pacing that is unique to DDD pacemakers.[7] Because the normal function of the pacemaker is to sense atrial activity and respond with a ventricular paced beat, retrogradely conducted P waves after premature ventricular systoles or ventricular paced beats can also potentially be sensed by the pacemaker and initiate ventricular pacing.

The paced beat then initiates another retrograde P wave and the cycle continues. Ventricular pacing then proceeds at the upper rate limit of the pacemaker (Fig. 16–6). Whenever a DDD pacemaker is seen to be functioning at its upper rate limit with the patient at rest, the possibility of PMT should be considered.

The causes of PMT include not only premature ventricular systoles, but also failure of atrial pacing and atrial oversensing. The potential for PMT is set up by any event that results in ventricular systole without a preceding P wave, thus allowing retrograde conduction.

Once PMT occurs, it can easily be terminated by applying an external magnet. This results in loss of atrial sensing, asynchronous pacemaker operation, and termination of the "endless loop" tachycardia. Programming the pacemaker to any mode other than DDD also terminates PMT, as does lengthening the atrial refractory period to encompass the ventriculoatrial (VA) conduction interval. The key to preventing PMT is to ensure that sensing of retrograde P waves does not occur, which is done by providing a long enough PVARP so that retrograde P waves are not sensed. This poses something of an engineering problem, however, since retrograde conduction is so slow in some patients that retrograde P waves appear as much as 400 milliseconds after the QRS complex. A fixed PVARP of this duration would limit the pacemaker's upper rate to 109 beats per minute, assuming an AV delay of 150 milliseconds. What is needed is a mechanism for extending the PVARP only after ventricular beats with no preceding atrial activity, and this is commonly provided as either an automatic extension of the atrial refractory period for one cycle or complete elimination of atrial sensing for one cycle following a PVC, resulting in DVI pacing for one beat.

INDICATIONS FOR PACING

Temporary Pacing

Although temporary pacing is often used before implantation of permanent pacing, the indications for temporary pacing do not necessarily parallel those for permanent pacing. Permanent pacemaker implantation should be performed as an elective procedure under carefully controlled circumstances. Some of the arrhythmias that require permanent pacing are true emergencies, however. In these situations, the arrhythmia requiring pacing is best controlled by the placement of a temporary pacing catheter until the patient's condition can be stabilized and permanent pacing implemented under elective conditions.

The necessity for temporary pacing should be dictated by either the presence of severe symptoms such as syncope or hypotension, or an association between the bradycardias and ventricular tachycardia or angina pectoris. Complete AV block, when associated with a slow ventricular escape rhythm, is an inherently unstable and unpredictable rhythm. Even though the patient may be relatively asymptomatic, the potential for the sudden development of asystole or ventricular tachycardia exists, and temporary pacing is indicated if any delay is anticipated in proceeding to permanent pacing.

Temporary pacing may also be indicated when conduction abnormalities are anticipated because of the patient's underlying cardiac condition. In these situations, permanent pacing may not become necessary if the patient's conduction abnormalities improve or do not progress. Typical clinical settings that may require temporary pacing include acute myocardial infarction with the development of either symptomatic sinus bradycardia unresponsive to atropine or bifascicular conduction block, and the postoperative cardiac patient in whom sinus node or AV nodal function is impaired. These patients may well improve with time and not require permanent pacing, but the hemodynamic instability associated with their immediate condition requires temporary pacing support, or the probability of progressing unexpectedly to complete AV block is high enough to warrant prophylactic pacing during the acute period.

The third group of patients requiring temporary pacing are those in whom pacing techniques are being used to suppress or terminate ventricular arrhythmias. Arrhythmias in the majority of these patients eventually are controlled by correction of a toxic or metabolic abnormality or by antiarrhythmic drugs, so that temporary pacing will no longer be required. A few require permanent pacing.

All patients with temporary pacemaker catheters should be monitored, not only to ensure continued normal pacemaker function, but because the presence of an unstable pacing catheter in the ventricle can lead to ventricular arrhythmias. Physical activity should be limited, although strict bed rest is not always necessary. The limitations on activity that should be imposed on a patient with a temporary pacing catheter depend on the stability of the pacing catheter and the indication for temporary pacing. The patient who is totally pacemaker-dependent (and thus at higher risk for asystole in the event of pacing failure) should be kept in bed until a permanent pacing system can be implanted.

Permanent Pacing

The indications for permanent pacing are frequently confusing and often controversial.[8] The decision to implant a pacemaker was once fairly straightforward: the major indication was complete AV block and virtually all patients being considered were extremely symptomatic. Advances in pacemaker technology, however, including smaller pacemakers, longer battery life, endocardial (transvenous) leads, and more physiologic pacemakers, have encouraged the use of pacemakers in many patients with less dramatic forms of bradycardia and with less clearcut symptoms. The decision to implant a pacemaker involves making two separate decisions: deciding whether to implant a permanent pacemaker, and deciding which type of pacemaker to use.

The indications for permanent pacing may be thought of in three groups: the presence of symptomatic bradycardia, prophylactic pacing in patients thought to be at high risk for the development of AV block, and rarely, the presence of bradycardia-associated ventricular arrhythmias. This oversimplification serves to stress the point that although specific forms of conduction-system disease may be listed as indications for pacing, any bradyarrhythmia that can be shown to be causing symptoms such as presyncope, syncope, dizziness, angina, congestive heart failure, exercise intolerance, or mental confusion can be treated with cardiac pacing. Conversely, asymptomatic bradyarrhythmias are not generally considered indications for permanent pacing, despite the specific diagnosis, except in the case of acquired complete AV block with a slow ventricular escape rhythm.

AV BLOCK

Atrioventricular block is classically divided into first-, second-, and third-degree (complete) AV block. First-degree AV block is not true conduction block at all, but rather a lengthening of the PR interval beyond 0.2 second. This may be the result of delayed conduction in the AV node, or below the node in the His-Purkinje system. Delayed conduction in the AV node is rarely associated with organic cardiac pathology, but rather is a functional abnormality that rarely progresses to higher grades of conduction block. Prolongation of His-Purkinje conduction, as assessed by a prolonged H-V interval, on the other hand, is usually associated with organic heart disease and is more likely to result in complete AV block, either intermittently or in the future. *Patients with symptoms* suggestive of bradycardia who display only marked prolongation of the H-V interval (greater than 100 milliseconds) may be considered for pacemaker implantation. It should be remembered, however, that a normal H-V interval does not preclude intermittent AV block in a patient with unexplained syncope (see Chapter 14).

Marked first-degree AV block may significantly impair cardiac hemodynamics owing to the loss of effective atrioventricular synchronization. In this unusual case, pacing to restore a more normal AV relationship may be indicated, no matter what the underlying pathology or site of conduction delay.

Second-degree AV block is the *intermittent* failure of AV conduction. Classic Wenckebach AV block is usually the result of conduction block in the AV node; most often it is not associated with significant AV node pathology and does not progress to complete AV block. In some patients it may be symptomatic enough to warrant pacing, but this is very unusual. Although rare, infranodal block can present with the typical Wenckebach periodicity of increasing PR intervals followed by failure of conduction of one or more P waves. Mobitz type-II AV block, an ECG pattern of abrupt failure of conduction of a P wave without any preceding lengthening of the PR interval, is associated with infranodal block, occurs in the setting of organic heart disease, and may progress to higher-grade AV block. The demonstration of Mobitz type-II block in a patient with symptoms such as syncope suggests that complete AV block may also be occurring intermittently.

A special situation is the occurrence of 2:1 AV conduction. His bundle studies define the site of block as either in the AV node or below the node. Classification of 2:1 block as Mobitz type I or II is impossible unless other tracings showing conduction of multiple sequential P waves are available, demonstrating typical Mobitz type-I or type-II patterns. Pacing is generally not indicated in these patients if they are asymptomatic. This form of conduction disturbance is often related to rate, however, and when 2:1 block develops during exercise, it limits the heart-rate response and leads to symptoms of exercise intolerance. In this instance pacing is beneficial.

Atrial fibrillation with a slow ventricular response is a common indication for pacing. Patients may be symptomatic at rest or may find that they are unable to increase their heart rate satisfactorily with exercise, leading to early fatigue. The possible effects of drugs acting on the AV node, such as digitalis, β-blockers, or other antiarrhythmic drugs, must be considered when evaluating such patients for pacemaker implantation.

Third-degree or complete AV block represents the complete failure of AV conduction. Usually a subsidiary junctional or ventricular pacemaker focus takes over and provides an escape rhythm. A distinction is made between patients with complete AV block and a narrow-QRS escape rhythm, which presumably arises high in the infranodal conduction system, often occurs at a faster rate, and tends to be more stable, and those with wide-QRS escape rhythms, which are usually slower and less reliable. The patient may be relatively asymptomatic, or severely symptomatic with syncope or congestive heart failure. Except for congenital AV block in asymptomatic children, complete AV block is almost always an indication for permanent pacing. This is especially true in the older adult with underlying cardiac disease, either valvular or ischemic. Patients with complete AV block are rarely truly asymptomatic, and although they may not give a history of syncope, they often have significant exercise intolerance or dizziness. The conduction abnormality and the symptoms may both develop gradually, so that the patient is not overly aware of these limitations and does not offer such complaints without careful questioning. Nevertheless, clear symptomatic improvement is usually evident after restoration of normal heart rate. Patients with complete AV block are also at risk for the development of ventricular tachycardia, which usually resolves with the institution of pacing.

SINUS BRADYCARDIA

The sick sinus syndrome (see also Chapter 13) is perhaps the most common indication for permanent pacing today. Sinus bradycardia, transient atrial arrhythmias, failure of normal heart-rate response to exercise, and AV conduction delays are all features of this syndrome, although all of these need not be present in any one patient. The concomitant use of antianginal medication or antiarrhythmic drugs to control atrial fibrillation may further exacerbate sinus node dysfunction. Asymptomatic sinus bradycardia is frequently detected by ambulatory monitoring but does not require permanent pacing.

An interesting variation on this theme is the *tachycardia-bradycardia syndrome*, in which atrial tachycardias (usually atrial flutter–fibrillation) are followed by prolonged pauses when they spontaneously terminate. The pause is due to suppression of the sinus node as well as other escape pacemakers in the atrium, AV junction, and ventricle during the tachycardia, and the patient classically gives a history of syncope preceded by palpitations that abruptly stop before loss of consciousness.

A difficult problem in patients with sick sinus syndrome, as well as in those with atrial fibrillation and a slow ventricular response, is the failure of the atrial or ventricular rate to increase with exercise. Although these patients may be asymptomatic at rest, they may experience a severe limitation in their exercise capacity due to fatigue or dyspnea. Such a failure of cardiac output to increase with exercise may be an indication for rate-responsive pacing.

CONDUCTION DISTURBANCES FOLLOWING ACUTE MYOCARDIAL INFARCTION

New conduction disturbances that develop during the course of acute myocardial infarction indicate damage to the conduction system. This is especially true in the case of anterior infarcts. Transient AV conduction block or sinus bradycardia may occur during acute inferior wall infarcts, and either of these disturbances usually resolves without evidence of permanent conduction-system damage. Complete AV block or second-degree AV block that persists after acute myocardial infarction, regardless of site, is an indication for permanent pacing. More controversial is the situation wherein transient AV block, either complete or incomplete (second-degree), resolves but leaves bifascicular or trifascicular block. In this case, some damage to the conduction system can be assumed and permanent pacing is generally indicated (see Chapter 14, pages 339 to 340).

SYNCOPE AND PRESYNCOPE

The potential causes of syncope are numerous. Many are cardiovascular, but not all of these are helped by cardiac pacing. Tachyarrhythmias may cause syncope and tend to occur in the same patient population as bradyarrhythmias. Other common causes include vascular and autonomic problems such as carotid sinus hypersensitivity, vasovagal reflexes, and orthostatic hypotension. When syncope or presyncope can be demonstrated to occur in association with bradycardia, pacing is indicated. In certain situations, however, bradycardia is associated with significant hypotension due to associated arteriolar vasodilatation, which may be the more important factor. This is often true in vasovagal reactions in which there is a vasodepressor component in addition to the cardioinhibitory component. Likewise in carotid sinus hypersensitivity, a reflex drop in blood pressure may accompany the slowing in heart rate or development of AV block; this hypotension cannot be prevented merely by maintaining the heart rate through pacing (see Chapter 13, pages 318 to 319).

Because many patients with *recurrent* unexplained syncope have intermittent conduction defects, the empiric implantation of a permanent pacemaker may be indicated if a thorough evaluation fails to result in a diagnosis. This is especially true in the patient with chronic bifascicular or trifascicular block.

REFERENCES

1. Rickards AF and Donaldson RM: Rate responsive pacing. Clin Prog Pacing Electrophysiol 1:12, 1983.
2. Parsonnet V, Furman S, Smyth NPD, and Bilitch M: Optimal resources for implantable cardiac pacemakers. Circulation 68:227A–244A, 1983.
3. Bernstein AD, Camm AJ, Fletcher RD, et al: The NASPE/BPEG generic pacemaker code for antibradyarrhythmia and adaptive-rate pacing and antitachyarrhythmia devices. PACE 10:794–799, 1987.
4. Furman S: Dual chamber pacemakers: Upper rate behavior. PACE 8:197–214, 1985.
5. Wish M, Fletcher RD, and Cohen A: Hemodynamics of AV synchrony and rate. J Electrophysiol 3:170–175, 1989.
6. Haskell RJ and French WJ: Optimum AV interval in dual chamber pacemakers. PACE 9:670–675, 1986.
7. Calfee RV: Pacemaker mediated tachycardia–engineering solutions. PACE 11(Suppl II):1917–1928, 1988.
8. Frye R, Collins J, DeSanctis R, et al (Report of Joint ACC/AHA Task Force on Assessment of Cardiovascular Procedures Subcommittee on Pacemaker Implantation): Guidelines for permanent cardiac pacemaker implantation, May 1984. J Am Coll Cardiol 4:434–442, 1984.

CHAPTER 17

Nonpharmacologic Therapy of Tachyarrhythmias

LAWRENCE D. GERMAN, MD

The nonpharmacologic therapy of cardiac arrhythmias implies the use of modalities (implantable pacemakers or defibrillators, external devices such as defibrillators, or surgical techniques) that do not involve pharmacologic agents, specifically antiarrhythmic drugs. Despite the very important role certain forms of nonpharmacologic therapy may play for some patients, however, most also require some form of pharmacologic therapy. Antiarrhythmic drugs remain the mainstay of antiarrhythmia prevention; many nonpharmacologic devices are designed to terminate arrhythmias once they occur, but are not effective in preventing their spontaneous occurrence. These devices and therapies should be thought of as adjuncts to the use of antiarrhythmic drugs, not as substitutes for them. Like many antiarrhythmic drugs, some of the devices or techniques discussed in this chapter are primarily suited for temporary or emergency treatment and are not practical for the long-term treatment of chronically recurring arrhythmias.

The use of pacemakers in patients with bradycardias is dealt with in Chapter 16; this chapter discusses the treatment of tachycardias.

DEFIBRILLATION AND CARDIOVERSION
Definitions

Both defibrillation and cardioversion involve the use of high-energy, direct-current electrical discharges through the chest to simultaneously depolarize a sufficient mass of myocardium to terminate an abnormal rhythm and to allow resumption of normal sinus rhythm. Standard defibrillators operate in either a synchronized or nonsynchronized mode. *Cardioversion* is used in dealing with rhythms such as ventricular tachycardia (VT), paroxysmal supraventricular tachycardia (PSVT or paroxysmal AV junctional tachycardia [PJT]), atrial fibrillation, or atrial flutter, in which the electrical discharge can be *synchronized* with the QRS complex. In the synchronized mode, the device monitors the patient's electrocardiogram (ECG) and automatically times the delivery of the electrical shock to occur during the QRS complex. This prevents the induction of ventricular fibrillation due to delivery of the shock during the vulnerable period of ventricular repolarization.

With some arrhythmias, however, such as those with very wide and slow QRS complexes, synchronization of the defibrillator may be difficult or impossible. Also, because during ventricular fibrillation there is no discrete ventricular activity with which to synchronize a defibrillatory shock, the defibrillator is used in these patients in the *nonsynchronized* mode, and the shock is delivered without regard for timing.

Indications

Transthoracic cardioversion or defibrillation may be used effectively to terminate both ventricular and supraventricular arrhythmias. Defibrillation is the treatment of choice and usually the only effective treatment for ventricular fibrillation and should be carried out immediately when this disturbance is identified.

In the case of VT, the clinical setting determines whether synchronized cardioversion or asynchronous defibrillation should be used. In patients with very rapid arrhythmias that have resulted in angina and loss of consciousness or other evidence of cerebral hypoperfusion, prompt termination of the arrhythmia is indicated. Delivery of a synchronized shock is preferable if possible, to avoid the potential induction of ventricular fibrillation, but if severe hemodynamic compromise is already present, time should not be lost in trying to set up a synchronized cardioversion. If the patient with VT is conscious and otherwise stable, it is desirable to take time to obtain assistance from someone skilled in airway management and to administer a short-acting anesthetic drug prior to cardioversion.

Supraventricular arrhythmias may also require the use of transthoracic cardioversion, which reliably terminates most forms of supraventricular tachycardia, including atrial fibrillation, atrial flutter, and the paroxysmal tachycardias due to reentry in the atrioventricular (AV) node or due to an accessory pathway (preexcitation syndromes). Synchronization of the shock is usually possible in these circumstances and is important to avoid the precipitation of an even more serious ventricular arrhythmia.

Some arrhythmias are not amenable to cardioversion. These include tachycardias due to abnormal automatic discharges from ectopic foci in the atria or AV junction, some forms of VT, atrial arrhythmias due to severe lung disease and hypoxemia (multifocal atrial tachycardia), and arrhythmias due to digoxin toxicity. In the acutely ill patient, sinus tachycardia is also often mistaken for atrial flutter.

Technique

The technique of transthoracic cardioversion is simple. Two metal paddles or large adhesive skin patches are applied to the chest in a configuration designed to deliver current through the thorax and the heart. An ECG cable is connected to electrode patches on the arms or torso to provide a surface ECG tracing for diagnostic use and also to time the shock when synchronized cardioversion is desired. In the emergency situation, where time is critical and synchronized cardioversion is not planned, connection of an ECG cable to monitor the patient's rhythm before defibrillation is not necessary. Most defibrillators can display an ECG tracing from the paddles once they are in contact with the chest, allowing a "quick-look" confirmation of the cardiac rhythm. Emergency defibrillation can be carried out using two hand-held paddles positioned over the upper right sternal border and the cardiac apex, respectively. The paddles are first coated with a layer of electrolytic paste, and firm pressure is applied to ensure good electrical contact. The most common cause of equipment failure in the emergency setting is for the defibrillator to be set in the synchronized mode when a nonsynchronized shock is desired. Without a sensed ECG signal with which to synchronize its shock, the defibrillator does not discharge.

An important part of the cardioversion procedure is adequate anesthesia. Personnel should be in attendance who are experienced in the administration of sedative medication, airway management, and ventilatory support. Short-acting anesthetic agents such as methohexital (Brevital) are preferred over drugs such as diazepam (Valium), because their respiratory depressant effects are shorter and the onset of anesthesia is more rapid. It is usually possible to achieve complete anesthesia without complete suppression of spontaneous respiration, so that the patient has no recollection of the shock but does not need artificial ventilation. Oxygen should be administered immediately before the procedure and during any period of hypoventilation that ensues. The use of a noninvasive pulse oximeter to monitor oxygen saturation is highly recommended.

The success of cardioversion or defibrillation depends on delivering an adequate current density to the myocardium to depolarize a sufficiently large tissue mass, thus terminating the arrhythmia. The proper function of the defibrillator depends not only on the size of the electrodes (paddles or patches) through which current is delivered, but also on the resistance to current flow from the electrodes to the patient. To optimize electrical conduction and current flow through the skin when metal paddles are used, they are first coated with an electrolytic jelly.

A more efficient and the recommended method is the use of disposable adhesive patches which can be positioned on the thorax and kept in place easily for long periods if repeated cardioversions are likely to be necessary. These patches are pre-jelled and eliminate the need to apply electrode jelly and defibrillator paddles to the patient every time a shock is to be delivered. Good contact between the electrodes and the patient also minimizes the chances of causing skin burns.

The amount of energy required for cardioversion varies from approximately 20 to 400 J, depending on the size of the patient and the arrhythmia being treated. In general, it is desirable to use the lowest amount of energy possible to restore sinus rhythm, minimizing possible thermal injury to the myocardium, the precipitation of worse arrhythmias, and burns to the skin. The ease with which ventricular fibrillation is terminated also depends on the duration of the arrhythmia, however, so that prompt termination of arrhythmia by using maximum energy is better than by attempting to use lower energies that may be ineffective and require repeated shocks. If recurrences of the arrhythmia over a short period of time make it apparent that multiple shocks are required, then attempts to find the lowest successful energy are warranted. Atrial tachyarrhythmias can often be terminated with relatively low energies (20 to 50 J), presumably because the mass of depolarized myocardium necessary to interrupt reentry is small.

Complications

Complications from cardioversion are relatively few and, with proper precaution, can be minimized. Probably excessive pain is the most frequent. This is the result of inadequate sedation before cardioversion. Skin burns are also preventable in most cases by the proper use of electrolyte jelly or prejelled adhesive pads. The precipitation of more serious arrhythmias such as ventricular fibrillation is always possible, even during synchronized cardioversion, so that the operator should be prepared to recharge the defibrillator immediately and deliver an unsynchronized shock if this happens. The need for constant ECG monitoring during the procedure is obvious in this regard. Lastly, the possibility of excessive bradycardia after conversion of the tachyarrhythmia should be kept in mind. Intense vagal discharge accompanies cardioversion and may result in transient bradycardia. In some patients with *sick sinus syndrome*, conversion from atrial flutter or fibrillation may be associated with complete atrial asystole. These transient bradyarrhythmias are usually not of great importance; when prolonged, they can be corrected by administration of atropine. Rarely, temporary pacing is required, but should it be necessary, facilities for noninvasive pacing should be available nearby.

Elective Cardioversion

Cardioversion of chronic, stable tachyarrhythmias (usually atrial fibrillation or flutter) is often done electively. Although not hemodynamically unstable or otherwise life-threatening, these arrhythmias may resist medical therapy and require cardioversion to restore sinus rhythm.

In the elective cardioversion setting, careful preparation is made to provide adequate ECG monitoring, appropriate anesthesia, airway management in the event of transient apnea, and temporary pacing should cardioversion result in asystole. The procedure should always be carried out with full resuscitation equipment and trained personnel present. If anesthesia is to be used, it is mandatory that the patient fast to prevent aspiration of stomach contents should vomiting occur. Informed consent should also be obtained.

The need for anticoagulation prior to the elective cardioversion of patients with chronic atrial fibrillation is not clearcut, but most physicians believe that anticoagulation with coumarin for at least 2 to 3 weeks is desirable to minimize the risk of embolism from an atrial clot when atrial contractions resume in sinus rhythm. Similarly, it is common practice to begin an antiarrhythmic agent such as quinidine or procainamide prior to cardioversion, to enhance the probability of maintaining sinus rhythm. This decision must be made on an individual basis, depending on the patient's history; the physician should bear in mind that many experienced cardiologists believe that the risk of ventricular arrhythmias in patients starting on quinidine (or any class Ia drug) mandates hospitalization (see Chapter 10, page 228, and Chapter 15, pages 353 and 358 to 362).

It has long been thought that the risk of precipitating ventricular arrhythmias during cardioversion increases in patients loaded with digitalis. In practice, this does not seem to be a significant problem, and the presence of the usual therapeutic levels of digitalis are not a contraindication to cardioversion. Toxic levels, on the other hand, should be recognized prior to elective cardioversion, and the procedure deferred until the levels have fallen.

Serum electrolyte derangements such as hypokalemia similarly should be corrected before the procedure.

TEMPORARY TRANSVENOUS PACING FOR THE TREATMENT OF TACHYARRHYTHMIAS

Temporary pacing techniques to treat or to prevent tachyarrhythmias may be thought of in terms of the prevention of bradycardia-dependent ventricular arrhythmias and the termination, by special pacing techniques, of supraventricular or ventricular tachyarrhythmias.

Indications

Extreme bradycardia, due to either sinus node dysfunction or high-grade AV block, produces abnormal ventricular repolarization with inhomogeneous refractoriness throughout the myocardium, and may lead to the development of ventricular tachycardia. In patients with other causes of abnormal repolarization such as the long-QT syndrome, bradycardia aggravates the electrophysiologic abnormality and may also result in torsades de pointes. Pacing to provide a closer to normal heart rate is usually effective in eliminating the ventricular arrhythmias due solely to bradycardia (e.g., in patients presenting with new-onset complete AV block) until a permanent pacemaker can be implanted. Pacing to maintain a faster-than-normal heart rate (100 to 110 beats per minute) in patients with torsades may help to control the arrhythmia until a precipitating factor such as hypokalemia or drug toxicity can be corrected.

Pacing to terminate other tachyarrhythmias is somewhat more complicated and often requires special equipment. Most reentrant tachyarrhythmias, including many forms of AV junctional reentry tachycardia (PSVT) and ventricular tachycardia, can be interrupted by correctly timed stimuli that produce local refractoriness in one part of the reentrant circuit (Fig. 17–1).[1] The success of pacing in the termination of these arrhythmias depends on several factors, including the rate of the tachycardia, the size of the reentrant circuit, the proximity of the pacing site to the reentrant circuit, and the electrophysiologic properties of the cardiac tissue involved in the reentrant circuit. Knowledge of the mechanism of the arrhythmia and the electrophysiology of the cardiac tissues involved is helpful in determining which cardiac chamber to pace and how the pacing stimuli should be delivered.

To be suitable for pacing termination, a tachyarrhythmia must be caused by a mechanism that can be interrupted by pacing. Many common tachycardias such as atrial fibrillation, multifocal atrial tachycardia, junctional tachycardias (e.g., digitalis toxicity), and ventricular flutter or fibrillation cannot be terminated by pacing. Secondly, the arrhythmia should be hemodynamically well tolerated, to allow time for the pacing procedure to take place. Patients with severe hemodynamic compromise are better treated by prompt cardioversion or defibrillation. In some hospitalized patients with recurrent VT, a temporary pacing catheter can be positioned and used rapidly to terminate arrhythmias that otherwise would require cardioversion. This spares the patient the discomfort and risk of repeated higher-energy shocks. Pacing to terminate episodes of tachycardia of unknown origin may have the additional advantage of providing diagnostic information at the same time. Finally, the use of pacing techniques to terminate episodes of PSVT or VT avoids exposure to intravenous drugs that may precipitate unwanted cardiovascular side effects or allergic reactions.

Techniques

The techniques of temporary pacing to terminate arrhythmias often are not available or are not used because they require more sophisticated equipment and more highly trained personnel than other forms of therapy. Although temporary pacing catheters are available that can be placed without the aid of fluoroscopy, this technique is unreliable and often may not be possible. Temporary pacing catheters

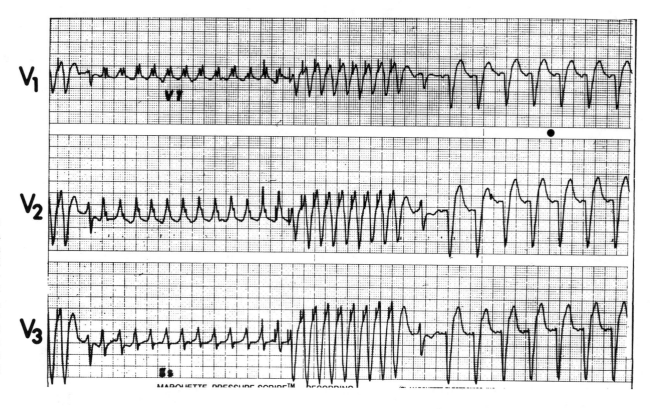

FIGURE 17–1. Termination of ventricular tachycardia (VT) by pacing. An 11-pulse burst of pacing at a fixed cycle length is delivered during an episode of VT. The first two pulses fail to capture, and the second results in a fusion beat. The subsequent eight pulses all result in ventricular capture; sinus rhythm is restored following the burst.

are introduced transvenously, usually through a femoral vein, an antecubital vein, the subclavian vein, or an internal jugular vein. The chamber paced is usually the right atrium or the right ventricle, depending on the arrhythmia to be treated. Ventricular pacing is generally necessary for the treatment of ventricular arrhythmias, although some forms of VT can be terminated by atrial overdrive pacing. Reentrant atrial arrhythmias often can be terminated by either atrial or ventricular pacing, but atrial pacing is safer; atrial flutter can only be terminated by atrial pacing. Special pacing catheters to be positioned in the right atrial appendage are available and can often be used without the aid of x-ray, although the ability to record the intracavitary electrogram from the catheter is helpful in ensuring proper positioning.

The actual pacing modality employed depends on the type of tachyarrhythmia being treated. Atrial flutter may often be terminated by a period of atrial pacing at rates somewhat faster than the rate of the flutter waves. Progressively faster rates may be used if initial pacing attempts are unsuccessful. Occasionally, it may not be possible to terminate atrial flutter directly, but conversion to atrial fibrillation may occur, with subsequent spontaneous conversion to sinus rhythm. Pacing at rates faster than the tachycardia rate may also be effective in terminating PSVT, or these tachycardias may be terminated by critically timed single or double premature stimuli from specially designed pacing devices. Premature stimuli are also frequently effective in terminating episodes of VT.

Complications

Whenever pacing during tachycardia is attempted, the possibility of accelerating the arrhythmia or producing fibrillation must be kept in mind. This is usually of little significance in treating atrial arrhythmias, except for the preexcitation syndromes, where rapid conduction over the accessory pathway during atrial flutter or fibrillation can cause severe hypotension or can precipitate ventricular fibrillation. When treating ventricular tachyarrhythmia, however, it is especially important to have the means for defibrillation readily at hand.

Further risks of temporary pacing include infection, hemorrhage, cardiac perforation, and sepsis. For these reasons, pacing for arrhythmia termination should be performed by physicians experienced in invasive cardiac procedures, and in a controlled, sterile environment. As with elective cardioversion, written consent should be obtained.

ESOPHAGEAL PACING FOR THE TREATMENT OF TACHYARRHYTHMIAS

A technique that is similar to transvenous temporary pacing involves pacing the atria from a catheter positioned in the esophagus.[2] Ventricular pacing from the esophagus, though possible in some patients, is rarely accomplished. Because only atrial pacing is usually possible, only atrial tachyarrhythmias benefit from treatment with esophageal pacing.

Indications

Esophageal pacing may be used in the atrial tachyarrhythmias potentially treatable by temporary pacing from the transvenous route. Diagnostic information about the mechanism of an arrhythmia can also be obtained from the esophageal lead (Fig. 17–2). The success rate of esophageal pacing in terminating tachycardias is less than that of transvenous pacing, however, because adequate atrial pacing cannot be obtained from the esophagus in some patients.

Techniques

The advantage of esophageal pacing over transvenous pacing is the elimination of the need for an intravenous or intracardiac catheter. The technique is therefore much safer. The disadvantages are that higher currents are required to pace the heart through the esophagus, making it more painful. Specialized equipment must also be used to perform esophageal pacing, because standard temporary pacemakers usually do not generate enough energy. Stimulators must be able to provide pulses with a pulse duration of 10 milliseconds and currents of up to 20 to 30 mA. Special esophageal electrode catheters are now commercially available.

Positioning of the esophageal lead is critical for successful atrial pacing. The most efficient method is to record the atrial electrograms from the electrodes of the lead as it is advanced or pulled back in the esophagus. The position that optimizes the sensed atrial electrogram usually results in the best pacing thresholds, although some trial-and-error positioning may be required.

Complications

Complications of esophageal pacing are uncommon. The most frequent is pain during pacing. Discomfort during positioning of the lead is common, but is mild and can be minimized by the use of an an-

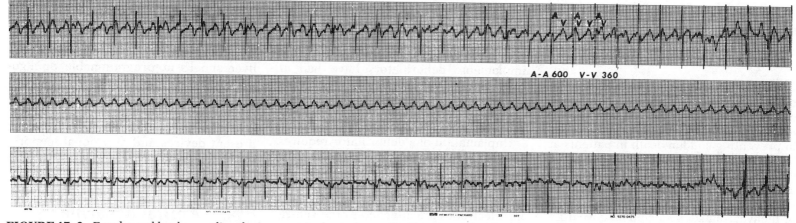

A-A 600   V-V 360

FIGURE 17–2. Esophageal lead recording during ventricular tachycardia. The top tracing shows a combination of surface electrocardiogram (ECG) lead and the esophageal lead atrial recording. The second tracing is the surface ECG lead alone, and the third is the atrial recording. Ventricular activity at a rate of 167 beats per minute (cycle length 360 milliseconds) is evident from the surface ECG. Slower, regular atrial activity at a cycle length of 600 milliseconds recorded from the esophageal lead allows the detection of atrioventricular (AV) dissociation and proves the diagnosis of ventricular tachycardia.

esthetic jelly such as viscous lidocaine. The pain of pacing is related to the amount of current required, so obtaining the best electrode positioning, thereby reducing the pacing threshold, is helpful. Positioning of the esophageal lead in the trachea is not infrequent but usually results only in cough. Likewise, the lead may coil in the nasopharynx. The use of electrogram monitoring during the positioning of the lead ensures proper positioning in the esophagus. Perforation or injury of the esophagus is possible, especially if the catheter is inappropriately stiff, but is rare when soft, flexible catheters are used.

IMPLANTABLE DEVICES FOR THE CONTROL OF RECURRENT TACHYARRHYTHMIAS

To this point in the chapter, the methods presented have been primarily intended for the treatment of emergencies or the temporary treatment of tachyarrhythmias in an acute setting. The real promise of nonpharmacologic forms of antiarrhythmic therapy, however, has been for the patient with medically refractory, recurrent tachyarrhythmias. Much effort has gone into the development of

devices that can be permanently implanted for control of tachyarrhythmias. Such devices are still in the early stages of development, but great progress has been made.

Implantable devices can be thought of in two groups: those that function like pacemakers, delivering timed pacing stimuli to interrupt reentrant tachycardias (in the same manner as discussed for temporary pacing), and those whose function is to deliver a higher-energy shock in an attempt to terminate ventricular tachyarrhythmia or fibrillation (i.e., implantable defibrillators). Neither type of device alone is optimal, and efforts continue to produce a device that can perform both functions.

Implantable Defibrillators

The development of implantable defibrillators has been the goal of a number of physicians who have recognized the limited effectiveness of antiarrhythmic drugs in preventing sudden death in patients at high risk for ventricular tachycardia or ventricular fibrillation. Such devices are able to distinguish potentially lethal arrhythmias from normal or benign forms of tachycardia such as sinus tachycardia or atrial fibrillation, and then respond with a shock similar to that used by external or transthoracic defibrillators. The device is small enough to implant permanently in the body, yet it contains the electronic circuitry needed to store and deliver sufficient energy to defibrillate the human heart automatically, a process with much greater energy requirement than pacing alone.

INDICATIONS

The indications for implantable defibrillators are governed by their limitations as well as by the potential for serious arrhythmia.[3] Patients are considered candidates for implantable defibrillators if they are believed to have a significant risk for a life-threatening tachyarrhythmia based on their underlying cardiac condition, a past history of tachyarrhythmia, and prior failed attempts to control ventricular arrhythmias induced during electrophysiologic studies or occurring spontaneously with medication. Most patients receiving implantable defibrillators have had at least one spontaneous episode of VT or fibrillation requiring resuscitation.

TECHNIQUE

Implantation of a defibrillator requires an open-chest procedure. Two electrodes in the form of wire-mesh patches are placed over the epicardial surfaces of the heart, and two additional myocardial pacing electrodes are attached to the ventricles. The patch electrodes are used to deliver the defibrillatory impulse to the heart, whereas the pacing electrodes (in the initial commercially available device) merely sense the cardiac rhythm. These four electrodes are then connected to the defibrillator itself, a large pacemaker-like device, which is buried subcutaneously in the abdomen (Fig. 17–3).

To avoid false recognition of sinus tachycardia or other supraventricular tachyarrhythmias, arrhythmia detection is a complicated procedure in some of these devices, requiring not only that a predefined heart rate be exceeded, but also that other characteristics of ventricular tachycardia or fibrillation be met. Once the arrhythmia detection criteria have been met, however, the device charges and delivers a shock of up to 30 J. Careful testing of the defibrillation threshold at the time of implantation is required to be sure that the patient's tachycardia can be converted reliably with this fixed amount of energy. Newer devices can deliver shocks at programmable or algorithm-driven variable energy levels, and also have the capability for antitachycardia and standby pacing.

Despite problems with the size of the present devices and occasional inappropriate shocks due to false arrhythmia recognition, the implantable defibrillator has undoubtedly saved many lives.

Antitachycardia Pacemakers

Implantable antitachycardia pacemakers have been developed to get around several of the problems with the implantable defibrillator.[4] In size and ease of transvenous implantation, these devices resemble the pacemakers for bradyarrhythmias described in Chapter 16. They contain sophisticated circuitry for the recognition and pacing termination of tachyarrhythmias. Because they pace rather than shock, these devices do not have to contain unusually large batteries, and arrhythmia termination is much more comfortable to the patient, who may not even be aware of the operation of the device.

Although many patients can have their ventricular tachycardia terminated by pacing, at some point most experience an acceleration of their arrhythmia or its de-

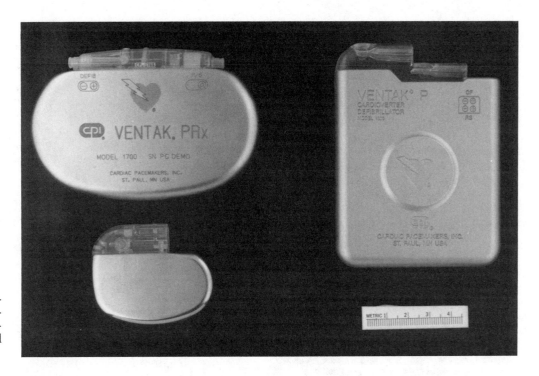

FIGURE 17–3. Size comparison of a commercially available programmable implantable defibrillator (top left); an older, nonprogrammable implantable defibrillator (right); and a standard-sized permanent pacemaker (bottom left).

generation to fibrillation with pacing. Clearly, the use of a pacing device for the ambulatory treatment of their arrhythmia occasionally might precipitate an even more deadly tachyarrhythmia. Because of this, the use of antitachycardia pacemakers has been limited largely to the treatment of supraventricular tachyarrhythmias. The use of antitachycardia pacemakers for ventricular tachycardia

has been eliminated by the development of defibrillators that incorporate antitachycardia pacing technology.

INDICATIONS

The indications for implantation of an antitachycardia pacemaker include medically refractory reentrant atrial tachyarrhythmias in which no propensity to degenerate to atrial fibrillation with pacing

has been found. This typically includes patients with PSVT due to one of the preexcitation syndromes or due to reentry in the AV node. The arrhythmias must be sufficiently stable hemodynamically to allow the patient to remain conscious long enough for the pacemaker to terminate the tachycardia, a procedure that could take several minutes. Certain patients with VT may be candidates for such a pacemaker if extensive testing reveals that the arrhythmia is well tolerated, can reliably be terminated by pacing, and does not degenerate to ventricular fibrillation. Often, concomitant antiarrhythmic therapy is necessary to slow the tachycardia and to increase the chances of pacing termination.

TECHNIQUES

The technique of implantation of antitachycardia pacemakers is not significantly different from that of antibradycardia pacemakers (see Chapter 16), but the electrophysiologic testing required before implantation is extensive. Testing during the implantation procedure is also needed, to demonstrate the effectiveness of arrhythmia sensing and termination from the actual site of the permanent pacing electrode.

ABLATIVE TECHNIQUES FOR ARRHYTHMIA CONTROL

Surgical Techniques

One of the most appealing forms of therapy for cardiac arrhythmias is the surgical removal of the abnormal region of myocardium responsible for the initiation or propagation of an arrhythmia, while preserving normal cardiac conduction and function. The successful application of surgical techniques to cardiac arrhythmias depends on our ability to understand the mechanism of the arrhythmia and to localize the region or site of arrhythmia origin. Furthermore, this site must be surgically accessible without damaging normal structures.

In the case of supraventricular tachycardias, the mechanisms of arrhythmia are well understood, and diagnostic electrophysiologic techniques for localization of anatomic structures (such as accessory AV pathways or functionally abnormal areas, as in the case of atrioventricular nodal reentry and ectopic atrial tachycardias) are accurate and highly developed. Surgery for supraventricular tachycardias is usually predicated on the presence of an accessory AV conduction pathway that can be divided, or an area of functionally abnormal atrial or AV nodal tissue that can be directly destroyed. Surgical techniques directed at specific sites can be performed with the help of intraoperative electrophysiologic mapping. Techniques for approaching the sites of supraventricular arrhythmias have also been developed to allow successful operation without undue danger of damage to important cardiac structures.

Ventricular tachycardias are much less well understood. The mechanisms of arrhythmia formation may vary from patient to patient, and diagnostic techniques to localize the origin of VT are more difficult. Many ventricular tachyarrhythmias are felt to arise from subendocardial sites in the left ventricle, requiring a surgical approach through the ventricular wall itself. It may be difficult or impossible to pinpoint a focal area responsible for the development of ventricular tachyarrhythmia, and the surgical resection of the areas involved may damage the remainder of the ventricle, impairing its hemodynamic functions.

INDICATIONS

Surgery for tachycardia is indicated in two broad categories: supraventricular arrhythmias and ventricular arrhythmias. The most common supraventricular arrhythmias treated surgically are forms of PSVT due to the preexcitation syndrome. In these patients, interruption of the accessory pathway eliminates tachycardia and usually obviates the need for further antiarrhythmic therapy. Atrial fibrillation frequently occurs in the same patients, however, and may be present postoperatively, because elimination of the accessory pathway does not directly affect the cause of atrial fibrillation. Surgical techniques to correct reentry in the AV node have also been developed, as have techniques for treatment of ectopic atrial tachycardias in some patients.

Ventricular tachycardia is an indication for surgery when it occurs in the setting of coronary artery disease, especially after myocardial infarction. Classically, patients with left ventricular aneurysms have been considered candidates for endocardial resection guided by intraoperative mapping. The presence of an aneurysm is not required for success, but a region of ventricle that can be opened without destroying normally functioning myocardium is desirable. An arrhythmia that can be reliably induced for mapping, both preoperatively and intraoperatively, is also highly favorable.

Much less frequent are patients with forms of VT that arise from ectopic foci in the left or right ventricles without underlying coronary disease. In these cases, surgical ablation of the focus, guided by intraoperative mapping, is highly successful.

Catheter Ablation

Catheter ablation techniques have become standard forms of therapy for some arrhythmias, and new technologies involving more controlled sources of energy are rapidly evolving. Electrical energy delivered through an electrode catheter to a selected site to destroy normal or abnormal tissue has been used to treat a variety of supraventricular and ventricular tachycardias.[5] More recently, radio-frequency energy delivered via catheters has been used in patients with paroxysmal atrioventricular nodal reentry and atrioventricular reciprocating tachycardias, with an extremely high success rate.[6,7]

INDICATIONS

High-energy electrical catheter ablation using direct current shock has been shown effective in creating complete AV block through destruction of the AV nodal region. Thus, any supraventricular arrhythmia can be controlled through the indirect creation of complete AV block. Permanent ventricular pacing is then required and the arrhythmia itself continues without affecting the ventricular rate. This technique has been used extensively in patients with atrial fibrillation who have not been controllable medically. Ectopic atrial tachycardias can also be controlled indirectly in this way.

The radio-frequency catheter techniques allow better control of the ablative current and are extremely effective in patients with AV nodal reentry or accessory AV pathways (Wolff-Parkinson-White syndrome) a "cure" rate that exceeds 90%. Because the delivered energy can be more carefully controlled and its effects closely monitored during its application (as compared with the burst of energy delivered with electrical ablation), AV conduction remains intact at the end of the procedure in the vast majority of patients.[6,7]

Direct approaches to atrial tachyarrhythmias themselves have also been used. Focal ablation of ectopic tachycardias is sometimes possible, especially in the right atrium, and ablation of posterior septal or right-sided accessory pathways in the Wolff-Parkinson-White syndrome has been accomplished.

Catheter ablation of VT is also possible, although much more difficult and less successful than ablation of the AV junction. The thick and scarred endocardium and endocardial clot often present in the left ventricle after infarction, combined with difficulties in pinpointing the site of tachycardia origin, limit the usefulness of this technique. Focal VTs arising in the right ventricle are the best suited for catheter ablation.

TECHNIQUES

The technique of electrical catheter ablation is relatively simple. Most commonly, electrical energy from a standard defibrillator is delivered through an electrode catheter positioned at the site desired (e.g., at the His bundle region for AV junctional ablation). Energies in the range of 200 to 400 J are delivered through the catheter. A temporary pacing catheter must be placed prior to the procedure so that ventricular pacing can be performed if complete AV block is achieved.

The radio-frequency technique also uses an intracavitary electrode positioned in either the left or right side of the heart, depending on the patient's problem (e.g., atrioventricular nodal reentry versus the site of an accessory pathway). The indifferent electrode is a patch on the anterior chest wall. The multiple other electrodes typical of an electrophysiologic study are also present and allow mapping of the important characteristics of the baseline tachycardia and its response to the radiofrequency energy. Other techniques being developed include the use of laser radiation through fiber-optic catheters.

COMPLICATIONS

The complications of electrical catheter ablation are surprisingly few. Any intracardiac electrical shock can result in ventricular fibrillation. Bradycardia due to either AV block or sinus bradycardia is also possible. Emboli occurring following ablation procedures in the left heart have been reported but are preventable with adequate anticoagulation. Minor, transient chest pain may occur, and VT developing from the site of ablation is seen occasionally during the 24 hours after the procedure. Close ECG monitoring during this period is necessary.

REFERENCES

1. German LD and Strauss HC: Electrical termination of tachyarrhythmias by discrete pulses. PACE 7:514–521, 1984.
2. Gallagher JJ, Smith WM, Kerr CR, et al: Esophageal pacing: A diagnostic and therapeutic tool. Circulation 65:336–341, 1982.
3. Mirowski M: The automatic implantable cardioverter-defibrillator: An overview. J Am Coll Cardiol 6:461–466, 1985.
4. Fisher JD, Johnston DR, Kim SG, Furman S, and Mercando AM: Implantable pacers for tachycardia termination: Stimulation techniques and long-term efficacy. PACE 9 (Suppl II):1325–1333, 1986.
5. Gallagher JJ, Svenson RH, Kasell JH, et al: Catheter techniques for closed chest ablation of the atrioventricular conduction system. A therapeutic alternative for the treatment of refractory supraventricular tachycardia. N Engl J Med 306:194–200, 1982.
6. Jackman WM, Wang X, Friday KJ, et al: Catheter ablation of accessory atrioventricular pathways (Wolff-Parkinson-White syndrome) by radiofrequency current. N Engl J Med 324:1605–1611, 1991.
7. Calkins H, Sousa J, El-Atassi R, et al: Diagnosis and cure of the Wolff-Parkinson-White syndrome or paroxysmal supraventricular tachycardias during a single electrophysiologic test. N Engl J Med 324:1612–1618, 1991.

APPENDIX

YOUR FAST HEARTBEAT: WHAT IT MEANS AND HOW TO STOP IT

You Have a Condition Called Paroxysmal Tachycardia. *Paroxysmal* means that it comes intermittently or occasionally, and *tachycardia* means "fast heartbeat." What all these fancy words mean is that you occasionally have a fast heart action, which starts suddenly and ends suddenly. A lot of fancy words to describe a problem that is not serious. Your tachycardia generally comes on for no particular reason. Sometimes when it starts you may feel a little lightheaded for 10 to 15 seconds. Usually, all you feel is a rapid heart action or fluttering in your neck, chest, or throat. When it stops, it stops abruptly, which means that one minute it is there, and the next minute it is gone. It does not gradually slow down. We are all aware of our heart action sometimes. If we are asked to stand up and suddenly give a speech, for example, our heart rate may suddenly speed up, but it gradually slows down. In contrast, your episodes of tachycardia occur spontaneously and can last for just a few seconds or may last many hours.

Does Tachycardia Mean I Have Heart Disease? No, it most certainly does not. A tachycardia represents an abnormal heart rhythm. It does *not* mean that you have any form of serious heart disease. A tachycardia also does not lead to any serious heart problems. People may have hundreds of episodes of tachycardia and are never left with any heart damage. A tachycardia does not have to be frightening once you understand that it is not serious and that there are ways to stop it. Most important, your tachycardia may go away or come less often as you get older.

Why Does It Start? Usually it comes on without warning. Sometimes when you are very tired or have been drinking or smoking excessively, you may notice your tachycardia comes on more easily. Sometimes it occurs during exercise. There may be some days when you feel as if you are going to have an episode of tachycardia. You may feel your heart "flip-flop" in your chest, a feeling that comes from extra beats that sometimes can trigger an episode of tachycardia. All of us have extra beats at one time or another. Just because you have them, they do not necessarily lead to an episode of tachycardia. On some days the irregular beats are more frequent than others. On those days you should avoid drinking coffee or taking stimulants such as cold medicine or alcohol. Not all patients experience this pattern, however. Some folks have one episode of tachycardia a year. If you are one of those folks, you really do not need to concern yourself about those days when you have extra beats.

How Can I Stop a Tachycardia? On some occasions, an episode of a tachycardia may last longer than a few seconds or minutes and does not seem to break by itself. You can stop such an episode yourself by attempting to perform the following maneuvers. These maneuvers work best if you are lying on your back with your feet slightly elevated.

1. *Deep Breathing.* While sitting quietly, take an extremely deep breath to the point where you can no longer take an additional amount of air; then exhale very rapidly. It is not enough to simply breathe deeply; you must take as deep a breath as you possibly can.

2. *Straining.* In this maneuver, sit quietly or lie down as described previously. Take a deep breath in and hold it. Then, without letting air escape, push the air against your abdomen and chest muscles. The strain of not exhaling any of the air you have taken in will increase the pressure in your chest and stop the tachycardia. This maneuver is identical to what you do when you are trying to force a bowel movement or have a baby. Maintain as forceful a strain of your stomach and chest muscles as you can for approximately 10 or 20 seconds and then release the air rapidly, and you probably will find that the episode of tachycardia will break shortly thereafter. This maneuver may make you feel lightheaded.

3. *Squatting.* Assume a squatting position and try to tuck your arms right into your chest in an effort to curl

your body up into a ball-like position. Remain in this position for 1 or 2 minutes. If the attack is going to break, it will probably terminate within this period of time. When you get up, do so carefully, as you may feel lightheaded.

4. *Coughing.* While sitting comfortably, force yourself to begin a series of strong and even violent coughing spells. Even though you may not have a natural tendency to cough at this time, try to build up a cough until you are making rather strong efforts, of the type you might make if you had a severe chest cold. Again, you might feel somewhat lightheaded at the end of your coughing spell.

5. *Sneezing.* Induce a forceful sneeze by one of several methods. The simplest might be to gently tickle the inside of one or another nostril with a soft, blunt object such as a cotton swab. A second method might involve inhaling some pungent, finely ground pepper, especially when it is held very close to your nostril. Remember, a very forceful sneeze is required.

6. *Head Down.* While in a sitting position, bend the trunk of your body forward until your head is down between your knees. Hold your head in this position for approximately one minute. Another method of achieving the same result involves lying horizontally across a bed and bringing your head and shoulders rapidly over the edge of the bed, allowing them to touch the floor. In this way, your abdomen and legs are on the bed while your head and shoulders are down on the floor. Maintain this position for 1 to 2 minutes.

7. *Cool Immersion.* Fill a sink basin or other suitable large container with cool water. Place yourself in front of it. Take a deep breath in and hold your breath while submerging your face in the water. Hold your face in the water for as long as you possibly can (30 seconds or more).

Cold water can be helpful in another way. Fill a large container or basin with extremely cold (ice) water. Immerse one or both of your arms up to the shoulder in this cold water. Hold your immersed arms in the water for approximately one and a half minutes.

8. *Gagging.* Sit quietly in a chair, and using a blunt, flat, long object such as the handle of a fork, slide the object along the tongue in a backward direction until it reaches far enough to cause you to gag. Repeat this maneuver until you gag rather forcefully.

9. *Carotid Sinus Massage.* Beneath the angle of your jaw on either side you can feel a prominent pulsation in your neck. This pulsation is created by the carotid artery. If you gently run your finger along your neck just beneath the angle of your jaw, you will not only feel a pulse in your artery, you will also note a small but distinctive swelling in this structure. This is normal and is present in all people. Using whichever finger is convenient for you, apply firm pressure over this swelling for approximately 3 to 5 seconds and then release. You should try applying this pressure on either side of your neck. Do not compress the artery on both sides of your neck at the same time. This maneuver works best if you are lying flat.

10. *Medication.* You may have been given a prescription for or already take a drug called digoxin (Lanoxin).

    a. IF YOU DO NOT TAKE DIGOXIN, and you have an episode of tachycardia that does not go away with these maneuvers, you should do the following:

    1) Take digoxin (Lanoxin), 2 tablets immediately. Each tablet is 0.25 mg, and you should take a total of 0.5 mg.

    2) If the tachycardia is still present after 1 hour, try repeating one or more of the maneuvers and take another 0.25-mg tablet. Very often, if you lie down for about an hour or so and then perform the maneuvers outlined previously, the tachycardia will break with the help of digoxin.

3) If it is still there an hour later (two hours after it began), take another 0.25-mg tablet and repeat the maneuvers. If after this time the tachycardia does not break, you should call your doctor for further advice.

b. IF YOU REGULARLY TAKE DI-GOXIN:

1) If you have *not* taken any digoxin (Lanoxin) in the past 4 hours, take 0.5 mg immediately. (Take two tablets of 0.25 mg.) If the tachycardia is still present an hour later, take one more 0.25-mg tablet of digoxin and repeat the maneuvers outlined previously.

2) If you *have* taken a dose of digoxin within the past 4 hours, only take *one* tablet of 0.25 mg as a first dose. If the tachycardia is still present an hour later, take a second 0.25-mg dose of digoxin, and repeat the maneuvers.

When Should I Call My Doctor or Come to the Emergency Room? Call your doctor before you go to the emergency room because he or she may be able to suggest an alternative. You should definitely call your doctor if any of the following are noted:

1. You passed out or you feel as if you might do so.
2. You are having chest pains or shortness of breath.
3. Your episode of tachycardia does not go away within 2 to 3 hours.

This information has been provided to make you feel more comfortable with your problem and to give you a strategy for dealing with it.

INDEX